Management of Myocardial Reperfusion Injury

Juan Carlos Kaski • Derek J. Hausenloy
Bernard John Gersh • Derek M. Yellon
Editors

Management of Myocardial Reperfusion Injury

Springer

Editors
Juan Carlos Kaski, DSc, DM(Hons), M.D., FRCP, FACC, FAHA, FESC
Cardiovascular Sciences Research Centre
Division of Clinical Sciences
St George's, University of London
Cranmer Terrace
SW17 ORE London
United Kingdom

Derek J. Hausenloy, BSc, MBChB, PhD, FRCP, FESC, FACC
Institute of Cardiovascular Science
University College London
The Hatter Cardiovascular Institute
67 Chenies Mews
WC1E 6HX, London
United Kingdom

Bernard John Gersh, MB, ChB, D.Phil, FRCP, Ph.D. (Hon Causa)
Mayo Clinic
Mayo Graduate School of Medicine
Dept. Cardiovascular Diseases
First Street SW. 200
55905 Rochester Minnesota
USA

Derek M. Yellon, D.Sc., FESC, FACC
Institute of Cardiovascular Science
University College London
The Hatter Cardiovascular Institute
67 Chenies Mews
WC1E 6HX, London
United Kingdom

ISBN 978-1-4471-5813-4 ISBN 978-1-84996-019-9 (eBook)
DOI 10.1007/978-1-84996-019-9
Springer Dordrecht Heidelberg New York London

Printed on acid-free paper

Springer is part of Springer Science+Business Media (www.springer.com)

Foreword

During my training in the 1950s and in my early years as a clinical and research cardiologist before 1961, acute myocardial infarction (AMI) was by far the most frequent cause of death in industrialized nations. Usually it occurred quite unexpectedly, like the proverbial "bolt out of the blue" which struck down unsuspecting persons. Most of the patients with AMI died before they reached the hospital, and of those who did, fully one-third succumbed before discharge. Among hospital survivors, more than half died, or were hospitalized for heart failure or a recurrent myocardial infarction within the next year.

It has been my privilege to observe – and in a few instances participate – in what has been an extraordinary series of advances which have transformed the approach to this deadly condition. Two giant steps have been taken. The first evolved from a short sole-authored paper by Desmond Julian, then a registrar in cardiology, describing the concept of the coronary care unit, the use of which immediately reduced the mortality of AMI by half by essentially eliminating death from ventricular fibrillation and other life-threatening arrhythmias.

By 1964, the remaining in-hospital mortality – approximately 15% – occurred primarily in patients whose large infarcts caused left ventricular pump failure. Experimental efforts were then directed towards attempting to reduce infarct size by increasing oxygen supply and/or reducing oxygen demand. The former proved to be the key. The second giant step in reducing mortality began in 1975 with Chazov's seminal demonstration of successful opening of an occluded coronary artery by the intracoronary infusion of streptokinase. In the ensuing 37 years, myocardial reperfusion techniques have improved progressively and now consist of bringing the patients to the hospital as rapidly as possible (to limit the duration of ischemia) and taking them immediately to the catheterization laboratory where they undergo balloon angioplasty followed by insertion of a coronary stent, followed, if possible, by catheter-based thrombectomy. These mechanical procedures are accompanied by appropriate and ever improving adjunctive anti-platelet and anticoagulant therapy as well as beta adrenergic blockers. Timely application of these measures that constitute this second step has improved outcomes substantially, but mortality rates in community-based registries seem to have plateaued at 8–10%.

While early reperfusion clearly reduces ischemic myocardial necrosis, it is not without adverse effects. In studies on experimental myocardial reperfusion as early as the 1960s, Jennings observed that this intervention was often accompanied by microvascular damage, swelling of capillary endothelial cells and of myocytes. In combination, these changes caused what has been termed the "no reflow" phenomenon. Moreover, rapid reperfusion of severely ischemic myocardium also causes lethal myocardial injury. Thus, by 1985, reperfusion following severe ischemia was considered to be a "double-edged sword." Substantial effort has been devoted to reducing infarct size in animal models of coronary occlusion and reperfusion. Many investigators have studied a large variety of interventions. Although there have been promising leads, often the observations were not reproducible in other laboratories, in other animal species, and most importantly, until recently, none have been reproduced consistently in patients.

There has been one promising lead – preconditioning of the myocardium. This phenomenon was first described by Murry and collaborators who noted in dogs that repetitive, brief occlusions of a coronary artery protected the myocardium from a subsequent prolonged occlusion. Preconditioning has now been reproduced in many species, including man. Although useful in patients in whom the timing of ischemia could be controlled, such as patients undergoing cardiac surgery or percutaneous coronary intervention, it has not been useful in patients developing myocardial infarction, because the timing of the coronary occlusion is not known. Interestingly, preconditioning can be remote, i.e. repetitive brief occlusions of an artery can reduce necrosis caused by subsequent prolonged occlusion of an artery perfusing a second (remote) vascular bed. Another key observation was that the repetitive brief remote occlusions could commence *after* the start of the prolonged occlusion of an artery feeding the target organ, referred to as remote ischemic preconditioning or postconditioning. Furthermore, there have now been several encouraging pilot studies in patients with AMI.

These observations open a new era in the several-decade-long effort to reduce lethal myocardial reperfusion injury, an era that is well described in *Myocardial Reperfusion Injury*, a book that has been very ably edited by a quartet of scientific and clinical leaders in the field – Kaski, Yellon, Hausenloy, and Gersh. This comprehensive volume begins with a section which summarizes current knowledge of pathophysiology of myocardial perfusion injury and of the challenges to translating cardioprotective strategies in the animal model into clinical therapy. The second section turns to the clinical features of reperfusion injury and describes the advantages and limitations of various imaging techniques – angiography, echocardiography, nuclear scanning, and magnetic resonance imaging – in assessing myocardial injury and tissue salvage. The third section describes various forms of conditioning, including a number of novel treatment strategies.

The editors have selected expert authors from Western Europe and North America and have produced a lucid book that will be welcomed by current investigators in the field. It is likely to be both a useful reference for and a source of inspiration to trainees who will contribute to taking the third giant step in reducing further the morbidity and mortality resulting from AMI.

USA Eugene Braunwald, M.D.

Preface

Early and successful myocardial reperfusion with thrombolytic therapy or primary percutaneous coronary intervention (PCI) remains the most effective therapeutic strategy for reducing the size of a myocardial infarct, preserving left ventricular systolic function, and improving clinical outcomes in patients presenting with an ST-elevation myocardial infarction (STEMI). However, restoring coronary blood flow to the acutely ischemic myocardium can in itself result in deleterious effects. This phenomenon, which has been termed "myocardial reperfusion injury," can therefore mitigate the beneficial effects of myocardial reperfusion, and its prevention and treatment remains one of the last uncrossed frontiers in the management of acute STEMI patients.

The potentially detrimental aspects of myocardial reperfusion injury include reversible forms of myocardial injury such as myocardial stunning, microvascular dysfunction, and reperfusion arrhythmias, which are amenable to management in the clinical setting. However, irreversible forms of myocardial reperfusion injury, which include microvascular obstruction and lethal myocardial reperfusion injury, are more difficult to manage. Lethal myocardial reperfusion injury, which refers to the reperfusion-induced death of cardiomyocytes which were viable at the time of resolution of ischemia, can increase myocardial infarct size by 30–40%, and may in part explain why, despite optimal myocardial reperfusion strategies using PPCI, the rate of death after an STEMI approaches 10%, and the incidence of heart failure after an acute myocardial infarction is almost 25% although there does appear a discordance between the magnitude of these effects as demonstrated in the experimental animal as opposed to the clinical setting.

Although the processes of myocardial reperfusion continue to be improved with the recent developments in PCI technology and the discovery of novel anti-platelet and anti-thrombotic therapies for maintaining the patency of the infarct-related coronary artery, there currently exists no effective therapy for preventing myocardial reperfusion injury.

Much has been written about myocardial reperfusion injury and the controversies surrounding its existence and clinical relevance in the past 20–30 years, but unfortunately the information has been generally presented in the form of original specialist papers, and until now little if any integral publication exists on the topic, summarising and analysing the clinical impact of the condition and its management. The pathophysiology and molecular mechanisms of myocardial reperfusion injury are complex and, regarding diagnosis, individual diagnostic techniques have been proposed but without a proper assessment of the relative values of these methods. The management of this condition has also been problematic, as therapeutic strategies that have been demonstrated to prevent myocardial reperfusion injury in the experimental models have not translated into beneficial treatment strategies for patients. In this book, leading cardiovascular researchers and cardiologists systematically address these issues relating to myocardial reperfusion injury in a comprehensive and critical manner. Novel therapeutic strategies for preventing myocardial reperfusion injury are discussed, which in the future, may result in new treatments for further reducing myocardial infarct size and improving clinical outcomes in patients presenting with acute myocardial infarction.

Juan Carlos Kaski, DSc, DM(Hons), M.D., FRCP, FESC, FACC, FAHA
Derek J. Hausenloy, BSc, MBChB, PhD, FRCP, FESC, FACC
Bernard John Gersh, MB, ChB, D.Phil, FRCP, Ph.D. (Hon Causa)
Derek M. Yellon, D.Sc., FESC, FACC

Acknowledgment

We are grateful to the authors of the book for their time and dedication in bringing this book to fruition.

Contributors

Jeroen J. Bax, M.D., Ph.D. Cardiology Department, Leiden University Medical Center, Leiden, The Netherlands

Michael V. Cohen, M.D. Department of Medicine, University of South Alabama Medical Center, Mobile, AL, USA

Department of Physiology, University of South Alabama, College of Medicine, Mobile, AL, USA

Victoria Delgado, M.D., Ph.D. Cardiology Department, Leiden University Medical Center, Leiden, The Netherlands

James M. Downey, Ph.D. Department of Physiology, University of South Alabama, Mobile, AL, USA

Meyer Elbaz, M.D., Ph.D. Department of Cardiology, Service de Cardiologie, Hôpital Rangueuil, University Paul Sabatier, Toulouse, France

Matthias G. Friedrich, M.D. Department of Cardiac Sciences and Radiology, Foothills Medical Centre, Calgary, AB, Canada

Christopher B. Granger, M.D. Department of Cardiology, Division of cardiovascular medicine, Duke University Medical Center, Duke Clinical Research Institute, Durham, NC, USA

Rong Jiang, M.D., Ph.D. Department of Surgery, Emory Children's Center, Atlanta, GA, USA

Robert A. Kloner, M.D., Ph.D. Department of Medicine, Division of cardiovascular medicine, Keck School of Medicine at University of Southern California, Los Angeles, CA, USA

The Heart Institute, Good Samaritan Hospital, Los Angeles, CA, USA

Division of Cardiology, Keck School of Medicine, University of Southern California, Los Angeles, CA, USA

Mitchell W. Krucoff, M.D., FACC, FAHA Department of Medicine, Division of Cardiology, Duke University Medical Center, Durham, NC, USA

Wichert J. Kuijt, M.D. Department of Cardiology, Academic Medical Center – University of Amsterdam, Amsterdam, The Netherlands

Andreas Kumar, M.D., M.Sc. Department of Cardiology, The Quebec Heart and Lung Institute, Laval University, Hopital Laval, Pavillon de Recherche, Quebec, QC, Canada

Olivier Lairez, M.D., Ph.D. Department of Cardiology, Service de Cardiologie, Hôpital Rangueuil, University Paul Sabatier, Toulouse, France

Nathan Mewton, M.D., Ph.D. Department of Cardiology and Clinical Research, Inserm U 1060 (CARMEN), Lyon, France

Service d'Exploration Fonctionnelles Cardiovasculaires, Hospices Civils de Lyon, Université Claude Bernard Lyon1, Lyon, France

Mariana Mirabel, M.D. Department of Cardiology, The Heart Hospital, University College London, London, UK

Paris Cardiovascular Research Center, Paris, France

Michel Ovize, M.D., Ph.D. Department of Cardiology and Clinical Research, Inserm U 1060 (CARMEN), Lyon, France

Service d'Explorations Fonctionnelles Cardiovasculaires, Hospices Civils de Lyon, Université Claude Bernard Lyon1, Lyon, France

Hôpital Louis Pradel, Lyon, France

University of Lyon, Lyon, France

Denis Pellerin, M.D., Ph.D. Department of Cardiology, The Heart Hospital, University College London Hospitals, London, UK

Christophe Piot, M.D., Ph.D. Department of Cardiology, Inserm U661, Montpellier, France

Hopital Arnaud de Villeneuve, Université de Montpellier I and II, Montpellier, France

Abhiram Prasad, M.D., FRCP, FACC Department of Medicine, Division of Cardiovascular Diseases, Mayo Clinic, Rochester, MN, USA

Thorsten Reffelmann, M.D. Klinik und Poliklinik für Innere Medizin B, Universitätsklinik der Ernst-Moritz-Amdt-Universität Greifswald, Greifswald, Germany

Gilles Rioufol, M.D., Ph.D. Department of Cardiology, Inserm U 1060 (CARMEN), Lyon, France

Interventional of Cardiology, Hospices Civils de Lyon, Université Claude Bernard Lyon1, Lyon, France

Matthew T. Roe, M.D., MHS Division of Cardiovascular Medicine, Duke University Medical Center, Duke Clinical Research Institute, Durham, NC, USA

François Roubille, M.D., Ph.D. Department of Cardiology, Inserm U661, Montpellier, France

Hopital Arnaud de Villeneuve, Université de Montpellier I and II, Montpellier, France

Arend F.L. Schinkel, M.D., Ph.D. Department of Cardiology, Thoraxcenter, Erasmus MC, Rotterdam, The Netherlands

Division of Pharmacology, Vascular and Metabolic Diseases, Department of Internal Medicine, Erasmus MC, Rotterdam, The Netherlands

Weiwei Shi, M.D., Ph.D. Division of Cardiothoracic Surgery, Department of Surgery, Emory University Hospital Midtown, Atlanta, GA, USA

Eva von Schmilowski, M.D., Ph.D. Department of Cardiology, The Royal Brompton Hospital, Sydney street, London, UK

Howard Swanton, M.A., M.D., FRCP, FESC, FACC Department of Cardiology, The Hearth Hospital, University College London Hospitals, London, UK

Jakob Vinten-Johansen, M.S., Ph.D. Department of Surgery, Division of Cardiothoracic Surgery, Emory University School of Medicine, Emory University Hospital Midtown, Atlanta, GA, USA

Cardiothoracic Research Laboratory, Carlyle Fraser Heart Center, Atlanta, GA, USA

Judson Williams, M.D., MHS Department of Surgery, Division of Cardiac Surgery, Duke University, Durham, NC, USA

Kai-Hang Yiu, M.B.B.S. Cardiology Department, Leiden University Medical Center, Leiden, The Netherlands

Amanda J. Zatta, B.Sc. (Hons), Ph.D. Department of Epidemiology and Preventive Medicine, The Alfred Centre, Monash University, Melbourne, VIC, Australia

Part I
Introduction

Chapter 1
Myocardial Reperfusion Injury as a New Frontier for Clinical Therapy

Derek J. Hausenloy, Juan Carlos Kaski, Bernard John Gersh, and Derek M. Yellon

Abstract Ischemic heart disease (IHD) is the leading cause of death and disability worldwide. A major manifestation of IHD is a ST-elevation myocardial infarction (STEMI), the optimal treatment for which is early myocardial reperfusion using primary percutaneous coronary intervention (PPCI). However, the process of myocardial reperfusion comes at a price, as restoring coronary blood flow to ischemic myocardium can in itself induce cardiomyocyte injury and death, a phenomenon which has been termed myocardial reperfusion injury. The presence of myocardial reperfusion injury mitigates the full benefits of PPCI in terms of myocardial salvage as it can be responsible for 40–50% of the infarct. Currently, there is no effective treatment for protecting the heart against myocardial reperfusion injury. Therefore, novel therapeutic strategies, which can be administered as adjuncts to PPCI and are capable of preventing myocardial reperfusion injury, are required to further limit infarct size, preserve left ventricular function and improve clinical outcomes in patients with IHD.

Keywords Myocardial reperfusion injury • Cardioprotection • Percutaneous coronary intervention • ST-segment elevation myocardial infarction

---

D.J. Hausenloy, BSc, MBChB, PhD, FRCP, FESC, FACC (✉) • D.M. Yellon, D.Sc., FESC, FACC
UCL Institute of Cardiovascular Science,
The Hatter Cardiovascular Institute, University College London Hospital,
67 Chenies Mews, London WC1E 6HX, UK
e-mail: d.hausenloy@ucl.ac.uk; d.yellon@ucl.ac.uk

J.C. Kaski, DSc, DM(Hons), M.D., FRCP, FACC, FAHA, FESC
Department of Clinical Sciences, Cardiovascular Sciences Research Centre, St. George's, University of London, Cranmer Terrace, London SW17 0RE, UK
e-mail: jkaski@sgul.ac.uk

B.J. Gersh, MBChB, D.Phil., FRCP, Ph.D. (Hon Causa)
Division of Cardiovascular Diseases, Mayo Clinic, First Street SW, Rochester 55902, MN, USA

Medicine Department, Mayo Clinic College of Medicine, Rochester, MN, USA
e-mail: gersh.bernard@mayo.edu

J.C. Kaski et al. (eds.), *Management of Myocardial Reperfusion Injury*,
DOI 10.1007/978-1-84996-019-9_1, © Springer-Verlag London 2012

Introduction

Ischemic heart disease (IHD) is the leading cause of death and disability worldwide. Timely and effective myocardial reperfusion by primary percutaneous coronary intervention (PPCI) is the treatment of choice for limiting myocardial infarct (MI) size, preserving left ventricular (LV) systolic function and improving clinical outcomes in patients presenting with an acute ST-segment elevation myocardial infarction (STEMI). Paradoxically, the process of myocardial reperfusion is a 'double-edge sword' [1] and comes at a price, as it can in itself paradoxically inflict further injury to the myocardium – a phenomenon which has been termed 'myocardial reperfusion injury' [1, 2]. Although, the process of myocardial reperfusion continues to be optimized with recent advances in PCI technology and anti-platelet and anti-thrombotic therapy, there is currently no effective therapy for reducing myocardial reperfusion injury. Therefore, novel therapeutic interventions, which are capable of preventing myocardial reperfusion injury and can be administered as adjunctive therapy to PPCI, are needed to improve clinical outcomes in STEMI patients undergoing IHD. In order to achieve this, robust reliable methods for detecting and quantifying the presence of myocardial reperfusion injury in PPCI patients need to be available. In this book, the pathophysiology, diagnosis and management of myocardial reperfusion injury are reviewed by leading experts in the research field of cardioprotection.

The Discovery of Myocardial Reperfusion Injury

Over 50 years ago, Jennings et al. [3] first documented in the canine heart the histological changes which occurred on reperfusing ischemic myocardium – these comprised contracture of myofibrils, disruption of the sarcolemma and the appearance of intra-mitochondrial calcium phosphate particles, features which appeared within minutes of myocardial reperfusion and which differed from those induced by myocardial ischemia alone, confirming myocardial reperfusion injury as a distinct pathological entity. However, the significance of these pathological findings only become apparent in the 1980s and 1990s when myocardial reperfusion by thrombolytic therapy and primary PCI was introduced as a therapy for STEMI patients. Clearly, myocardial reperfusion was shown to be essential for myocardial salvage, but it soon emerged that the presence of myocardial reperfusion injury diminished the benefits of thrombolysis and PPCI in terms of MI size limitation. The reversible effects of myocardial reperfusion injury include myocardial stunning (a term which describes the 'mechanical dysfunction that persists after reperfusion despite the absence of irreversible damage and despite restoration of normal or near-normal coronary flow' [4]) and reperfusion arrhythmias, both of which are reversible and are easily managed in the clinical setting. The more serious irreversible effects of myocardial reperfusion injury include microvascular obstruction and lethal myocardial reperfusion injury. In Chap. 2, James M. Downey and Michael

Cohen provide a comprehensive account of the pathophysiology of myocardial reperfusion injury.

Microvascular Obstruction

Microvascular obstruction was first described in 1966 by Krug et al. [5] in the feline heart as the 'inability to reperfuse a previously ischemic region'. The actual cause of MVO remains unclear, although its major pathophysiological features include capillary damage with impaired vasodilatation, external capillary compression by endothelial cell and cardiomyocyte swelling, micro-embolization of friable material released from the atherosclerotic plaque, platelet microthrombi and neutrophil plugging [6]. The process is dynamic, is believed to be initiated during myocardial ischemia and is exacerbated during reperfusion. The presence of coronary no-reflow at the time of PPCI is often treated with intracoronary adenosine or nitrates, although the efficacy of these therapeutic agents is unclear. Importantly, up to 60% of STEMI patients with normal coronary flow (TIMI 3) post-PPCI may still have evidence of MVO on cardiac MRI, the presence of which is associated with impaired LV systolic function, adverse LV remodelling and worse clinical outcomes. Therefore, a large proportion of STEMI patients may benefit from being administered at the time of PPCI, a therapeutic intervention capable of reducing the incidence and extent of MVO. In Chap. 3, Thorsten Reffelmann and Robert A. Kloner give a comprehensive overview of this irreversible form of myocardial reperfusion injury.

Lethal Myocardial Reperfusion Injury

The existence of lethal myocardial reperfusion injury as a distinct entity, which is capable of independently inducing cardiomyocyte death following a sustained episode of myocardial ischemia, has been hotly debated over the years. Part of the problem has been the inability to directly demonstrate that the actual process of reperfusion induces the death of cardiomyocytes which were viable at the end of the ischemic episode. Indirect evidence for the existence of myocardial reperfusion injury has been provided by the large number of pre-clinical animal studies, demonstrating 40–50% reductions in MI size with therapeutic interventions applied at the onset of myocardial reperfusion [2]. This data would suggest that myocardial reperfusion injury may account for 40–50% of the final MI size. The pathophysiology of lethal myocardial reperfusion injury is closely related to the abrupt effects of myocardial reperfusion on mitochondrial function: the re-energization of the electron transport chain, the production of oxidative stress, mitochondrial calcium and phosphate overload, the rapid restoration of physiological pH and the opening of the mitochondrial permeability transition pore (mPTP), a critical mediator of cardiomyocyte death in reperfused hearts. In Chap. 4, Jakob Vinten-Johansen and colleagues provide a comprehensive account of lethal myocardial reperfusion injury.

Clinical Relevance of Myocardial Reperfusion Injury

Among clinical cardiologists, the idea that myocardial reperfusion by thrombolysis or PPCI, which is essential for myocardial salvage in STEMI patients, may actually have detrimental effects on the heart appears implausible. After all, restoring coronary blood flow and maintaining the patency of the infarct-related artery are the major priorities of this therapeutic approach. The evidence that lethal myocardial reperfusion injury exists in man and may actually be relevant to the clinical setting was first provided in a small proof-of-concept clinical study published in 2005 by Staat et al. [7, 8]. These authors demonstrated that a therapeutic intervention applied to STEMI patients at the time of PPCI could reduce MI size by 38% (measured by 72 h area under the curve total CK) [7]. This therapeutic intervention, ischemic postconditioning (IPost), had been demonstrated in pre-clinical animal studies to reduce lethal myocardial reperfusion injury [9] and comprised the interruption of coronary blood flow with four 1-min low-pressure angioplasty balloon inflations/deflations within the infarct-related artery [7]. Subsequent clinical studies have confirmed the beneficial effects of IPost using myocardial nuclear scanning [10], echocardiography [10] and cardiac MRI [11]. Taken together, these clinical cardioprotection studies suggest that in STEMI patients undergoing PPCI, about 40% of the final MI is due to lethal myocardial reperfusion injury. Therefore, by applying a therapeutic intervention to prevent lethal myocardial reperfusion injury in STEMI patients at the time of PPCI may result in a further 40% reduction in MI size.

Myocardial Reperfusion Injury as a Therapeutic Target

Until the discovery of IPost, the translation of a large number of therapeutic interventions, which had been shown to reduce myocardial reperfusion injury in pre-clinical animal MI studies, had failed in the clinical setting. This problem may be overcome in the future with more rigorous testing of novel cardioprotective interventions in the pre-clinical setting (with the use of more clinically relevant animal MI models and the formation of multi-centre research networks for randomized controlled double-blinded testing of cardioprotective interventions in large animal MI models) [12] and more careful design of the clinical studies [13]. The topic of failed clinical translation of cardioprotection is covered in Chap. 5 by Michel Ovize and colleagues.

The diagnosis and treatment of myocardial reperfusion injury in PPCI patients is critically dependent on the ability to detect and quantify its presence in PPCI patients. In Chaps. 6, 7, 8, 9 and 10, the diagnosis of myocardial reperfusion injury in the cardiac catheter laboratory, using echocardiography, myocardial nuclear scanning and cardiac MRI, are reviewed. There are a number of promising therapeutic interventions for reducing myocardial reperfusion injury including cyclosporin A (an mPTP inhibitor) [14, 15], exenatide (a glucagon-like protein 1 agonist) [16] and remote ischemic perconditioning (four 5-min cycles of upper limb ischemia/reperfusion induced by cuff inflation/deflation) [17, 18], which have been demonstrated in proof-of-concept clinical studies to reduce MI size in STEMI patients when administered prior to PPCI. Large multi-centre clinical trials are now required to determine whether preventing lethal myocardial reperfusion injury can improve clinical outcomes in STEMI patients treated with PPCI. These emerging therapeutic strategies for reducing myocardial reperfusion injury in PPCI patients are reviewed in Chaps. 11 and 12.

In summary, this book provides a comprehensive review and critical analysis of the pathophysiology, diagnosis and management of myocardial reperfusion injury. Importantly, novel therapeutic interventions capable of reducing myocardial reperfusion injury in IHD patients are explored.

References

1. Braunwald E, Kloner RA. Myocardial reperfusion: a double-edged sword? J Clin Invest. 1985;76(5):1713–9.
2. Yellon DM, Hausenloy DJ. Myocardial reperfusion injury. N Engl J Med. 2007;357(11):1121–35.
3. Jennings R, Sommers H, Smyth G, Flack H, Linn H. Myocardial necrosis induced by temporary occlusion of a coronary artery in the dog. Arch Pathol. 1960;70:68–78.
4. Braunwald E, Kloner RA. The stunned myocardium: prolonged, postischemic ventricular dysfunction. Circulation. 1982;66(6):1146–9.
5. Krug A, Du Mesnil de Rochemont W, Korb G. Blood supply of the myocardium after temporary coronary occlusion. Circ Res. 1966;19(1):57–62.
6. Reffelmann T, Kloner RA. The no-reflow phenomenon: a basic mechanism of myocardial ischemia and reperfusion. Basic Res Cardiol. 2006;101(5):359–72.
7. Staat P, Rioufol G, Piot C, Cottin Y, Cung TT, L'Huillier I, Aupetit JF, Bonnefoy E, Finet G, Andre-Fouet X, Ovize M. Postconditioning the human heart. Circulation. 2005;112(14):2143–8.
8. Yellon DM, Opie LH. Postconditioning for protection of the infarcting heart. Lancet. 2006;367(9509):456–8.
9. Zhao ZQ, Corvera JS, Halkos ME, Kerendi F, Wang NP, Guyton RA, Vinten-Johansen J. Inhibition of myocardial injury by ischemic postconditioning during reperfusion: comparison with ischemic preconditioning. Am J Physiol Heart Circ Physiol. 2003;285(2):H579–88.
10. Thibault H, Piot C, Staat P, Bontemps L, Sportouch C, Rioufol G, Cung TT, Bonnefoy E, Angoulvant D, Aupetit JF, Finet G, Andre-Fouet X, Macia JC, Raczka F, Rossi R, Itti R, Kirkorian G, Derumeaux G, Ovize M. Long-term benefit of postconditioning. Circulation. 2008;117(8):1037–44.
11. Lonborg J, Kelbaek H, Vejlstrup N, Jorgensen E, Helqvist S, Saunamaki K, Clemmensen P, Holmvang L, Treiman M, Jensen JS, Engstrom T. Cardioprotective effects of ischemic postconditioning in patients treated with primary percutaneous coronary intervention, evaluated by magnetic resonance. Circ Cardiovasc Interv. 2010;3(1):34–41.
12. Schwartz LL, Kloner RA, Arai AE, Baines CP, Bolli R, Braunwald E, Downey J, Gibbons RJ, Gottlieb RA, Heusch G, Jennings RB, Lefer DJ, Mentzer RM, Murphy E, Ovize M, Ping P, Przyklenk K, Sack MN, Vander Heide RS, Vinten-Johansen J, Yellon DM. New horizons in cardioprotection: recommendations from the 2010 national heart, lung, and blood institute workshop. Circulation. 2011;124(10):1172–9.

13. Hausenloy DJ, Baxter G, Bell R, Botker HE, Davidson SM, Downey J, Heusch G, Kitakaze M, Lecour S, Mentzer R, Mocanu MM, Ovize M, Schulz R, Shannon R, Walker M, Walkinshaw G, Yellon DM. Translating novel strategies for cardioprotection: the Hatter Workshop Recommendations. Basic Res Cardiol. 2010;105(6):677–86.
14. Piot C, Croisille P, Staat P, Thibault H, Rioufol G, Mewton N, Elbelghiti R, Cung TT, Bonnefoy E, Angoulvant D, Macia C, Raczka F, Sportouch C, Gahide G, Finet G, Andre-Fouet X, Revel D, Kirkorian G, Monassier JP, Derumeaux G, Ovize M. Effect of cyclosporine on reperfusion injury in acute myocardial infarction. N Engl J Med. 2008;359(5):473–81.
15. Mewton N, Croisille P, Gahide G, Rioufol G, Bonnefoy E, Sanchez I, Cung TT, Sportouch C, Angoulvant D, Finet G, Andre-Fouet X, Derumeaux G, Piot C, Vernhet H, Revel D, Ovize M. Effect of cyclosporine on left ventricular remodeling after reperfused myocardial infarction. J Am Coll Cardiol. 2010;55(12):1200–5.
16. Lønborg J, Vejlstrup N, Kelbæk H, Bøtker HE, Kim WY, Mathiasen AB, Jørgensen E, Helqvist S, Saunamäki K, Clemmensen P, Holmvang L, Thuesen L, Krusell LR, Jensen JS, Køber L, Treiman M, Holst JJ, Engstrøm T. Exenatide reduces reperfusion injury in patients with ST-segment elevation myocardial infarction. Eur Heart J. 2011 Sep 14. [Epub ahead of print]
17. Botker HE, Kharbanda R, Schmidt MR, Bottcher M, Kaltoft AK, Terkelsen CJ, Munk K, Andersen NH, Hansen TM, Trautner S, Lassen JF, Christiansen EH, Krusell LR, Kristensen SD, Thuesen L, Nielsen SS, Rehling M, Sorensen HT, Redington AN, Nielsen TT. Remote ischaemic conditioning before hospital admission, as a complement to angioplasty, and effect on myocardial salvage in patients with acute myocardial infarction: a randomised trial. Lancet. 2010;375(9716):727–34.
18. Rentoukas I, Giannopoulos G, Kaoukis A, Kossyvakis C, Raisakis K, Driva M, Panagopoulou V, Tsarouchas K, Vavetsi S, Pyrgakis V, Deftereos S. Cardioprotective role of remote ischemic periconditioning in primary percutaneous coronary intervention: enhancement by opioid action. JACC Cardiovasc Interv. 2010;3(1):49–55.

Part II
The Pathophysiology of Myocardial Reperfusion Injury: From a Pre-clinical Phenomenon to a New Target for Cardioprotection

Chapter 2
Pathophysiology of Myocardial Reperfusion Injury

James M. Downey and Michael V. Cohen

Abstract The debate over the existence and nature of lethal reperfusion injury has been sustained by the fact that we do not know exactly why an ischemic insult kills cells in the first place. While the mechanism of lethal ischemia is far from fully understood, much is known about it, and it is not simply a matter of cells starving to death from lack of nutrition. In practical terms, ischemia must be treated by reperfusion. But for many years, scientists suspected that reperfusion itself causes a component of injury and reasoned if that injury could be eliminated, the outcome of reperfusion therapy would be improved. In this chapter, we will explore some of the proposed theories of reperfusion injury, including membrane failure from swelling, calcium overload, free radical attack, inflammation, and mitochondrial permeability transition pores. We will explore how each theory originated and the evidence supporting each.

Keywords Cardioprotection • Free radicals • Mitochondrial permeability transition pore • Myocardial infarction • Myocardial ischemia • Stunned myocardium

J.M. Downey, Ph.D. (✉)
Department of Physiology, University of South Alabama, College of Medicine, Room 3074, Medical Science Building, Mobile, AL 36688, USA
e-mail: jdowney@usouthal.edu

M.V. Cohen, M.D.
Department of Medicine, University of South Alabama Medical Center, Mobile, AL, USA

Department of Physiology, MSB3050, University of South Alabama, College of Medicine, Mobile, AL, USA
e-mail: mcohen@usouthal.edu

J.C. Kaski et al. (eds.), *Management of Myocardial Reperfusion Injury*,
DOI 10.1007/978-1-84996-019-9_2, © Springer-Verlag London 2012

Why Has Lethal Reperfusion Injury Been So Hard to Identify?

Reperfusion injury refers to a form of injury specifically caused by the act of reperfusing an ischemic tissue. In this chapter, we will focus on lethal reperfusion injury of the heart. Both scientists and clinicians have hotly debated exactly what constitutes a reperfusion injury, what its mechanism is, and, until recently, if it even exists. The nature of ischemia/reperfusion models themselves causes our initial uncertainty. One can easily create myocardial ischemia by obstructing an animal's coronary artery. The amount of tissue death will be proportional to the length of time the artery is obstructed. If it is never reperfused, then virtually all of the ischemic cells will die. If it is reperfused after, for example, 30 min, then much of the previously ischemic myocardium will survive. While reperfusion is by definition needed to cause reperfusion injury, it is also needed to terminate the ischemia and salvage the tissue. The most obvious experiment to reveal the existence of any reperfusion injury would be comparison of cells that have been reperfused for only a minute or two to cells that have not been reperfused. The problem, however, is that it is not easy to distinguish if the cells are dead or alive. We tend to think of death as a black or white issue, but it actually includes many shades of gray. The brain-dead individual can donate a very viable heart. Intestines removed from a cow at the slaughter house can provide a scientist with living visceral smooth muscle cells for many days after the steaks have been consumed. So exactly when does the cardiomyocyte die? When its ATP is depleted? When its membrane ruptures? When striations disappear? When pro-apoptotic factors have been activated? Because we cannot always determine if a cell is dead or alive, the alternative approach has been to reperfuse it and see if it recovers [1]. If the cell recovers, then it must not have been dead. But, of course, reperfusion also initiates the destructive reperfusion injury. This conundrum has fueled debate for many decades.

A much more powerful approach to identifying reperfusion injury has focused on finding an intervention that would eliminate it. If an intervention were given at the time of reperfusion that resulted in a smaller infarct, then one could reason that the component of injury that was prevented was that which would be the product of a reperfusion injury. That approach was hampered until recently by the absence of any intervention that unambiguously reduced infarct size when administered at or after the time of reperfusion.

The debate about the existence and nature of lethal reperfusion injury has been sustained by the realization that we do not know exactly why ischemia kills cells in the first place. In this chapter, we will explore what is known about the mechanisms whereby ischemia can kill a cell. The mechanism of lethal ischemia is far from fully understood, but much is known about it and it is not simply a matter of cells starving to death from lack of nutrition. We will then explore some of the proposed theories of reperfusion injury, how they originated, and the evidence supporting each.

Oncosis: Death by Swelling

In the 1960s, Robert Jennings' laboratory [2] began studying ischemic myocardium with a newly developed research tool, the electron microscope. He and his colleagues noted that tissue swells when it is ischemic. They proposed that swelling resulted from a defect in volume regulation in these ischemic cells [3]. Mammalian cells are surrounded by membranes that have a high permeability to water and very little structural rigidity. Cells must maintain their volume through an osmotic equilibrium across their outer membrane. They are filled with osmotically active constituents like proteins and nucleotides that cannot traverse the membrane. If a cardiomyocyte were placed in pure water, it would quickly swell and burst. So how does it survive in the aqueous milieu of the body? Nature has cleverly solved that problem by making the cell's membrane very impermeable to sodium and using membrane sodium pumps to force sodium out of the cell against a concentration gradient such that the extracellular sodium can balance the pull of everything else inside the cell. The transmembrane sodium gradient is not needed just for generating action potentials, and even cells that do not generate action potentials must extrude sodium to create osmotic balance.

Thus the sodium–potassium ATPase in the membrane is the bilge pump that keeps the cell afloat. If the power to a leaky ship's bilge pump is interrupted for too long, the ship will fill with water and sink. The same is true about the cell's sodium pump. During ischemia, the ATP level can quickly fall below that required to run the ion pumps so that any sodium that leaks in can no longer be pumped out. As more sodium accumulates in the cell, more water is pulled in after it. If enough swelling occurs, there will be inevitable catastrophic rupture of the outer cell membrane with rapid loss of vital soluble cytosolic enzymes, nuceotides, and cofactors. This condition is called necrosis (or more correctly oncosis). The commonly used supravital tetrazolium staining method used to differentiate live from dead tissue is based on the loss of dehydrogenase enzymes and cofactor that ordinarily change the tetrazolium to a colored product [4, 5]. If those constituents have been lost, the tissue will not stain, and it can be considered to be dead.

Other factors besides a loss of the sodium gradient contribute to ischemic swelling. For example, metabolism of ATP ultimately results in one molecule of AMP plus 2 molecules of inorganic phosphate. Since none of these molecules can diffuse through the membrane, the osmotic pull they exert has been essentially tripled from that of ATP alone (osmotic pressure is proportional to the molar concentration of the substance and is independent of its molecular size). The ATP concentration is approximately 5 mM in the myocyte, and each mM of an osmolyte exerts 19 mmHg of osmotic pressure. Thus, depletion of ATP alone would increase the osmotic pressure in the cell by a substantial 190 mmHg! Cleaving proteins into many small peptides by proteases will have a similar effect.

One of the earliest suggestions of a reperfusion injury was made by Kloner et al. [3] when they noted that swelling was greatly accelerated during reperfusion.

They described this as "explosive swelling" at reperfusion (Fig. 2.1). During ischemia, sodium leaks from the interstitial space into the cell. Because the interstitial compartment in the heart is small compared to the intracellular compartment, only a small amount of fluid can shift into the cells. But during reperfusion, the extracellular fluid is replenished with an endless supply of isotonic fluid which then passes into the cells causing them to quickly swell. Furthermore, a large amount of sodium moves into the cells in the first minutes of reperfusion presumably through the membrane exchangers (see below) [6]. Is the fluid shift a reperfusion injury? In a sense it is. Reperfusion with a hypertonic perfusate in an attempt to blunt swelling reportedly does prevent some necrotic death [7].

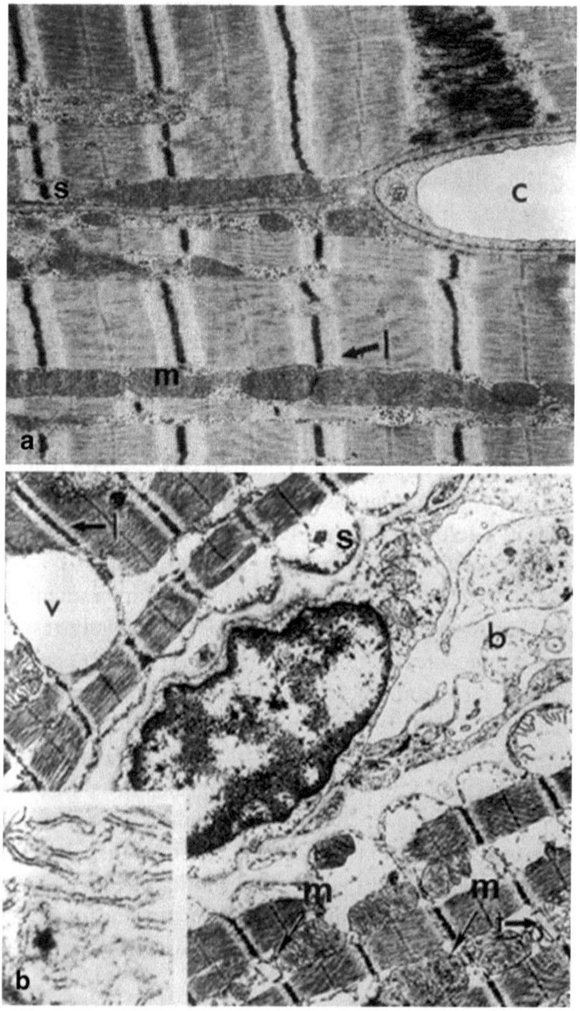

Fig. 2.1 (**a**) Electron micrograph of normal canine myocardium. Note regular sarcomeres separated by dense mitochondria (*m*). The sarcolemma (*s*), I bands (*I*, see *arrow*), and a capillary (*c*) can also be seen. (**b**) Shows the heart after 40 min of ischemia. Note how the cells are swollen. The mitochondria (*m*) and inset (see *arrows*), are enlarged and less electron-dense. The sarcolemma (*s*) is pushed away from the cell and tethered only by its z-line attachments. A large water-filled vacuole (*v*) and bleb in the capillary endothelium (*b*) are also seen. The transverse tubule (*t*) is intact (see *arrows*). (**c**) Shows a biopsy taken 30 min after reperfusion. The sarcomeres have shortened into irreversible contraction bands (*cb*). The sarcolemma (*s*) is no longer continuous so that cytosolic contents have been lost (see *arrows*) (From Kloner et al. [3]. Used with kind permission from Elsevier)

Fig. 2.1 (continued)

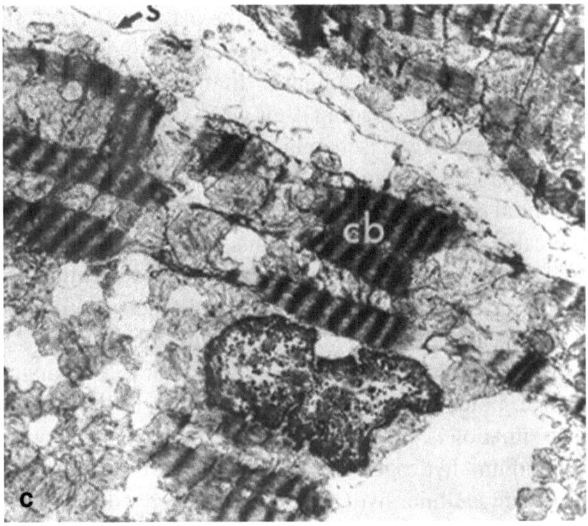

Calcium Overload

It is well known that calcium is an important intracellular signaling molecule. As a result, the behavior of many enzymes and proteins is modulated by the presence of calcium. In the heart, calcium triggers contraction by causing actin and myosin filaments to slide past each other. The muscle then relaxes when calcium is removed from the cytosol during diastole. During ischemia, cardiac muscle goes into a state of continuous contraction. Two factors account for this. The first is depletion of ATP, which is required to break the cross bridges between the actin and myosin molecules. This is termed rigor. The second factor is elevated calcium in the cytosol, which binds to troponin and continuously activates cross bridge cycling, termed contracture. A variety of calcium-sensitive probes has demonstrated that the calcium level is greatly increased during reperfusion [8].

This high calcium level is thought to be responsible for the contraction band form of necrosis seen in reperfused hearts in which ultrashort sarcomeres appear [3]. A similar pattern of contraction band necrosis also accompanies the calcium paradox [9]. In the calcium paradox, perfusion of a heart for a few minutes with calcium-free buffer paradoxically makes the heart become very sensitive to calcium. When calcium is reintroduced, the heart promptly goes into contracture and dies.

The source of the intracellular calcium has long been a matter of debate. Some of the increase in calcium has been attributed to activity of the sodium–hydrogen exchanger. During ischemia, the heart tries to maintain ATP production by anaerobic glycolysis of its glycogen. Although anaerobic glycolysis is not sufficiently robust to completely sustain all of the heart's functions, it does help. In the process, hydrogen ions are produced and the pH drops. The sodium–hydrogen exchanger in the membranes of cardiomyocytes detects the fall in pH and extrudes hydrogen ion in exchange for extracellular sodium. Thus, while trying to maintain a neutral pH, the cell is actually loading itself with sodium, which appears to be a somewhat paradoxical response to ischemia.

In the healthy cardiomyocyte, most of the calcium that enters during an action potential is subsequently removed by the sodium–calcium exchanger [10]. Normally, the calcium and sodium gradients are such that any small rise in cytosolic calcium will in turn lead to a favorable exchange for extracellular sodium. The sodium is then quickly pumped out by the membrane's sodium–potassium ATPase. However, if the transmembrane sodium gradient falls as occurs with sodium loading during ischemia, then intracellular sodium starts to exchange with extracellular calcium. Hence, potentially toxic calcium is brought into and accumulates within the cell. The situation is greatly exacerbated by reperfusion, which accelerates the actions of the sodium–hydrogen exchanger by neutralizing the extracellular pH [8]. Thus even more intracellular hydrogen ion is exchanged for extracellular sodium. Again, this would appear as a reperfusion injury. While giving a sodium–hydrogen exchange blocker before or during ischemia is very protective against infarction, it is much less so when given at the time of reperfusion [11].

Calcium can also enter via defects in the membrane caused by swelling. The increased intracellular calcium concentration is high enough to cause contracture and activate a number of calcium-dependent enzymes. The relative contribution of membrane failure versus pump- and exchanger-mediated calcium loading has never been resolved, but they are intimately related. It is also unknown whether sodium–hydrogen exchange blockers ultimately protect by preventing osmotic swelling or calcium entry. Both are possible.

Free Radicals

When most biologists think of reperfusion injury, they usually think of free radicals as the instruments of that damage. In the 1970s, it was noted that there were a variety of sources of reactive oxygen species (ROS) when an ischemic organ was reperfused. Those sources included injured mitochondria [12], xanthine oxidase activity [13], and leukocytes [14]. Many of the ROS species belong to the chemical class of "free radicals," molecules with unpaired electrons in their outer shell, which makes them very reactive. These include superoxide and hydroxyl radicals and peroxynitrite. However, not all biologically important ROS are radicals, hydrogen peroxide being a prime example.

The description by David Hearse et al. [15] of the oxygen paradox was one of the earliest observations suggesting that ROS are injurious in myocardial ischemia. Hearse and colleagues subjected an isolated rat heart to a prolonged period of perfusion with hypoxic buffer. When they switched back to oxygenated buffer, the heart promptly went into contracture [16] and released a massive quantity of its intracellular enzymes [15], thus recalling what was seen with the calcium paradox. Hearse, therefore, termed this phenomenon the oxygen paradox. They did not know the cause of the injury, but they speculated that one possible mechanism was production of free radicals, and this turned out to be the correct choice. The beauty of the study was the simplicity of its design. In ischemia/reperfusion, there are many things that are changing in addition to oxygen delivery. In the experiments in which the oxygen paradox was documented, only the pO_2 of the buffer was altered, and yet this produced a most dramatic result.

Stunning Versus Infarction

Since Hearse's original study, there has been a great deal of work investigating the role of ROS in myocardial ischemia. The primary tools for that work have been the free radical scavengers. A variety of chemicals have been developed that can neutralize many of the ROS species. And they have been studied in a variety of ischemia models. Before we can discuss the effects of radical scavengers, we must make an important point about the models that were being used to evaluate an intervention's cardioprotective potential.

In the 1970s, two models of myocardial ischemia were being extensively used. The first was the "recovery-of-function" model. In the latter, a small animal's heart was removed, and the isolated heart was perfused with a crystalloid buffer. Some parameter of the heart's mechanical function (e.g., developed ventricular pressure) would be measured, and then the heart would be subjected to a global ischemic insult for a prolonged period of time. During ischemia, the heart quickly stopped contracting and became quiescent. The heart would then be reperfused, and the degree to which the mechanical function recovered was noted. Anything that would increase that recovery was considered to be cardioprotective. In the second model, a coronary arterial branch of an open-chest animal would be first occluded for a set period (the index ischemia) and then reperfused after which the heart would be sliced into serial sections and the volume of the infarcted zone measured. Anything that reduced necrosis would again be considered to be cardioprotective. These two models were assumed to measure the same thing, the extent of myocardial tissue death. The prevalent assumption was that the depressed function simply reflected the loss of contraction of infarcted cells in the heart and that was backed up by the appearance of cytosolic enzymes in the venous effluent.

Unfortunately the above assumption proved to be false. Much of the depressed postischemic function results from a phenomenon termed myocardial stunning [17]. Stunning is largely the result of ROS attack on the heart's contractile proteins which occurs when the heart is reperfused [18]. Unlike the lethal injury of infarction, stunning is fully reversible after an extended (hours to days) period of reperfusion. On the other hand, infarction is not reversible and the role of free radicals in infarction is much less obvious. Because scavengers were very effective in recovery-of-function models, they were quickly popularized by the research and clinical communities. Unfortunately, the scavengers were much less effective in the infarct models. And as the infarct models became more and more refined, scavengers performed less and less well. To date, there is little credible evidence that a free radical scavenger can salvage ischemic myocardium in any species [19–22].

The Surgeon Versus the Cardiologist

Two branches of cardiac medicine are concerned with cardioprotection. The surgeon makes the heart globally ischemic when he operates on it and then must reperfuse the heart when it is disconnected from the bypass pump. If the heart is stunned at that time, it may be unable to support the circulation and the surgeon is suddenly faced with having to deal with major adverse hemodynamic and prognostic consequences. An anti-stunning treatment would be very desirable in that setting. In contrast, in acute ST-segment elevation myocardial infarction, ischemia is usually regional and in the distribution of the occluded artery. When the occluded artery is reperfused, nonlethal stunning in the ischemic region is usually not a pressing issue since the unaffected myocardium is capable of maintaining the circulation, although this may not be the case in the setting of prior infarction at other sites. Any stunned muscle will eventually recover. What is important is the amount of tissue that was lost to infarction. Since the heart lacks the ability to regenerate myocardium, that loss will be permanent, and the heart's work load will have to be carried by the surviving tissue. If that load is too great, the overworked muscle will remodel itself, and there will likely be eventual progression to heart failure—what would be helpful is the ability to reduce the degree of infarction if this is possible.

The needs of the surgeons and cardiologists differ in one other important aspect. The surgeon has access to the patient prior to ischemia and, therefore, can pretreat, but because stunning occurs at reperfusion and scavengers given at that time are very effective, pretreatment is seldom needed. However, the cardiologist only sees the patient with acute myocardial infarction after ischemia has begun. Since the discovery of ischemic preconditioning in 1986 [23], it has been proven that it is possible to make the heart muscle resistant to infarction if one can treat prior to the onset of ischemia. Ironically, for years the surgeons had treatments that protected against stunning when given at reperfusion, while the cardiologists had anti-infarct interventions that only worked as pretreatments. The cardiologists desperately needed something that would protect against infarction once ischemia had begun. But the only way that could be possible was if myocardium were being killed by a lethal reperfusion-type injury. Hence, there was great excitement when the theory that free radicals at reperfusion were killing a significant amount of myocardium was introduced. Although free radicals do contribute to myocardial stunning, a nonlethal form of reperfusion injury, they sadly appear to have little direct effect on the process of infarction.

Inflammation

A twist on the free radical theory was that leukocytes were invading the reperfused myocardium and were killing viable myocardium. The evidence was clear—leukocytes were seen wherever the myocardium was infarcted. One of the major weapons in the leukocyte's cytotoxic arsenal is superoxide radical generated by NADPH oxidase. Leukocytes start to invade the infarcted myocardium several hours after reperfusion has begun [24], and by 5 h, they are present in great numbers [25]. Of course, this delayed attack would be unaffected by any antioxidant treatment confined to only the first minutes of reperfusion. The problem with the leukocyte hypothesis is that it is difficult to establish a cause-and-effect relationship between the presence of leukocytes and the infarct. Leukocytes naturally home in on necrotic tissue to remove dead cells so scar formation can commence. The important question was whether they would also attack injured but salvageable tissue.

One might argue that failure of free radical scavengers to prevent infarction would imply that leukocytes are not a factor in this process. However, leukocytes may injure myocardium by a mechanism not involving free radicals. More than 25 years ago, Engler et al. [26] proposed that leukocytes might impair reflow by mechanically occluding the microcirculation leading to a no-reflow situation. That issue has not been resolved, and there is still great interest in promoting improved patency of the coronary tree of patients undergoing angioplasty and stenting [27]. So are leukocytes killing the heart muscle or is dead muscle attracting the leukocytes? The data provide mixed signals. A number of anti-inflammatory agents have been subjected to clinical trials, but so far none has been effective at decreasing infarction (see Chap. 12) [21].

The most common method for measuring infarction in the animal models has been supravital tetrazolium staining. Tetrazolium stains only living tissue because membrane failure in necrotic tissue has caused it to lose the dehydrogenase enzymes and cofactor that reacts with tetrazolium to form the red formazan pigment. Most investigators have reported that the full extent of infarction can be reliably measured with tetrazolium after only 2 h of reperfusion [5]. But that would have preceded most of the leukocyte invasion. We found that infarct size measured by tetrazolium staining 3 h after reperfusion was no different from that measured after several days of reperfusion in rat or rabbit (Fig. 2.2) [28]. However, one recent report does describe an appreciable difference between infarct size measured several hours after reperfusion and that measured after 24 h of reperfusion in a canine heart model of ischemia/reperfusion [29].

Does the leukocyte attack constitute a reperfusion injury? The answer is unclear since the leukocytes invade many hours after reperfusion. One could argue that they are simply homing in on tissue that was injured by the ischemia. Where does the reperfusion phase end and the recovery phase begin? Does every detrimental thing that happens to a patient after he is reperfused constitute reperfusion injury? But this is only a matter of semantics, and the distinction may be unimportant. If leukocyte attack does account for an appreciable amount of tissue death, then it should be feasible to prevent the latter in the patient with acute myocardial infarction and salvage more myocardium.

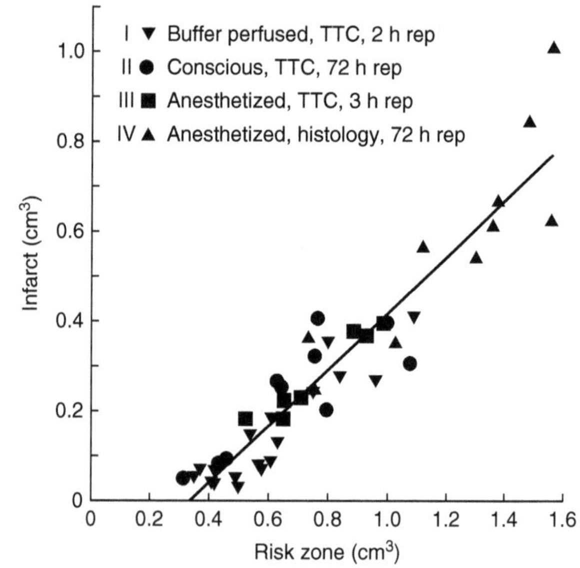

Fig. 2.2 A plot of infarct size versus ischemic (risk) zone size in rabbit hearts exposed to 30 min of ischemia. The infarct sizes were similar in anesthetized, conscious, or isolated buffer-perfused hearts. Also, the infarct size was the same in 2- or 72-h reperfusion models, suggesting that in rabbit hearts the ultimate infarct size had been reached after only 2 h of reperfusion (Adapted from Ytrehus et al. [28]. Used with kind permission from The American Physiological Society)

Myocardial Effects of Preconditioning

In the 1990s, most experts were convinced that ischemic preconditioning had a direct protective effect on the myocardium, although the actual mechanism was elusive. The team [23] that first described ischemic preconditioning originally proposed that it was suppressing mitochondrial ATPase [30]. The mitochondria generate ATP by extruding hydrogen ions from the matrix. This makes the matrix very basic and provides a strong pH gradient across the inner mitochondrial membrane. Located in the membrane is F_1 ATP synthase which is actually an ATP-driven pump that can pump hydrogen ions out of the matrix. If the ion gradient is high enough, hydrogen ions will be forced backward through the pump and into the matrix which amazingly turns the pump into a generator of ATP rather than a consumer. By that method, the mitochondria phosphorylate ADP to make ATP. During ischemia, electron transport ceases along with hydrogen ion extrusion. Soon, the transmembrane hydrogen ion gradient falls. With no gradient, F_1 synthase reverts to its pump mode and switches from generation to consumption of ATP. It is reported that about 35% of the ATP consumed by ischemic myocardium is through this pathway [31]. The prevailing hypothesis at that time was that preconditioning somehow prevented this mitochondrial ATPase activity which would preserve ATP and extend viability. Unfortunately, the evidence supporting that theory was not forthcoming [32]. The ATP-sparing theory was finally abandoned when it was shown that a vigorous preconditioning protocol could deplete so much ATP that a protected heart could end up with a lower ATP level than the unprotected control heart [33].

Another theory was that preconditioning opened ATP-sensitive potassium channels, which would shorten action potential duration and spare ATP [34]. However, when action potential shortening from cromakalim was blocked with dofetilide, protection was not aborted [35]. It was subsequently observed that K_{ATP} channel opening acts as a trigger of preconditioning's signal transduction pathways rather than as an end-effector of protection [36]. We tested whether preconditioning might have altered the antioxidant status of the heart [37] but found no differences. One theory even suggested that the sodium–hydrogen exchanger was blocked during ischemia by preconditioning [38]. The problem with all of these hypotheses was that the underlying assumption that preconditioning was protecting against injury during ischemia was incorrect. Everyone was looking for the protective change at the wrong time.

Proof of Reperfusion Injury

Yellon's group had noted that some agents such as TGF-β(beta) could protect against infarction when given at reperfusion [39]. More importantly, they noted that TGF-β(beta)'s protection could be blocked by an ERK inhibitor. Eventually, Hausenloy et al. [40] tested kinase inhibitors against ischemic preconditioning in an isolated rat heart. They administered the inhibitors to ERK or PI3-kinase at the end of the index ischemia. Either one could completely block protection. They also reported that both Akt (a down-stream target of PI3-kinase) and ERK in tissue sampled just after reperfusion were more phosphorylated at their activation sites in preconditioned than in non-preconditioned hearts (Fig. 2.3). They concluded that these

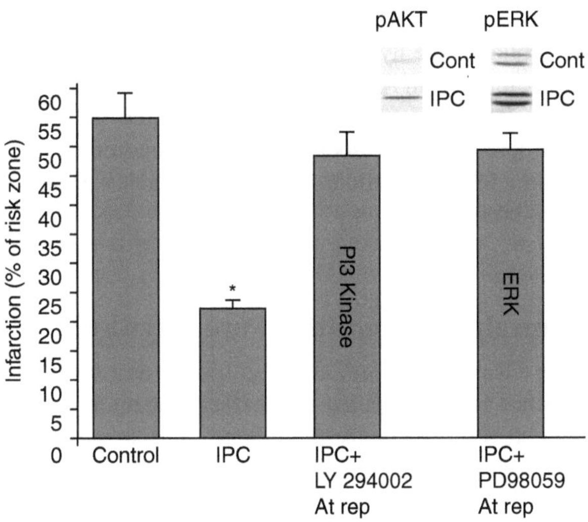

Fig. 2.3 Infarct size in rat hearts exposed to 35-min ischemia. Ischemic preconditioning is very protective when compared to hearts that were not preconditioned (control). When LY 294002 (PI3-kinase inhibitor) or PD 98059 (ERK inhibitor) was given to a preconditioned heart just prior to reperfusion, protection was lost, indicating that protection occurred at or after reperfusion. The *insets* are western blots which show that the activation sites of AKT (target for PI3-kinase) or ERK were preferentially phosphorylated in preconditioned hearts at reperfusion (Adapted from data presented in Hausenloy et al. [40])

adjacent cell explodes and drenches it in cytoplasm. The confluent nature of necrosis allows us to assess infarct size with gross techniques like tetrazolium staining or magnetic resonance imaging. On the other hand, hearts attacked by apoptosis would be expected to look more like Swiss cheese with scattered microscopic holes where the condemned myocytes formerly were. In theory, tetrazolium staining should not detect changes in apoptosis in the tissue because these cells are scattered among intact cells, and they never break open to disgorge intracellular contents.

In 2000, the Nobel Prize for Physiology or Medicine was awarded to Brenner, Horvitz, and Sulston for their work on apoptosis, which suddenly made everyone aware of this phenomenon. The obvious question was whether apoptosis could be contributing to injury following ischemia/reperfusion. Indeed, caspase activation was seen in reperfused hearts along with endonuclease attack of their chromatin [51]. Clearly, ischemia/reperfusion triggers apoptosis. But was apoptosis contributing to the infarct? Necrotic cells in their death throes may also activate apoptosis, but that probably would be the least of their problems. But consider another scenario. Transition pores release cytochrome C, a potent trigger of apoptosis in the cell. Cells that have enough functioning mitochondria to avoid necrosis may still have released enough cyctochrome C to trigger the slow cell death process of apoptosis that may kill the cell in a day or two. Perhaps, extensive apoptosis occurs outside the necrotic infarct that is undetected by the tetrazolium stain but nevertheless insidiously weakens the heart muscle.

Ischemic preconditioning greatly reduces apoptosis in hearts exposed to ischemia/reperfusion. One obvious link is the transition pores whose opening triggers apoptosis through cytochrome C release. Since preconditioning or drugs that protect through preconditioning's mechanism suppress transition pore formation, it is reasonable to propose that fewer apoptotic cells should be seen in a preconditioned heart. But the connection may be more direct than that. Several reports claim that infarct size can be reduced by a direct blocker of caspase activity [52] or by expression of antiapoptotic proteins like Bcl2 [53].

Is Ischemia or Reperfusion the Real Villain?

Transition pores at reperfusion are not the only factors killing myocardium. Ischemia also is lethal. It causes swelling as mentioned above, and depletion of ATP will eventually starve the cell to death. Reperfusion will induce transition pores, but only if the heart has first sustained ischemic injury. Patients routinely undergo elective angioplasty in which a coronary artery is occluded for up to a minute and then reperfused with no untoward effects. Again, it comes down to a question of semantics. Is reperfusion good for the patient? Yes! Reimer and Jennings [54] showed that infarct size in dogs was proportional to the duration of ischemia. They noted that as the duration of the ischemic period was prolonged, the infarct enlarged, but they never found an ischemic time after which reperfusion made the infarct larger than that seen with permanent occlusion. This observation forms the scientific basis for recommending reperfusion therapy for all patients with acute myocardial infarction who present within 6–12 h of the onset of symptoms.

Can reperfusion be improved upon? Yes again! We can safely conclude that inclusion of a maneuver to suppress transition pores can greatly limit infarction in either animals [55] or humans [56]. We now believe that there are four populations of cells in the reperfused heart. There are those that were killed from ischemia alone. Those probably constitute the small infarct seen in a preconditioned heart. Then, there are those that survived the ischemia but will be killed soon after reperfusion by transition pore formation. This population seems to be surprisingly large as evidenced by the salvage obtained by postconditioning or cyclosporin A. The third population includes those cells that would have survived ischemic injury and transition pore formation only to be killed many hours after reperfusion by inflammation or apoptosis. The fourth population includes those lucky cells that survive the gauntlet of all of the above injuries and would represent the long-term survivors seen in a reperfused heart without any anti-infarct treatment.

Concluding Remarks

In this chapter, we have reviewed the prevailing theories of lethal injury seen in ischemia/reperfusion in the heart and how our concept of lethal reperfusion injury has evolved over the years. At present, we believe that mitochondrial transition pores contribute greatly to lethality at the time of reperfusion. Whether there are other components of cell death following reperfusion such as inflammation or calcium overload is still not clear. Preventing cell death with pre- or postconditioning does not eliminate all necrosis in the reperfused heart, indicating that other factors are contributing to cell death. Future studies are needed to dissect out the different processes that contribute to cell death in ischemia/reperfusion so that hopefully a combination therapy will emerge that can eventually eliminate them one by one.

References

1. Jennings RB, Sommers HM, Smyth GA, Flack HA, Linn H. Myocardial necrosis induced by temporary occlusion of a coronary artery in the dog. Arch Pathol. 1960;70:68–78.
2. Herdson PB, Sommers HM, Jennings RB. A comparative study of the fine structure of normal and ischemic dog myocardium with special reference to early changes following temporary occlusion of a coronary artery. Am J Pathol. 1965;46(3):367–86.
3. Kloner RA, Ganote CE, Whalen Jr DA, Jennings RB. Effect of a transient period of ischemia on myocardial cells. II. Fine structure during the first few minutes of reflow. Am J Pathol. 1974;74(3):399–422.
4. Fishbein MC, Meerbaum S, Rit J, et al. Early phase acute myocardial infarct size quantification: validation of the triphenyl tetrazolium chloride tissue enzyme staining technique. Am Heart J. 1981;101(5):593–600.

49. Weiss JN, Korge P, Honda HM, Ping P. Role of the mitochondrial permeability transition in myocardial disease. Circ Res. 2003;93(4):292–301.
50. Argaud L, Gateau-Roesch O, Chalabreysse L, et al. Preconditioning delays Ca^{2+}-induced mitochondrial permeability transition. Cardiovasc Res. 2004;61(1):115–22.
51. Gottlieb RA, Burleson KO, Kloner RA, Babior BM, Engler RL. Reperfusion injury induces apoptosis in rabbit cardiomyocytes. J Clin Invest. 1994;94(4):1621–8.
52. Mocanu MM, Baxter GF, Yellon DM. Caspase inhibition and limitation of myocardial infarct size: protection against lethal reperfusion injury. Br J Pharmacol. 2000;130(2):197–200.
53. Zhao Z-Q, Budde JM, Morris C, et al. Adenosine attenuates reperfusion-induced apoptotic cell death by modulating expression of Bcl-2 and Bax proteins. J Mol Cell Cardiol. 2001;33(1): 57–68.
54. Reimer KA, Jennings RB. The "wavefront phenomenon" of myocardial ischemic cell death. II. Transmural progression of necrosis within the framework of ischemic bed size (myocardium at risk) and collateral flow. Lab Invest. 1979;40(6):633–44.
55. Hausenloy DJ, Duchen MR, Yellon DM. Inhibiting mitochondrial permeability transition pore opening at reperfusion protects against ischaemia-reperfusion injury. Cardiovasc Res. 2003;60(3):617–25.
56. Piot C, Croisille P, Staat P, et al. Effect of cyclosporine on reperfusion injury in acute myocardial infarction. N Engl J Med. 2008;359(5):473–81.

Chapter 3
Microvascular Obstruction: The No-Reflow Phenomenon in Animal Models of Myocardial Ischemia and Reperfusion

Thorsten Reffelmann and Robert A. Kloner

Abstract In animal models of coronary artery occlusion and reopening of the epicardial artery, perfusion defects within the area at risk may develop during reperfusion despite complete reopening of the epicardial artery. These anatomical areas of no-reflow are confined to areas of myocardial necrosis and substantially expand during ongoing reperfusion. This reperfusion injury at the microvascular level may be related to ultrastructural alterations of the microvasculature, production of reactive oxygen species during reperfusion, leukocyte accumulation, and release of vasoconstrictive agents. Myocardial infarct size appears to be the major determinant of no-reflow, and cardioprotective interventions leading to smaller infarcts result in reduced microvascular obstruction in most of the models. Several therapeutic strategies have been developed to reduce no-reflow; however, in most of these investigations it was difficult to dissociate no-reflow from infarct size. Transfer to the clinical setting of myocardial infarction shows many similarities, but additional mechanisms such as coronary microembolization significantly contribute to clinical no-reflow.

Keywords Microvascular obstruction • No-reflow • Ischemia • Reperfusion Myocardial blood flow

---

T. Reffelmann, M.D. (✉)
Klinik und Poliklinik fur Innere Medizin B,
Universitatsklinik der Ernst-Moritz-Amdt-Universitat Greifswald,
Friedrich-Loffler-Str.23a, Greifswald 17485, Germany
e-mail: thorstenreffelmann@web.de

R.A. Kloner, M.D., Ph.D.
Department of Medicine, Division of Cardiovascular Medicine,
Keck School of Medicine at University of Southern California,
Los Angeles, CA, USA

The Heart Institute, Good Samaritan Hospital, Los Angeles, CA, USA

Division of Cardiology, Keck School of Medicine, University of Southern California,
1225 Wilshire Blvd., Los Angeles 90017-2395, CA, USA
e-mail: rkloner@goodsam.org

J.C. Kaski et al. (eds.), *Management of Myocardial Reperfusion Injury*,
DOI 10.1007/978-1-84996-019-9_3,

Definition: Microvascular Obstruction: No-Reflow Phenomenon

Acute myocardial infarction occurs when blood supply to the myocardial tissue is not sufficient for survival of myocardial tissue over a critical period of time. In the majority of cases, this is the result of an occlusive epicardial coronary artery thrombus, compromising blood flow below a critical level [1]. In animal models of myocardial infarction, ligation of a coronary artery is most frequently used to induce myocardial ischemia to simulate pathophysiological alterations of the clinical syndrome of myocardial infarction [2].

Reperfusion of the ischemic myocardial tissue as early as possible is effective in reducing myocardial infarct size, the degree of myocardial contractile dysfunction, and also long-term mortality, as demonstrated in basic animal research as well as large-scale clinical trials [3, 4]. However, it has become increasingly recognized that complete reopening of an occluded epicardial coronary artery does not necessarily mean complete reperfusion of the myocardial tissue. After restoration of epicardial coronary artery flow, be it by thrombolysis or acute coronary angioplasty in the clinical setting or release of the coronary artery ligation in the animal model, tissue perfusion critically depends on microvascular integrity [5, 6].

Initially, the term "no-reflow-phenomenon" was coined to describe compromised microvascular perfusion despite reopening of the epicardial coronary artery in animal models of myocardial ischemia and reperfusion [7, 8]. Later, this expression was transferred to the clinical setting to describe microvascular obstruction in spite of successful restoration of epicardial artery diameters by acute coronary angioplasty or thrombolysis [9–11].

While reperfusion of the occluded epicardial coronary artery is necessary for the occurrence of no-reflow by definition, ongoing reperfusion itself appears to significantly contribute to the occurrence and degree of microvascular obstruction. As outlined below, no-reflow may therefore be regarded as a form of reperfusion injury at the microvascular level.

The following paragraphs will delineate major characteristics and determinants of microvascular obstruction with a particular emphasis on basic science findings from animal research.

Animal Models of Ischemia and Reperfusion

In 1966, Krug et al. first described the "no-reflow" phenomenon after coronary artery ligation and reopening of the occlusion in a cat model of myocardial infarction [6]. Distinct anatomical zones of severely depressed tissue perfusion developed within the myocardium supplied by the coronary tree which had been temporarily occluded by the ligation. In subsequent studies, various dyes, injected into the circulation to stain perfused tissue, were used to visualize these zones of hypoperfusion (Fig. 3.1). Perfusion defects after temporary coronary artery ligation were

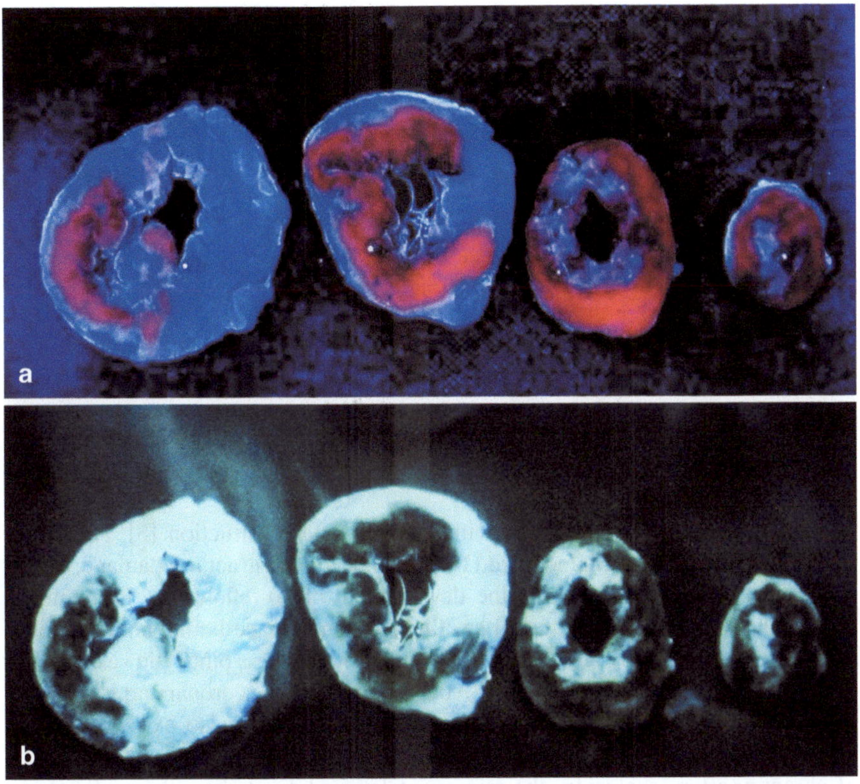

Fig. 3.1 Anatomical no-reflow, visualized in a rabbit model of coronary artery ligation and reopening of the epicardial ligation. The blue dye Uniperse Blue (**a**) and the fluorescent vital stain thioflavin S (**b**), photography under ultraviolet light) were injected into the left atrium after 120 min of coronary artery occlusion and 120 min of reperfusion. Both dyes leave a substantial part of the left ventricle unstained, indicating areas of no or low perfusion no-reflow (From Reffelmann and Kloner [2], with permission)

visualized as zones not stained by the dye, presenting so-called zones of anatomical no-reflow within the myocardial tissue at risk [8].

In a canine model, injection of the dyes, carbon black (particulate black dye), and thioflavin S (fluorescent vital stain) after 40 min of coronary occlusion with subsequent reopening of the coronary artery resulted in homogeneous staining of the myocardium [8]. However, after 90 min of coronary occlusion followed by reperfusion, distinct areas not stained by the two dyes were identified, which were predominantly located in the subendocardium. These areas of "no-reflow" were characterized by very low regional myocardial blood flow between 0.13 ml/g/min and 0.39 ml/g/min (at the time of perfusion staining), as determined by the radioactive microsphere technique. In the dog heart, normal myocardial flow amounts to approximately 1.0 ml/g/min. In this study, these areas of no-reflow were first systematically examined by electron microscopy, which allowed the description of the

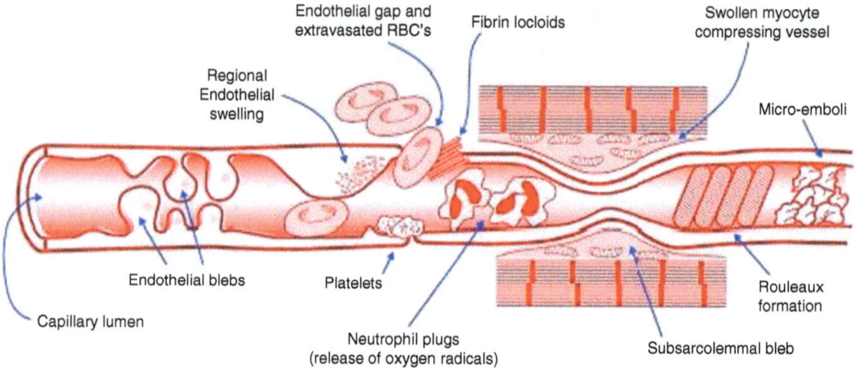

Fig. 3.2 Schematic figure, summarizing different mechanisms, involved in the development of no-reflow, and accompanying ultrastructural alterations of the microvascular bed (*RBC* red blood cell) (From Reffelmann and Kloner [2], with permission)

ultrastructural changes associated with microvascular obstruction [8]. Areas not stained by the dye were characterized by pronounced ultrastructural damage, which might also be a causal factor in the development of no-reflow, and intraluminal endothelial protrusions, endothelial swelling, and membrane-bound bodies (blebs) were observed (Fig. 3.2). The endothelial cells contained less pinocytic vesicles and demonstrated chromatin margination. After reopening of the coronary artery, packed red blood cells (rouleaux formation), and after some time also extravasation of erythrocytes along with endothelial gaps, were characteristic findings. After 40 min of coronary artery occlusion, the microvasculature did not show these ultrastructural characteristics.

Fishbein et al. demonstrated a very close spatial correlation of microvascular damage and myocardial hemorrhage [12]. Zones of hemorrhage were always confined to areas of vascular damage in these investigations. Zones of hemorrhage were located in the subendocardium and most importantly were closely correlated with areas of myocardial necrosis. The close correlation of microvascular obstruction and hemorrhage was also shown in the rabbit heart [13].

Unlike the canine heart, which is characterized by significant collateral flow to the ischemic myocardium once the coronary artery has been occluded, rat or rabbit hearts, which were studied extensively in models of ischemia and reperfusion, have negligible collateral flow to the ischemic myocardium, when the epicardial coronary artery has been occluded. Simultaneous injection of two dyes, thioflavin S and Uniperse blue (particulate blue dye), after coronary artery occlusion and reperfusion in the rabbit, led to closely correlating areas not stained by the two dyes after various durations of occlusion and reperfusion (Fig. 3.1). The thioflavin S negative tissue was always slightly smaller but confined to areas not stained by Uniperse Blue regardless of the duration of occlusion and reperfusion. Thus, the ability of the dye, used for perfusion staining, to penetrate into the tissue with compromised reflow determines the size of visualized zones of microvascular obstruction [2].

Vascular function is also altered after ischemia and reperfusion: Various vasodilatatory stimuli, in particular those involving release of nitric oxide, are compromised after conditions of ischemia and reperfusion [14, 15]. In rat coronary arteries, for example, vasodilatatory responses to acetylcholine were markedly reduced after ischemia and reperfusion, however, not after ischemia alone [14]. Of note, these functional abnormalities may persist over weeks.

Clinical Correlates of the No-Reflow Phenomenon

Along with the increasing clinical use and scientific validation of reperfusion therapy for acute myocardial infarction, it became clear that microvascular integrity might also limit myocardial tissue perfusion after adequate restoration of epicardial flow in the clinical realm. Based on coronary angiograms, TIMI (Thrombolysis in Myocardial Infarction) flow grade was defined (0–3) [2]. While TIMI 3 flow grade refers to complete reperfusion, and TIMI 2 means partial reperfusion, TIMI 1 is characterized by minimal flow to the distal coronary artery bed, and TIMI 0 means no flow at all. Both in acute percutaneous coronary angioplasty interventions for myocardial infarction and also in elective coronary angioplasty, a TIMI grade of less than 3 may occur despite epicardial vessel patency. This so-called angiographic no-reflow is suggestive of microvascular obstruction. The incidence may be as high as 11.5% in acute myocardial infarction [16]. Angiographic no-reflow (TIMI grade < 3) was shown to be a strong predictor of major cardiac events, such as heart failure, arrhythmia, and cardiac death after myocardial infarction [10].

Myocardial contrast echocardiography allows visualization of myocardial tissue perfusion by intracoronary or intravenous injection of special contrast media, which results in enhanced echocardiographic contrast in perfused myocardium. Thereby, perfusion defects may become visible. Ito et al. showed that even when reperfusion therapy for acute myocardial infarction results in TIMI grade 3 flow, perfusion defects were detectable in 16% of the patients by contrast echocardiography [17]. In TIMI grade 2 patients, perfusion defects were visualized in every patient. These perfusion defects on contrast echocardiography were shown to have relevant prognostic significance [18, 19].

Zones of microvascular obstruction were also visualized by magnetic resonance imaging (MRI) as areas with less contrast enhancement after injection of contrast medium. In a canine model, the size of these areas was validated against anatomical zones of no-reflow, as assessed by thioflavin S perfusion staining, demonstrating a close correlation between both methods [20]. Evidence for prognostic significance of microvascular obstruction assessed by MRI techniques was also provided [9, 21, 22].

Other measures of microvascular obstruction used in the clinical realm are based on parameters determined in the catheterization laboratory, like TIMI-frame count, myocardial blush grade, and intracoronary blood flow velocity measurement using

Doppler-wire technique [11], or simply on analysis of ST-segment resolution over time after reperfusion therapy in acute coronary syndromes [2].

In the clinical realm, no-reflow shares many characteristics of the phenomenon first described in animal research. Nonetheless, it becomes increasingly recognized that additional mechanisms, such as coronary microembolization, activation of platelets, and several vasoconstrictive pathways, significantly contribute to microvascular dysfunction in patients with reperfused myocardial infarction [5, 23–26]. Most of the clinical issues will be discussed in detail in other chapters of this book.

Major Determinants of No-Reflow

In the following paragraphs, major determinant of no-reflow as seen in animal models of coronary artery ligation and reperfusion will be described.

Infarct Size

Infarct size appears to be the major determinant of the occurrence and degree of no-reflow in many animal models of myocardial infarction and also in clinical circumstances. In the early studies, performed in the dog heart, it became clear that a certain duration of coronary occlusion was necessary for no-reflow to occur [8, 27]. After 40 min of occlusion and 20 min of reperfusion, no zones of microvascular obstruction were visualized; however, after 90 min and longer durations of coronary occlusion, substantial perfusion defects developed within the ischemic risk zone, in particular in the subendocardium. In the rabbit heart, which is characterized by negligible collateral flow to the ischemic tissue, regional myocardial blood flow in the risk zone after various durations of occlusion and reperfusion demonstrated a significant accordance with infarct size regardless of the duration of ischemia or reperfusion (Fig. 3.3) [28]. Infarct size appeared to be the major determinant of the degree of microvascular dysfunction in these experiments. Similarly, perfusion staining with thioflavin S in various experiments in the rabbit model demonstrated a close spatial accordance between infarct size and anatomical no-reflow [2, 6, 13, 29–31]. Notably, infarct size was always slightly larger than no-reflow. Several cardioprotective interventions, reducing myocardial infarct size, resulted in proportional reduction of anatomical no-reflow, again suggesting that infarct size is the main determinant of microvascular obstruction [31]. Interestingly, epicardial cooling started during late ischemia and continued during the reperfusion period resulted in smaller zones of no-reflow expressed as a percentage of the infarcted tissue. In this study, hypothermia disproportionately reduced the no-reflow zone in relationship to infarct size. In normothermic treated rabbits, 75% of the necrotic region developed no-reflow, whereas in hypothermic rabbits, only 36% of the necrotic region developed no-reflow [29].

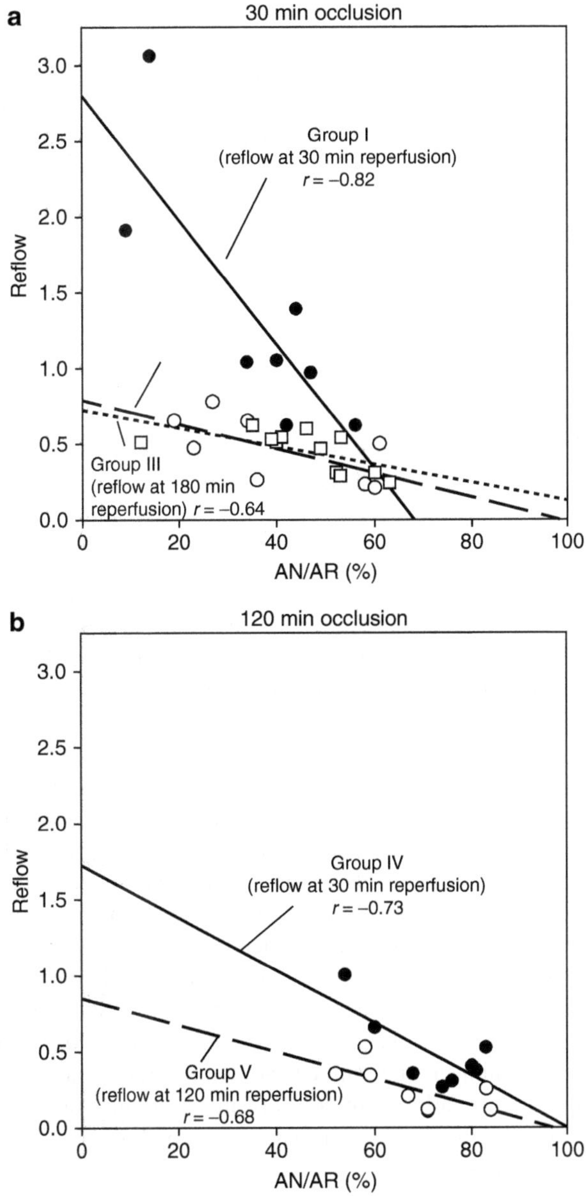

Fig. 3.3 (**a**, **b**) Linear regression between the area of necrosis as a percentage of the area at risk (AN/AR) and reflow (ratio of regional myocardial blood flow in the risk area and the nonischemic tissue, determined by the radioactive microsphere technique) in a rabbit open-chest model of coronary occlusion and reperfusion after different durations of occlusion and reperfusion. There was a close correlation between infarct size and regional myocardial blood flow in each of the five groups, regardless of the duration of ischemia and reperfusion (From Reffelmann et al. [28], with permission)

Duration of Reperfusion

Reperfusion itself appears to significantly contribute to size and degree of no-reflow. In the canine model, Ambrosio et al. [32] observed an approximately twofold increase in the size of anatomical no-reflow zone between 2 min of reperfusion and 3.5 h of reperfusion. These perfusion defects, not stained by thioflavin S, expanded from the subendocardium to the epicardium with ongoing reperfusion. Simultaneously, regional myocardial blood flow progressively decreased during reperfusion. In the rabbit heart, subjected to 30 min of coronary occlusion followed by 2, 30, 60, or 480 min of reperfusion, areas of no-reflow similarly expanded from 12.2% of the risk area after 2 min to 30.8% after 2 h and 34.9% after 8 h of reperfusion (Figs. 3.4 and 3.5) [13]. After 2 h of reperfusion, the expansion of no-reflow appeared to reach a plateau. Regional myocardial blood flow was hyperemic within the risk zone 2 min after release of the coronary occlusion and then progressively decreased to a plateau of approximately 0.9 ml/g/min within the risk area after 2–8 h of reperfusion (normal regional flow in the rabbit heart: approximately 2 ml/g/min, Fig. 3.5).

Relationship Between No-Reflow Zones and Myocardial Hemorrhage

Ultrastructural investigations of areas of microvascular damage demonstrated endothelial gaps and extravasation of erythrocytes with ongoing reperfusion (see Fig. 3.2). In the rabbit model of ischemia and reperfusion, a close spatial correlation between areas of microvascular damage and reddish zones within the risk zone, as visualized by macroscopic assessment, which may represent some form of macroscopic hemorrhage, is obvious (see Fig. 3.4) [13].

In the early investigations, when beneficial effects of reperfusion therapy were established in animal models of coronary artery ligation and reperfusion, a relevant question was whether intramyocardial hemorrhage, which appeared to be a consequence of reperfusion, might contribute to myocardial damage and extension of necrosis [33–36]. Most of these investigations described hemorrhagic transformation of myocardial infarcts confined to zones of preexisting myocardial necrosis and typically in zones of severely depressed flow [35, 36]. Therefore, the conclusion of most of these studies was that intramyocardial hemorrhage did not result in extension of myocardial necrosis, but rather occurred within the already severely damaged tissue. Similar to findings in the rabbit heart (Fig. 3.4) [13], systematic investigations in the canine heart demonstrated that hemorrhagic zones have a close spatial correlation with zones of microvascular obstruction [12, 35]. Most importantly, thrombolytic agents, such as streptokinase, did not seem to aggravate hemorrhagic transformation of infarcts [37].

With the introduction of MRI techniques to visualize intramyocardial hemorrhage in the clinical realm, some recent studies compared extent and spatial distribution of zones of microvascular obstruction with hemorrhagic zones in patients with reperfused myocardial infarction. Interestingly, a similarly close correlation between microvascular damage and intramyocardial hemorrhage was demonstrated in these clinical studies, which may again support the concept of translating the no-reflow phenomenon, characterized in animal research, to the clinical phenomenon of no-reflow and microvascular obstruction [38–40].

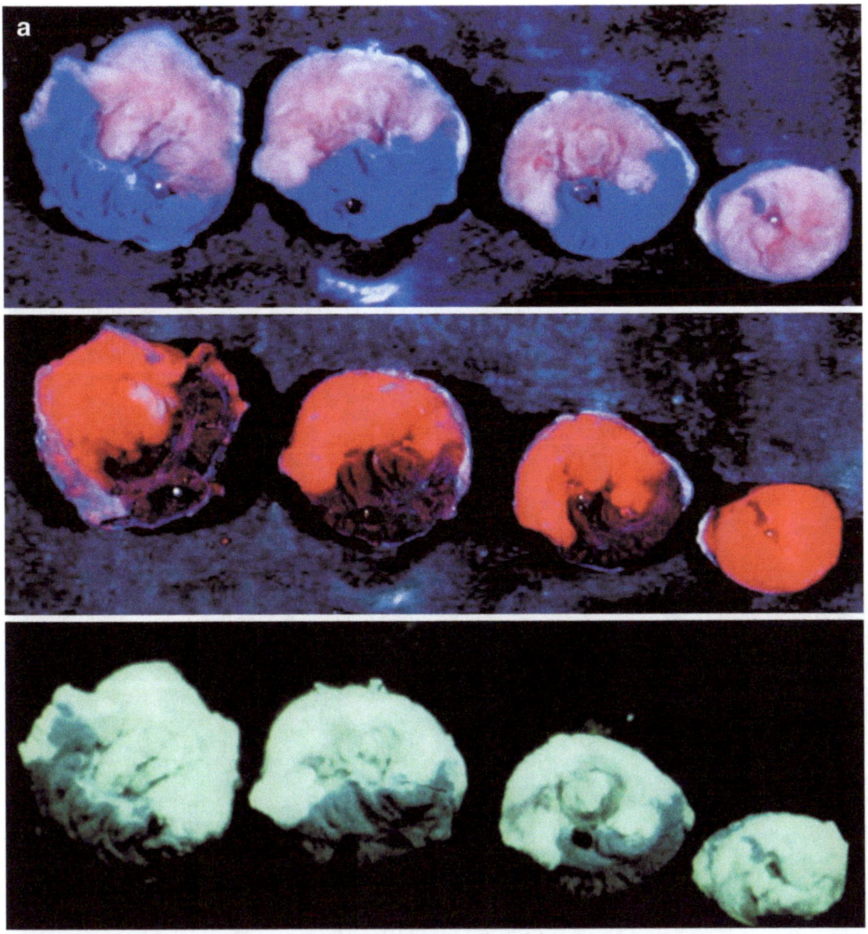

Fig. 3.4 In a rabbit model of coronary artery occlusion followed by different durations of reperfusion, anatomical no-reflow in relationship to infarct size and macroscopically visible hemorrhage was investigated: The picture shows the apical slices of hearts after 30 min of occlusion and 2 min of reperfusion (**a**) and 8 h of reperfusion (**b**). A fluorescent dye (thioflavin S) was injected at the end of the reperfusion period to stain perfused tissue, a blue dye after coronary reocclusion at the end of the experiment was used to delineate the area at risk (*not blue*). After slicing of the hearts, incubation in triphenyltetrazolium chloride (TTC) was used to stain vital myocardium red. Consequently, the infarct appeared pale. (**a**) After 2 min of reperfusion, there is no macroscopically visible hemorrhage in the risk area (*top*), the TTC-negative area is relatively small (*middle*), and only small zones within the risk area appear nonfluorescent under an ultraviolet light (*bottom*). (**b**) After 8 h of reperfusion, however, the risk area contains a substantial amount of brownish-red tissue, defined as the macroscopic hemorrhage (*top*). TTC staining leaves the necrotic tissue unstained, showing a pale color after 8 h of reperfusion (*middle*). Sizable nonfluorescent zones, the area of no-reflow, are visible after 8 h, which closely correlates with hemorrhage and necrosis (*bottom*). Within the nonischemic tissue, less fluorescence is visible due to the blue dye (From Reffelmann and Kloner [13], with permission)

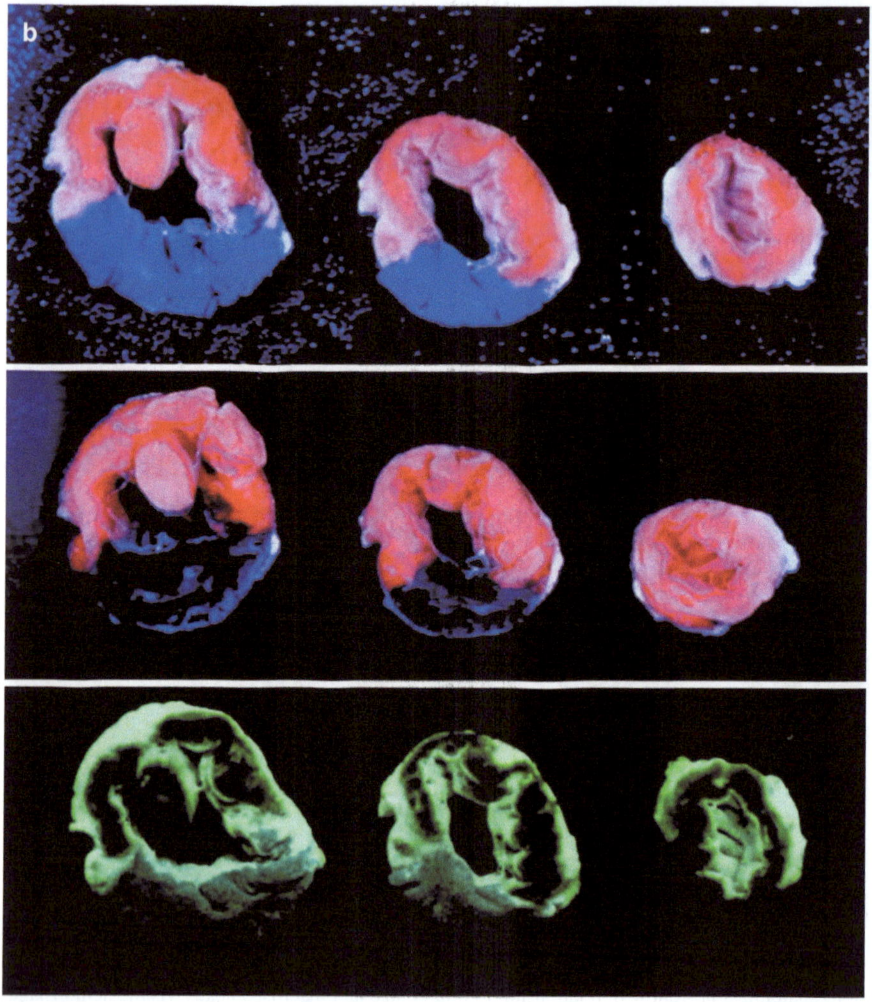

Fig. 3.4 (continued)

Pathophysiology and Mechanisms of No-Reflow

While coronary microembolization, be it from coronary thrombus formation or atherosclerotic debris, significantly contributes to microvascular obstruction in the clinical setting, most animal models of reperfused myocardial infarction used mechanical ligation and reopening of the coronary artery which is, in the majority of studies, not affected by significant atherosclerosis. Therefore, therapeutic strategies used to reduce no-reflow in the clinical setting, such as thrombus aspiration, distal microcirculatory protection, and others, target additional mechanisms of microvascular obstruction compared with no-reflow in animal research [24, 25].

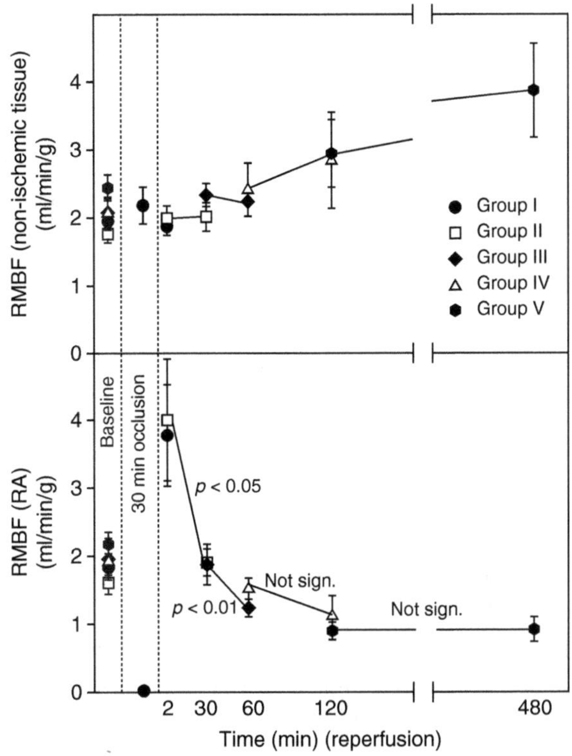

Fig. 3.5 Regional myocardial blood flow (*RMBF*) in nonischemic tissue (*top*) and within the RA (*bottom*) in the rabbit heart subjected to 30 min of coronary artery ligation followed by different durations of reperfusion (2, 30, 60, 120, 480 min). Regional myocardial blood flow progressively declined in the area at risk. Therefore, no-reflow may be regarded as a form of reperfusion injury at the microvascular level (From Reffelmann and Kloner [13], with permission)

The following paragraphs delineate pathophysiological concepts, put forward for the development of no-reflow in animal research, even if mechanisms of no-reflow remain incompletely understood.

Ultrastructural Changes of the Microvascular Bed After Ischemia/Reperfusion

Ultrastructural damage, such as endothelial protrusions, local endothelial swelling, and accumulation of tightly packed erythrocytes as a consequence of ischemia and reperfusion (as summarized in Fig. 3.2), presumably directly contribute to microvascular perfusion defects. The protrusions observed by electron microscopy may act to occlude the capillary lumen. With ongoing reperfusion, the increasing number of red blood cells within the capillary lumen with rouleaux formation demonstrates that some blood flow must have occurred immediately after reopening of the coronary artery, but thereafter, blood flow within the capillary bed ceases [8, 27, 37, 41].

Reactive Oxygen Species Early After Reopening of the Coronary Artery

Reactive oxygen species are produced during reperfusion, in particular within the first minutes after reopening of the coronary artery. At the same time, the superoxide dismutase pathway, responsible for the clearance of superoxide anions, may be impaired by myocardial ischemia. Various investigations studied the effect of oxygen radical scavengers on vascular function and no-reflow. Microvascular damage could be reduced by such interventions, for example, by application of superoxide dismutase and catalase in some studies, albeit contradictory results were also obtained in some investigations [42–44]. Therefore, oxygen radicals, derived from polymorphonuclear cells, mitochondria, or via the xanthine oxidase pathway, may significantly contribute to no-reflow, in particular to the deterioration of perfusion defects during reperfusion.

Mechanical Compression Due to Tissue Edema

Early morphological alterations after reopening of an occluded coronary artery include swelling of cardiomyocytes, and interstitial edema, which could lead to mechanical compression of the vascular bed and thereby contribute to perfusion defects [45]. These mechanisms may in part explain microvascular obstruction occurring within the early phase of reperfusion [46]. Nonetheless, intervention aimed at reducing tissue edema, for example, application of hypertonic solutions, did not significantly reduce perfusion defects in animal models of ischemia and reperfusion [47, 48].

Interaction of Leukocytes with the Endothelium, Platelets, and Cardiomyocytes

In the landmark study by Ambrosio et al. [32], zones of no-reflow substantially expanded during reperfusion which was accompanied by significant accumulation of neutrophils predominantly within the areas of no-reflow. Early animal investigations demonstrated leukocyte accumulation within the microvasculature after ischemia and reperfusion, which seemed to plug the capillary bed and could not be washed out by crystalloid solution [49]. Release of reactive oxygen species, proteolytic enzymes, and lipoxygenase products by polymorphonuclear cells may result in interaction with endothelial cells, platelets, and cardiomyocytes. Endothelial cells can modulate leukocyte function by altered expression of adhesion molecules and by release of soluble factors such as nitric oxide, prostacyclin, endothelin, and platelet activating factor. Platelets could affect endothelial cells and leukocytes by release of thromboxane A2, serotonin, adenosine, lipooxygenase products, and proteases. Thereby, the interaction between leukocytes, platelets, and the endothelium is complex and may involve also the complement system [50]. Animal models, investigating several methods of leukocyte depletion in myocardial ischemia and reperfusion, demonstrated reduced microvascular damage in several studies [51–53]. Nonetheless, even in Langendorff-hearts perfused with crystalloid, blood-free solutions, perfusion defects can be demonstrated after ischemia and reperfusion.

Coagulation, Platelets, Tissue Factor

Electron microscopy studies in the dog heart did not suggest that thrombus formation within the capillary bed is the major mechanism of no-reflow. Some investigations found rare microthrombi, others did not provide evidence for activation of the coagulation cascade [2, 8, 27]. Administration of acetylsalicylic acid, streptokinase, or plasminogen activator did not improve microvascular function in most of the animal studies of coronary artery ligation and release of the ligation [37, 41].

When the endothelium is damaged, tissue factor, exposed to flowing blood, might activate the coagulation cascade. In a rabbit model of infarction, active-site-blocked factor VIIa was shown to reduce no-reflow and infarct size [54, 55].

Vascular Dysfunction After Ischemia/Reperfusion

Ischemia and reperfusion result in vascular dysfunction, and many studies investigated whether vasodilator therapies could reduce microvascular obstruction [56, 57]. Of note, ischemic preconditioning not only reduces infarct size in animal models of ischemia and reperfusion but also reduces vascular dysfunction [14]. In some animal models of ischemia and reperfusion, vasodilator interventions, such as adenosine or calcium antagonists, were also shown to reduce no-reflow [58–62]. In particular, adenosine treatment, which, however, might have effects in addition to vasodilation, was examined in multiple animal trials with mixed results, some of them showing infarct size reduction along with reduction of no-reflow and some of them were negative [60–62]. Of note, verapamil, adenosine, and other vasodilatatory interventions were shown to be effective in treating no-reflow in specific clinical circumstances [63, 64]. As another vasodilator mechanism, pharmacological endothelin antagonism was also shown to reduce perfusion defects visualized by myocardial contrast echocardiography in a dog model of myocardial infarction [65]. From most of these, in part contradictory studies, it is not clear whether the interventions reduce no-reflow independently of infarct size or no-reflow as a proportion of the infarct.

Interventions to Reduce No-Reflow in Animal Models of Ischemia/Reperfusion

Many interventions to reduce no-reflow were examined in animal models as well as in the clinical setting. While most clinical treatment options, such as thrombus aspiration, distal microvascular protection, and vasodilatatory and antithrombotic therapies, will be discussed in other chapters, preclinical treatment studies will be the focus of the following paragraph.

Many therapeutic interventions, tested in animal models, had direct effects on myocardial necrosis and microvascular damage. Therefore, many strategies, resulting in reduced myocardial infarct size, resulted in proportional reduction of no-reflow. For example, in a rabbit model of ischemia/reperfusion, two independent cardioprotective interventions, ischemic preconditioning and pharmacological inhibition of the Na^+/H^+ exchange, by the agent cariporide, were tested with respect to their differential effect on infarct size and extent of anatomical no-reflow (Fig. 3.6) [31]. While both interventions reduced infarct size significantly, anatomic no-reflow was reduced proportionally with each intervention in this model. Therefore, as infarct size is the major determinant of no-reflow, reducing infarct size can be expected to be associated with reduced zones of no-reflow. Whether some interventions, such as hypothermia, intra-aortic balloon counterpulsation as hemodynamic support, or others, can dissociate no-reflow from necrosis is still under debate [29, 66]. Interestingly, a study that failed to demonstrated reduction of infarct size by a postconditioning protocol in the rabbit also did not demonstrate reduction of no-reflow [67].

Table 3.1 summarizes several interventions aimed at reducing microvascular obstruction tested in animal models. Interventions range from vasodilator agents, oxygen radical scavengers, and leukocyte depletion to antithrombotic treatment and support of the peripheral circulation by intra-aortic balloon counterpulsation [66, 68, 69]. Some results remain contradictory and may depend on the specific model used for the experiments. Notably, extent of collateral flow to the ischemic area might be a significant modifier in these experiments.

Prognostic Implications of No-Reflow

In the clinical setting, the occurrence and extent of no-reflow was demonstrated to have relevant prognostic impact in terms of myocardial contractile function, remodeling, and long-term morbidity and mortality [9, 10, 18, 19, 21, 22]. In a rat model of ischemia and reperfusion, reduced microvascular perfusion could be demonstrated for a period of 4 weeks after 60 min of coronary artery occlusion followed by reperfusion (Fig. 3.7) [70]. Similar to clinical investigations, showing an association of microvascular obstruction with left ventricular remodeling, histological examination of these 4-week-old reperfused infarcts demonstrates a close association of the amount of microvascular obstruction with thinning of the infarcted scar and infarct expansion, which might be a histological correlate of the prognostic impact (Fig. 3.8) [70].

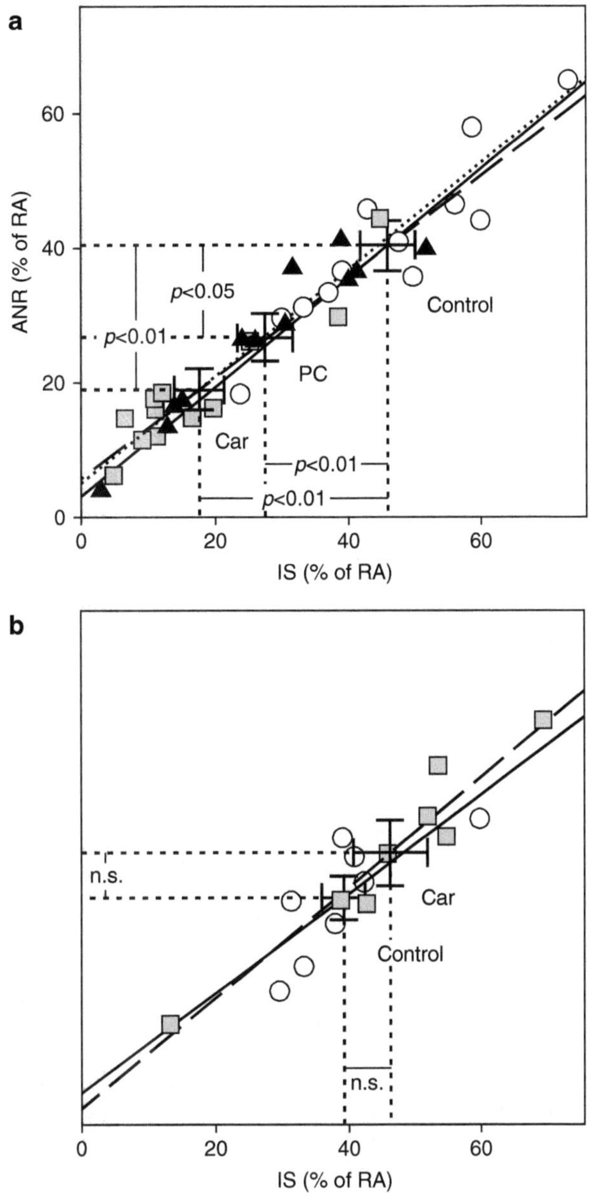

Fig. 3.6 Relationship between anatomical no-reflow (ANR) and infarct size (IS) with different cardioprotective interventions in a rabbit model of coronary artery ligation and reopening of the ligation (RA risk area). (**a**) Control group (○, *solid line*), the Na+/H+ exchange inhibitor Cariporide (*Car*) given before occlusion (□, *dashed line*), and ischemic preconditioning (*PC*) group (▲, *dotted line*) (nonlethal period of ischemia prior to ischemia). (**b**) Control group (○, *solid line*) and Cariporide (Car) given at reperfusion (□, *dashed line*). While cariporide prior to ischemia and ischemic preconditioning significantly reduced infarct, the relationship between infarct size and anatomical no-reflow was similar with each intervention (From Reffelmann and Kloner [31], with permission)

Clinical Perspective: Managing No-Reflow in the Clinical Realm

In the clinical setting of reperfusion therapy of myocardial infarction, the occurrence and extent of no-reflow was also shown to be of significant importance; however, mechanisms might differ from animal models, as arteries in patients with acute myocardial infarction are significantly affected by atherosclerosis and most often

Table 3.1 Interventions tested in animal models of ischemia and reperfusion aimed at reducing microvascular obstruction

Intervention	Description	Animal species	References
Adenosine during reperfusion	In canine models, improved regional blood flow ultrastructural microvascular preservation, and less leukocyte infiltration, in some studies accompanied by infarct size reduction	Dogs	[60–62]
	No reduction of anatomical no-reflow but reduced specific vascular resistance within the risk area	Rabbits	[56]
Adenosine-regulating agent	The adenosine-regulating agent GP531, given prior to coronary occlusion, reduced infarct size and no-reflow	Rabbits	[69]
Calcium-channel antagonists	Reduced area of no-reflow with nisoldipine in a model of global ischemia (isolated heart)	Rats	[59]
	Gallopamil during ischemia reduced infarct size and no-reflow	Rabbits	[58]
	No reduction of anatomical no-reflow but reduced specific vascular resistance within the risk area	Rabbits	[56]
Reactive oxygen species scavenging	Superoxide dismutase and catalase during reperfusion resulted in preservation of endocardial regional myocardial flow, less ultrastructural damage	Dogs	[43, 44]
Leukocyte depletion	Reperfusion with neutrophil-depleted blood	Dogs	[53]
	Leukocyte depletion by intraperitoneal mustin resulted in better coronary flow	Rat	[51]
	Intracoronary oxygenated perfluorochemicals reperfusion	Dogs	[52]
Interventions in the coagulation cascade/ platelet function	Plasminogen tissue activator or streptokinase did not alter no-reflow nor did they increase hemorrhagic transformation	Dogs	[37, 41]
	Active-site-blocked factor VIIa during reperfusion reduced infarct size and no-reflow	Rabbits	[54]
	Unlike aspirin/clopidogrel, tirofiban, an inhibitor of the platelet GP IIb/IIIa inhibitor, reduced no-reflow in a swine model of coronary occlusion and reperfusion	Pigs	[68]
Hypothermia	Epicardial cooling during late ischemia and reperfusion reduced infarct size and no-reflow (with more than proportional microvascular protection)	Rabbits	[29]
Endothelin-A-antagonist	Endothelin-A-antagonist during reperfusion reduced perfusion defects seen on myocardial contrast echocardiography	Dogs	[65]
Intra-aortic balloon counterpulsation (IABP)	IABP for 24 h after ischemia and reperfusion reduced microvascular obstruction, as assessed by MRI without reduction of myocardial necrosis	Dogs	[66]

are occluded by an epicardial thrombus. Many determinants related to myocardial ischemia and reperfusion are most likely similar, but microembolization of thrombotic material and atherosclerotic debris might be an additional mechanism in patients. Consequently, therapeutic strategies in patients focus on these characteristics, with thrombus aspiration before balloon inflation or distal protection during

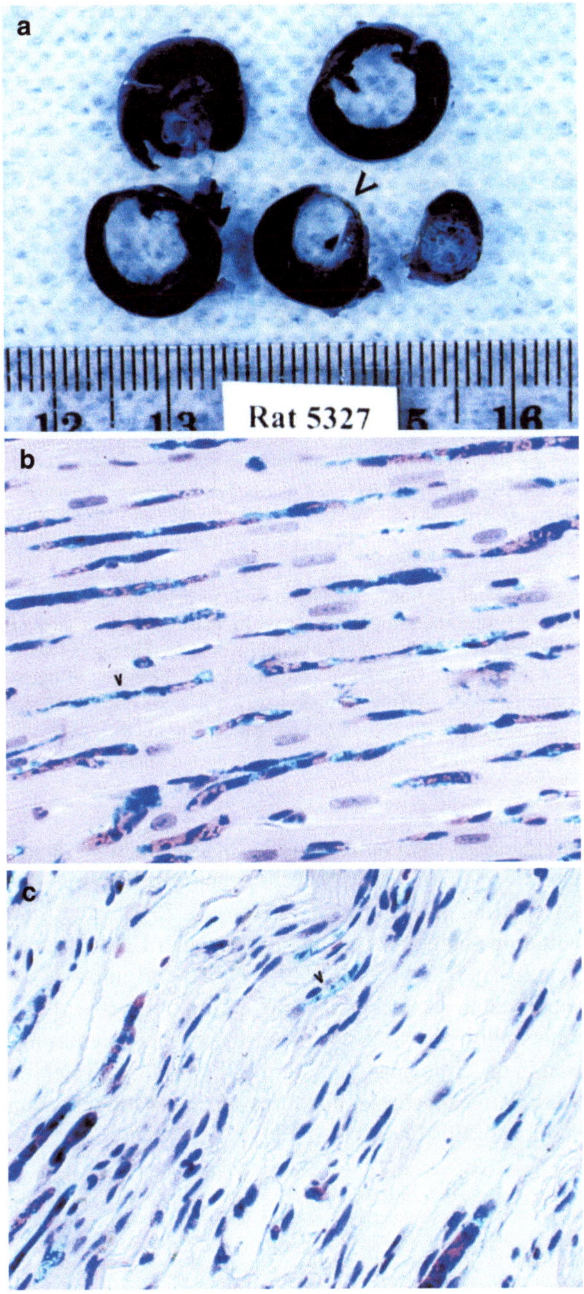

Fig. 3.7 After 60 min of coronary occlusion followed by reperfusion, the chest was closed, and the rat was examined after 4 weeks (injection of a particulate blue dye to stain perfused capillaries). (**a**) Sliced rat heart after 4 weeks of reperfusion showing macroscopic evidence of no-reflow, visible as tissue not stained by blue dye. Microscopically, a marked reduction of capillaries containing blue particles (*arrowhead*) after in vivo staining was visible in the infarcted tissue (**c**) compared with noninfarcted control (**b**) (40-fold magnification) (From Reffelmann et al. [70], with permission)

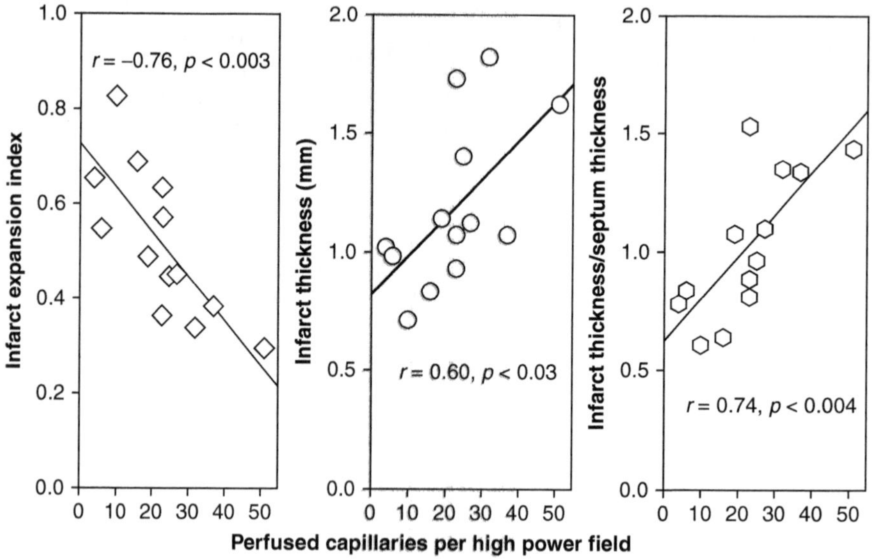

Fig. 3.8 Multiple linear regression analysis between the number of perfused capillaries within the infarcted zone and indices of left ventricular remodeling after 60 min of coronary occlusion and 4 weeks of reperfusion. A significant inverse correlation between the number of perfused capillaries in infarct zone (*abscissa*), as a measure of the extent of microvascular obstruction, and infarct expansion index (*left*) was apparent. This was the consequence of a positive correlation with the thickness of the infarct (*middle*) and ratio of infarct to septum thickness (*right*) (From Reffelmann et al. [70], with permission)

percutaneous interventions [23–26]. Mechanical devices designed to trap embolic debris during angioplasty were developed forming an umbrella-like or basket-like device distal in the coronary artery [23, 25]. Furthermore, antiplatelet interventions, including antagonists of the glycoprotein IIB/IIIa receptor appear to prevent detrimental sequelae of distal embolisation and improve microvascular perfusion [71]. In particular, intracoronary application of glycoprotein IIb/IIIa receptor antagonists could improve tissue perfusion in coronary syndromes [72]. Other interventions used in the clinical setting comprise vasodilator intervention (adenosine, verapamil, nicorandil, papaverine, nitroprusside, etc.) and others and will be discussed in other chapters of this book.

Summary

In animal models of coronary artery occlusion and reopening of the epicardial artery, perfusion defects within the area at risk may develop during reperfusion despite complete reopening of the epicardial artery. These anatomical areas of no-reflow are confined to areas of myocardial necrosis and substantially expand during ongoing reperfusion. This reperfusion injury at the microvascular level may be related to ultrastructural alterations of the microvasculature, production of reactive oxygen species during reperfusion, leukocyte accumulation, and release of vasoconstrictive agents. Infarct size appears to be the major determinant of no-reflow, and cardioprotective interventions leading to smaller infarcts result in reduced microvascular obstruction in most of the models. Several therapeutic strategies have been developed to reduce no-reflow; however, in most of these investigations it was difficult to dissociated no-reflow from infarct size. Transfer to the clinical setting of myocardial infarction shows many similarities, but additional mechanisms such as coronary microembolization significantly contribute to clinical no-reflow.

References

1. Davies MJ, Woolf N, Robertson WB. Pathology of acute myocardial infarction with particular reference to coronary thrombi. Br Heart J. 1976;38:659–64.
2. Reffelmann T, Kloner RA. The "no-reflow" phenomenon: basic science and clinical correlates. Heart. 2002;87:162–8.
3. The Gusto Investigators. An international randomized trial comparing four thrombolytic strategies for acute myocardial infarction. N Engl J Med. 1993;329:673–82.
4. Keeley EC, Boura JA, Grines CL. Primary angioplasty versus intravenous thrombolytic therapy for acute myocardial infarction: a quantitative review of 23 randomised trials. Lancet. 2003;361:13–20.
5. Bekkers SCAM, Yazdani SK, Virmani R, Waltenberger J. Microvascular obstruction. J Am Coll Cardiol. 2010;55:1649–60.
6. Reffelmann T, Kloner RA. The no-reflow phenomenon: a basic mechanism of myocardial ischemia and reperfusion. Basic Res Cardiol. 2006;101:359–72.
7. Krug A, de Rochemont WM, Korb G. Blood supply to the myocardium after temporary coronary artery occlusion. Circ Res. 1966;19:57–62.
8. Kloner RA, Ganote CE, Jennings RB. The "no-reflow" phenomenon after temporary coronary occlusion in dogs. J Clin Invest. 1974;54:1496–508.
9. Wu KC, Zerhouni EA, Judd RM, et al. Prognostic significance of microvascular obstruction by magnetic resonance imaging in patients with acute myocardial infarction. Circulation. 1998;97: 65–72.
10. Morishima I, Sone T, Okumara K, et al. Angiographic no-reflow as a predictor of adverse long-term outcome in patients treated with percutaneous transluminal coronary angioplasty for first myocardial infarction. J Am Coll Cardiol. 2000;36:1202–9.
11. Lepper W, Hoffmann R, Kamp O, et al. Assessment of myocardial reperfusion by intravenous myocardial contrast echocardiography and coronary flow reserve after primary percutaneous transluminal coronary angiography in patients with acute myocardial infarction. Circulation. 2000;101:2368–74.
12. Fishbein MC, Y-Rit J, Lando U, Kanmatsuse K, Mercier JC, Ganz W. The relationship of vascular injury and myocardial hemorrhage to necrosis after reperfusion. Circulation. 1980;62:1274–9.
13. Reffelmann T, Kloner RA. Microvascular reperfusion injury: rapid expansion of anatomic no reflow during reperfusion in the rabbit. Am J Physiol Heart Circ Physiol. 2002;283: h1099–107.
14. Kaeffer N, Richard V, Francois A, Lallemand F, Henry JP, Thuillez C. Preconditioning prevents chronic reperfusion-induced coronary endothelial dysfunction in rats. Am J Physiol Heart Circ Physiol. 1996;271:H842–9.

15. Kloner RA, Giacomelli F, Alker KJ, Hale SL, Mathey R, Bellows S. Influx of neutrophils into the wall of large epicardial coronary arteries in response to ischemia/reperfusion. Circulation. 1991;84:1758–72.
16. Piana RN, Paik GY, Mascucci M, et al. Incidence and treatment of 'no-reflow' after percutaneous coronary intervention. Circulation. 1994;89:2514–8.
17. Ito H, Okamura A, Iwakura K, et al. Myocardial perfusion patterns related to thrombolysis in myocardial infarction perfusion grades after coronary angioplasty for first acute myocardial infarction. Circulation. 1996;93:1993–9.
18. Ragosta M, Camarano G, Kaul S, et al. Microvascular integrity indicates myocellular viability in patients with recent myocardial infarction: new insights using myocardial contrast echocardiography. Circulation. 1994;89:2562–9.
19. Sakuma T, Hayashi Y, Sumii K, et al. Prediction of short and intermediate-term prognosis of patients with acute myocardial infarction using myocardial contrast echocardiography one day after recanalization. J Am Coll Cardiol. 1998;32:890–7.
20. Rochitte CE, Lima JA, Bluemke DA, et al. Magnitude and time course of microvascular obstruction and tissue injury after acute myocardial infarction. Circulation. 1998;98: 1006–14.
21. Gerber BL, Rochitte CE, Melin JA, et al. Microvascular obstruction and left ventricular remodeling early after acute myocardial infarction. Circulation. 2000;101:2734–41.
22. Weir RA, Murphy CA, Petrie CJ, et al. Microvascular obstruction remains a portent of adverse remodeling in optimally-treated patients with left ventricular systolic dysfunction after acute myocardial infarction. Circ Cardiovasc Imaging. 2010;3(4):360–7. Epub 2010 Mar 26.
23. Topol EJ, Yadav JS. Recognition of the importance of microembolization in atherosclerotic vascular disease. Circulation. 2000;101:570–80.
24. Silva-Orrego P, Colombo P, Bigi R, et al. Thrombus aspiration before myocardial reperfusion in acute myocardial infarction. The DEAR-MI (Dethrombosis to Enhance Acute Reperfusion in Myocardial Infarction) Study. J Am Coll Cardiol. 2006;48:1552–9.
25. Stone GW, Webb J, Cox DA, et al. Distal microcirculatory protection during percutaneous coronary intervention in acute ST-segment elevation myocardial infarction. A randomized controlled trial. JAMA. 2005;293:1063–72.
26. Roe MT, Ohman M, Maas ACP, et al. Shifting the open artery hypothesis downstream: the quest for optimal reperfusion. J Am Coll Cardiol. 2001;37:9–18.
27. Kloner RA, Rude RE, Carlson N, Maroko PR, DeBoer LWV, Braunwald E. Ultrastructural evidence of microvascular damage and myocardial cell injury after coronary artery occlusion. Which comes first? Circulation. 1980;62:945–52.
28. Reffelmann T, Hale SL, Li G, Kloner RA. Relationship between no reflow and infarct size as influenced by the duration of ischemia and reperfusion. Am J Physiol Heart Circ Physiol. 2002;282:H766–72.
29. Hale S, Dae MW, Kloner RA. Hypothermia during reperfusion limits 'no-reflow' injury in a rabbit myocardial infarct model. Cardiovasc Res. 2003;59:715–22.
30. Hale SL, Kloner RA. The antianginal agent, ranolazine, reduces myocardial infarct size but does not alter anatomic no-reflow or regional myocardial blood flow in ischemia/reperfusion in the rabbit. J Cardiovasc Pharmacol Ther. 2008;13:226–32.
31. Reffelmann T, Kloner RA. Is microvascular protection by cariporide and ischemic preconditioning causally linked to myocardial salvage? Am J Physiol Heart Circ Physiol. 2003;284:H1134–41.
32. Ambrosio G, Weissmann HF, Mannisi JA, Becker LC. Progressive impairment of regional myocardial perfusion after initial restoration of postischemic blood flow. Circulation. 1989;80: 1846–61.
33. Geft IL, Fishbein MC, Hashida J, et al. Effects of late coronary artery reperfusion after myocardial necrosis is complete. Am Heart J. 1984;107:623–9.
34. Garcia-Dorado D, Théroux P, Solares J, et al. Determinants of hemorrhagic infarcts. Histologic observations from experiments involving coronary occlusion, coronary reperfusion, and reocclusion. Am J Pathol. 1990;137:301–11.

35. Higginson LA, White F, Heggtveit HA, Sanders TM, Bloor CM, Covell JW. Determinants of myocardial hemorrhage after coronary reperfusion in the anesthetized dog. Circulation. 1982;65:62–9.
36. McNamara JJ, Lacro RV, Yee M, Smith GT. Hemorrhagic infarction and coronary reperfusion. J Thorac Cardiovasc Surg. 1981;81:498–501.
37. Kloner RA, Alker KJ. The effect of streptokinase on intramyocardial hemorrhage, infarct size, and the no-reflow phenomenon during coronary reperfusion. Circulation. 1984;70:513–21.
38. Ganame J, Messalli G, Dymarkowski S, Rademakers FE, van de Werf R, Bogaert J. Impact of myocardial haemorrhage on left ventricular function and remodeling in patients with reperfused acute myocardial infarction. Eur Heart J. 2009;30:1440–9.
39. Asanuma T, Tanabe K, Ochiai K, et al. Relationship between progressive microvascular damage and intramyocardial hemorrhage in patients with reperfused anterior myocardial infarction: myocardial contrast echocardiographic study. Circulation. 1997;96:448–53.
40. Beek AM, Nijveldt R, van Rossum AC. Intramyocardial hemorrhage and microvascular obstruction after primary percutaneous coronary intervention. Int J Cardiovasc Imaging. 2010;26:49–55.
41. Kloner RA, Alker K, Campbell C, Figures G, Eisenhauer A, Hale S. Does tissue-plasminogen activator have direct beneficial effects on the myocardium independent of its ability to lyse intracoronary thrombi? Circulation. 1989;79:1125–36.
42. Duilio C, Ambrosio G, Kuppusamy P, DiPaula A, Becker LC, Zweier JL. Neutrophils are primary source of O_2 radicals during reperfusion after prolonged myocardial ischemia. Am J Physiol Heart Circ Physiol. 2001;280:H2649–57.
43. Ambrosio G, Becker LC, Hutchins GM, Weisman HF, Weisfeldt ML. Reduction in experimental infarct size by recombinant human superoxide dismutase: insights into the pathophysiology of reperfusion injury. Circulation. 1986;74:1424–33.
44. Przyklenk K, Kloner RA. "Reperfusion injury" by oxygen-derived free radicals? Effect of superoxide dismutase plus catalase, given at the time of reperfusion, on myocardial infarct size, contractile function, coronary microvasculature, and regional myocardial blood flow. Circ Res. 1989;64:86–96.
45. Tranum-Jensen J, Janse MJ, Fiolet JWT, Krieger WJG, D'Alnoncourt CN, Durrer D. Tissue osmolality, cell swelling, and reperfusion in acute regional myocardial ischemia in the isolated porcine heart. Circ Res. 1981;49:364–81.
46. Manciet LH, Poole DC, McDonagh PF, Copeland JG, Mathieu-Costello O. Microvascular compression during myocardial ischemia: mechanistic basis for no-reflow phenomenon. Am J Physiol Heart Circ Physiol. 1994;266:H1541–50.
47. Willerson JT, Watson JT, Hutton I, Fixler DE, Curry CG, Templeton GH. The influence of hypertonic mannitol on regional myocardial blood flow during acute and chronic myocardial ischemia in anaesthetized and awake dogs. J Clin Invest. 1975;55:892–902.
48. Carlson RE, Aisen AM, Buda AJ. Effect of reduction in myocardial edema on myocardial blood flow and ventricular function after coronary reperfusion. Am J Physiol Heart Circ Physiol. 1992;262:H641–8.
49. Engler RL, Schmid-Schönbein GW, Pavelec RS. Leukocyte capillary plugging in myocardial ischemia and reperfusion in the dog. Am J Pathol. 1983;111:98–111.
50. Martin SE, Chenoweth DE, Engler RL, Roth DM, Longhurst JC. C5a decreases regional coronary blood flow and myocardial function in pigs: implications for a granulocyte mechanism. Circ Res. 1988;63:483–91.
51. Galinanes M, Lawson CS, Ferrari R, Limb GA, Derias NW, Hearse DJ. Early and late effects of leukopenic reperfusion on the recovery of cardiac contractile function studies in the transplanted and isolated blood-perfused rat heat. Circulation. 1993;88:673–83.
52. Kolodgie FD, Virmani R, Frab A. Limitation of no-reflow injury by blood-free reperfusion with oxygenated perfluorochemical (Fluoso-DA 20%). J Am Coll Cardiol. 1991;18:215–23.
53. Litt MR, Jeremy RW, Weisman HF, Winckelstein JA, Becker LC. Neutrophil depletion limited to reperfusion reduces myocardial infarct size after 90 minutes of ischemia. Evidence for neutrophil-mediated reperfusion injury. Circulation. 1989;80:1816–27.

54. Golino P, Ragni M, Cirillo P, et al. Recombinant human, active site-blocked factor VIIa reduces infarct size and no-reflow phenomenon in rabbits. Am J Physiol Heart Circ Physiol. 2000;278:H1507–16.
55. Golino P, Ragni M, Cirillo P, et al. Effects of tissue factor induced by oxygen free radicals on coronary flow during reperfusion. Nat Med. 1996;2:35–41.
56. Reffelmann T, Kloner RA. Effects of adenosine and verapamil on anatomic no-reflow in a rabbit model of coronary artery occlusion and reperfusion. J Cardiovasc Pharmacol. 2004;43:580–6.
57. Reffelmann T, Kloner RA. Effects of sildenafil on myocardial infarct size, microvascular function, and acute ischemic left ventricular dilation. Cardiovasc Res. 2003;98:275–84.
58. Villari B, Ambrosio G, Golino P, et al. The effects of calcium channel antagonist treatment and oxygen radical scavenging on infarct size and no-reflow phenomenon in reperfused hearts. Am Heart J. 1993;125:11–23.
59. Watt JA, Hawes EM, Jenkins SH, Williams TC. Effects of nisoldipine on the no-reflow phenomenon in globally ischemic rat hearts. J Cardiovasc Pharmacol. 1990;14:487–94.
60. Babbit DG, Virmani R, Forman MB. Intracoronary adenosine administered after reperfusion limits vascular injury after prolonged ischemia in the canine model. Circulation. 1989;80: 1388–99.
61. Pitarys CJ, Virmani R, Vildibill HD, Jackson EK, Forman MB. Reduction of myocardial reperfusion injury by intravenous adenosine administered during the early reperfusion period. Circulation. 1991;83:237–47.
62. Homeister JW, Hoff PT, Fletcher DD, Lucchesi BR. Combined adenosine and lidocaine administration limits myocardial reperfusion injury. Circulation. 1990;82:595–608.
63. Marzilli M, Orsini E, Marraccini P, Testa R. Beneficial effects of intracoronary adenosine as an adjunct to primary angioplasty in acute myocardial infarction. Circulation. 2000;101:2154–9.
64. Taniyama Y, Ito H, Iwakura K, et al. Beneficial effect of intracoronary verapamil on microvascular and myocardial salvage in patients with acute myocardial infarction. J Am Coll Cardiol. 1997;30:1193–9.
65. Galiuto I, DeMaria AN, del Balzo U, et al. Ischemia-reperfusion injury at the microvascular level treatment by endothelin-A selective antagonist and evaluation by myocardial contrast echocardiography. Circulation. 2000;102:311–3116.
66. Amado LC, Kraitchman DL, Gerber BL, et al. Reduction of "no-reflow" phenomenon by intra-aortic balloon counterpulsation in a randomized magnetic resonance imaging experimental study. J Am Coll Cardiol. 2004;43:1291–8.
67. Hale SL, Mehra A, Leeka J, Kloner RA. Postconditioning fails to improve no reflow or alter infarct size in an open-chest rabbit model of myocardial ischemia-reperfusion. Am J Physiol Heart Circ Physiol. 2008;294:H421–5.
68. Yang YJ, Zhao JL, You SJ, et al. Different effects of tirofiban and aspirin plus clopidogrel on myocardial no-reflow in a mini-swine model of acute myocardial infarction ad reperfusion. Heart. 2006;92:1131–8.
69. Hale SL, Kloner RA. Cardioprotection with adenosine-regulating agent, GP531: effects on no-reflow, infarct size, and blood flow following ischemia/reperfusion in the rabbit. J Cardiovasc Pharmacol Ther. 2010;15:60–7.
70. Reffelmann T, Hale SL, Dow JS, Kloner RA. No-reflow phenomenon persists long-term after ischemia/reperfusion in the rat and predicts infarct expansion. Circulation. 2003;108:2911–7.
71. Hamm CW, Heeschen C, Goldman B, et al. Benefits of abciximab in patients with refractory unstable angina in relation to serum troponin T levels. N Engl J Med. 1999;340:1623–9.
72. Deibele AJ, Jennings LK, Tcheng JE, Neva C, Earhart AD, Gibson CM. Intracoronary eptifibatide bolus administration during percutaneous coronary revascularization for acute coronary syndromes with evaluation of platelet glycoprotein IIb/IIIa receptor occupancy and platelet function: the Intracoronary Eptifibatide (ICE) Trial. Circulation. 2010;121:784–91.

Chapter 4
Lethal Myocardial Reperfusion Injury

Jakob Vinten-Johansen, Amanda J. Zatta, Rong Jiang, and Weiwei Shi

Abstract Early coronary artery reperfusion reduces infarct size and mortality and improves left ventricular contractile performance after myocardial ischemia compared to permanent occlusion. However, reperfusion itself causes either an acceleration of injury that is not present during ischemia or causes de novo reversible and lethal injury to heart tissue. In vitro and in vivo experimental data strongly suggest that reperfusion injury is initiated during the first few moments of reperfusion and proceeds over minutes to hours in a cascade involving numerous interactive mechanisms leading to damage or death of myocardium and coronary vascular endothelium. This reperfusion injury contributes to contractile dysfunction, metabolic derangements, and ultimately cell death by necrosis, apoptosis, and autophagy. The

J. Vinten-Johansen, M.S., Ph.D. (✉)
Department of Surgery, Division of Cardiothoracic Surgery,
Emory University School of Medicine, Emory University Hospital Midtown,
550 Peachtree Street, NE, Atlanta, GA 30308-2228, USA

Cardiothoracic Research Laboratory, Carlyle Fraser Heart Center,
Atlanta, GA, USA
e-mail: jvinten@emory.edu

A.J. Zatta, B.Sc. (Hons), Ph.D.
Department of Epidemiology and Preventive Medicine,
The Alfred Centre, Monash University,
99 Commercial Rd., Melbourne, VIC 3004, Australia
e-mail: amanda.zatta@monash.edu

R. Jiang, M.D., Ph.D.
Department of Surgery, Emory Children's Center,
2015 Uppergate Dr., Room 306, Atlanta 30322, GA, USA
e-mail: rjiang2@emory.edu

W. Shi, M.D., Ph.D.
Division of Cardiothoracic Surgery, Department of Surgery,
Emory University Hospital Midtown,
550 Peachtree St., Atlanta 30308, GA, USA
e-mail: wshi6@emory.edu

J.C. Kaski et al. (eds.), *Management of Myocardial Reperfusion Injury*,
DOI 10.1007/978-1-84996-019-9_4, © Springer-Verlag London 2012

mechanisms underlying lethal reperfusion injury include: (1) generation of ROS (oxygen paradox) from mitochondria, cytosolic and extracellular compartments, coronary vascular endothelium, and inflammatory cells such as neutrophils in a robust burst followed by sustained increased levels; (2) intracellular calcium accumulation (calcium paradox); (3) rapid normalization of tissue pH (pH paradox); (4) activation of proteolytic enzymes; (5) opening of the mitochondrial permeability transition pore; and (6) an inflammatory-like response. Although inflammatory cells and other cell types involved in inflammation (e.g., endothelium) contribute ROS and proinflammatory mediators during reperfusion, the role of inflammation in lethal reperfusion injury remains incompletely understood. ROS and calcium accumulation and rapid normalization of tissue pH which occur during the early moments of reperfusion create an environment in which the mitochondrial permeability transition pore opens, thereby promoting mitochondrial swelling and the release of proapoptotic substances which directs the cell to pursue a necrotic or an apoptotic pathway to death. Microvascular obliteration, a major physiological consequence of ischemia-reperfusion injury, may lead to no-reflow zones of myocardium and may also be involved in expansion of infarction as the duration of reperfusion increases and no-reflow zones expand. Age and gender may affect the heart's tolerance to ischemia such that lethal injury is more severe or occurs after shorter periods of ischemia; some mechanisms of reperfusion injury may be more exaggerated in older animal models but is known to occur in humans. Comorbidities such as hypertension, hypercholesterolemia, and diabetes may also exaggerate the response to ischemia-reperfusion by mechanisms that are relevant to reperfusion such as increased oxidant stress at reflow, preexisting endothelial cell dysfunction that limits the bioavailability of nitric oxide ($NO^{\bullet}$), or downregulation of the endogenous cardioprotective signaling pathways. Endogenous mechanisms exist that may combat reperfusion injury, such as the antioxidants glutathione and glutathione peroxidase, the autacoid adenosine, NO, and certain kinases (reperfusion injury salvage kinases, RISK). However, these are either not sufficiently stimulated or are rapidly overwhelmed. They can be enhanced by mechanical maneuvers such as postconditioning (a series of brief ischemia and reperfusion applied at the onset of reperfusion) or by pharmacological agents administered at the onset of reperfusion. Fully understanding the time course of reperfusion injury will help define and bracket the timing of effective reperfusion interventions. More fully understanding the mechanisms of reperfusion injury will help identify potential candidate therapies. Although previous clinical trials of drugs administered after percutaneous coronary interventions have revealed largely negative or inconclusive results, contemporary large-scale clinical trials should be undertaken with the immediacy and narrow window of reperfusion injury in mind, with the knowledge of effective concentrations of drugs at the target organ with consideration given to direct delivery to the target, and with appropriate duration of treatment to address immediate and delayed reperfusion injury.

Keywords Reactive oxygen species • Oxygen radicals • Superoxide anions Hydroxyl radical • Hypochlorous acid • Superoxide dismutase • Catalase Endogenous antioxidants • Nitric oxide • Endothelium • Endothelial dysfunction • Vasorelaxation responses • Nitric oxide synthase • Neutrophil adherence • Inflammation Neutrophils Survival kinases • Acute myocardial infarction • Necrosis • Apoptosis • Infarct size Coronary artery disease • Percutaneous coronary interventions • Toll-like receptors Diabetes • Senescence Hypercholesterolemia • Hypertension • Contractile stunning Cytokines • Tumor necrosis factor alpha • Complement • Interleukins Sarcoplasmic reticulum • Calcium overload • Antioxidants • Sodium/hydrogen exchanger • Sodium/ calcium exchanger

Introduction

On a global level, the major causes of mortality have changed from infectious diseases to noncommunicable type diseases, of which cardiovascular disease is a major category [1]. Cardiovascular disease is the leading cause of death worldwide, being responsible for 29% of all-cause mortality, and 80% of cardiovascular deaths are in the low- to middle-income countries. Coronary artery disease (CAD) is thought to be the cause of almost half of these deaths, numbering over seven million annually and being nearly equally divided between the male and female genders. CAD is the underlying cause of acute and chronic myocardial infarction. The incidence of acute myocardial infarction (AMI) will increase as a result of an escalating prevalence of diabetes, age, obesity, and hyperlipidemia, now being expressed collectively as metabolic syndrome. Infarct size has been linked to mortality, arrhythmias, and left ventricular dysfunction [1, 2]. In addition, heart failure is an increasingly common outcome of myocardial infarction and a frequent cause of cardiovascular morbidity and mortality [3]. In patients who survive an out of hospital AMI, the incidence of heart failure is inversely related to the amount of myocardium that is salvaged.

It was established early on that timely coronary artery reperfusion reduces infarct size [4, 5] and mortality, [6] and improves left ventricular contractile performance [2, 4]. However, reperfusion itself can cause either an acceleration of injury that is present during ischemia or can cause de novo injury to cells and their organelles, termed reperfusion injury. This reperfusion can cause reversible or irreversible injury. The first type of reversible injury includes myocardial stunning, i.e., impaired contractile function in the absence of irreversible injury (necrosis or apoptosis) despite restoration of blood flow [7]. Stunning, which clinically presents as regional myocardial dyskinesis, or global low cardiac output, persists for days to weeks. As with other aspects of ischemia-reperfusion injury, cardiomyocytes are not the only casualty of stunning; the coronary vascular endothelium in the postischemic myocardium can also suffer from transient dysfunction [8, 9] as well as irreversible injury. The pathophysiology and implications of this vascular dysfunction will be described below. Cardiac arrhythmias, which may occur after reperfusion of the myocardium that is stunned or undergoing evolving infarction, are another manifestation of reperfusion injury. Reperfusion has also been recognized to injure cardiomyocytes and endothelial cells irreversibly (lethal reperfusion injury). This chapter will discuss the manifestations, mechanisms, and implications of lethal myocardial reperfusion injury.

Lethal Reperfusion Injury

Lethal reperfusion injury occurs to cells that were viable at the end of ischemia. Whether this represents injury that occurs during ischemia but is not expressed until reperfusion (as holes in a hose do not leak until the faucet is turned on) or is a de novo injury is still debated. The event(s) that initiate the transition from reversibly injured to irreversibly injured cells are still not known. Furthermore, the biological characteristics of lethal reperfusion injury, i.e., the time course of its progression in a "reperfusion wavefront," the relationship of the previous ischemic duration and severity to the time course and extent of lethal reperfusion injury are also largely unknown. It is, however, clear that the lethal injury targets not only the cardiomyocyte but also the coronary vascular endothelium. There is a better understanding of the individual mechanisms involved in lethal reperfusion injury, but these mechanisms, determined in isolation, may act quite differently when integrated in the in vivo animal or human.

The concept of reperfusion injury originated from early seminal studies by Tennant and Wiggers [10] in 1935 who noted that ventricular fibrillation was a consequence of reperfusion in canine hearts; from the collective experience of many investigators, this may be a feature specific to canine hearts. Later, Jennings et al. [11] in 1960 suggested that reperfusion after prolonged ischemia was associated with myocardial injury not observed after ischemia alone. This study reported cell swelling, mitochondrial calcification, and the hallmarks of necrosis—myofibrillar contracture forming characteristic "contraction bands," sarcolemmal disruption, and flocculent densities thought to be calcium phosphate particles; these features were not apparent after ischemia alone. It was concluded that reperfusion "hastens" the progression of postischemic injury. Others have suggested that reperfusion may actually cause de novo lethal injury. Hearse et al. [12] reported that oxygenation of ischemic myocardium was accompanied by a robust release of cardiac enzymes indicative of necrosis. The cardiac surgeon Denton Cooley observed the contracture of the myocardium that occurred after reperfusion and that characterized the "stone heart" [13] from which the heart could not recover. Indeed, the existence of reperfusion injury has been (and still is) debated and thought to be a curiosity that was confined to the experimental laboratory with no clinical counterpart [14]. This debate is perpetuated by difficulties in identifying reperfusion injury using tools that cannot separate anatomopathological changes occurring during ischemia from those taking place during reperfusion, or by using pharmacological or mechanical interventions that incompletely inhibit the complex array of purported mechanisms of injury, and therefore incompletely inhibit the injury. It is a bit like gauging the size of an iceberg by the portion that is visible on the surface. These issues represent a challenge to scientists that should result in the development of better tools with which to characterize reperfusion injury, and to physicians to apply interventional tools in the clinical setting that attenuate reperfusion injury and thereby attain the full potential of cardioprotection which, at this time, is not fully known.

The observation that postischemic injury could be reduced by interventions applied at, or shortly before, the onset of reperfusion has provided compelling evidence that lethal reperfusion injury is a clinical entity that can be avoided or prevented, with a consequent reduction in infarct size and an increase in microvascular and contractile function [3, 15–21]. This evidence has been summarized in an excellent review by Yellon and Hausenloy [22]. The concept of modified reperfusion as a therapeutic approach arose from the understanding of the mechanisms underlying the pathophysiology of reperfusion and successfully applying reperfusion therapeutics in cardiac surgery [23, 24]. The reduction in infarct size has become a therapeutic end point because of its importance in the pathogenesis of postischemic complications, heart failure, and death.

Cell Death: Necrosis and Apoptosis

Necrosis is a disintegration of the cell caused by cell swelling and hypercontracture of the sarcomeres consistent with the contraction bands reported by Jennings et al. [11]. The mechanical stresses of contracture contribute to disruption of the sarcolemma [25] and subsequent release of the intracellular contents. Importantly, necrosis is a rapid process that occurs in the early moments of reperfusion [26, 27]. This type of "accidental" cell death prompts an inflammatory response. Apoptosis, on the other hand, is an "intentional" cell death brought about by signaling cascades that ultimately trigger the organized demise of the cell by condensation of cellular and nuclear contents and formation of apoptotic blebs which are phagocytozed by adjacent cells. In contrast to necrosis, apoptosis requires the expenditure of ATP. Studies suggest that apoptosis may be initiated during ischemia but executed at reperfusion [28–31].

Time Course of Reperfusion Injury: The Early Moments of Reperfusion Are Critical

The classic view on the time course of necrosis is that it progresses transmurally in the area at risk in a "wavefront" pattern starting at the most vulnerable subendocardial myocardium and advances toward the subepicardium [32] and whose progression could be tempered by collateral blood flow [33]. In the "wavefront" experimental studies [32], coronary occlusion was carried out in dogs for 40 min, 3 h, or 6 h, of ischemia, followed by 2–4 days of reperfusion. Infarct size increased progressively with time and was nearly transmural after 6 h of ischemia, with no further significant increase thereafter (Fig. 4.1); accordingly, the degree of salvageable myocardium reciprocally decreased as the ischemic duration increased. This time course is species dependent;

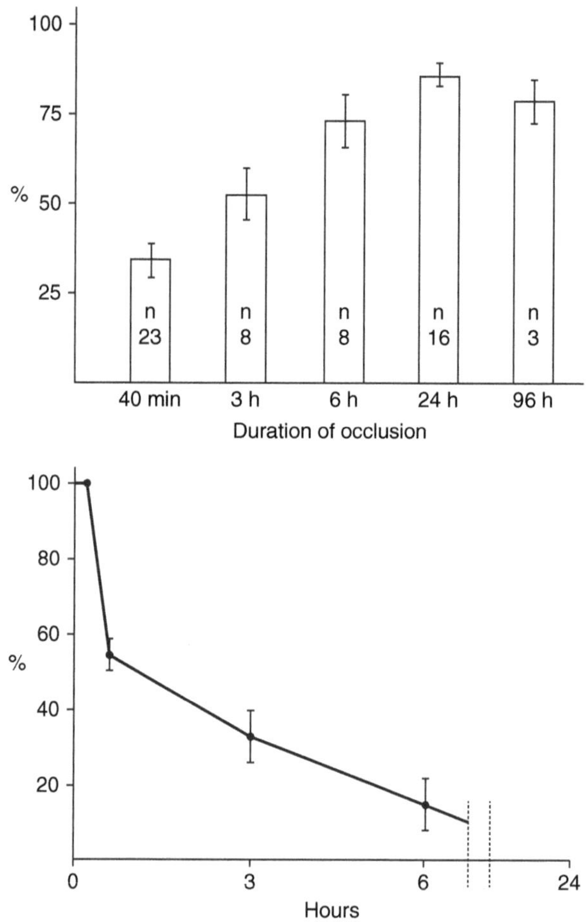

Fig. 4.1 The wavefront phenomenon as described by Reimer et al. (From Reimer et al. [32]. Reprinted with kind permission from Wolters Kluwer Health)

in pigs, the progression of necrosis is much faster compared to dogs [34], with transmural necrosis occurring after 90 min of occlusion [35], and in rodents transmurality of infarct is achieved in 1 h or less. Importantly, the ischemia-reperfusion protocol in those studies induced not only ischemic injury but also injury that was contributed by reperfusion. To date, the time course of ischemia-reperfusion injury has not been separated into its ischemia and reperfusion injury components. Ganz et al. [36] reported no extension of necrosis after various periods of reperfusion following 90–240 min of coronary artery occlusion; Miura et al. [37] suggested in an editorial to the paper by Ganz et al. [36] that advancing necrosis could be observed after longer periods of reperfusion or after shorter periods of ischemia. Other investigators also disputed the progressive nature of injury after reperfusion or reoxygenation (see the collections of opinions published by Przyklenk [38]).

However, in vitro and in vivo experimental data strongly suggest that lethal reperfusion injury occurs at the onset of reoxygenation or reperfusion and extends the severity of lethal injury beyond that observed after ischemia (or hypoxia/anoxia) alone [12, 39, 40]. Plasma creatine kinase (CK) activity is often used experimentally and clinically as a marker of necrosis. Plasma CK release is scant during ischemia but significantly and substantially increases during reperfusion (see Fig. 4.2). One interpretation of these data is that necrosis (vis-a-vis plasma CK activity) increases most predominantly during reperfusion, with little being released during ischemia. An alternative interpretation is that collateral blood flow is insufficient to wash out myocardial CK into the systemic circulation. However, the interpretation of these data is still controversial. Using radionuclide assessment of myocardial viability, Matsumura et al. [41] demonstrated that initially viable myocardium after 5 min of reperfusion was nonviable after 180 min of reperfusion, consistent with increasing necrosis during reperfusion. Zhao and colleagues [29, 42], using the canine model of ischemia-reperfusion, reported that infarct size indeed increased with the duration of reperfusion after a fixed duration (1 h) of coronary artery occlusion (Fig. 4.2).

Evidence also suggests that apoptosis also increases during reperfusion [30, 43, 44]. Necrosis may be a rapid "explosive" response to reperfusion that comes to completion relatively quickly (hours), while apoptosis at least in the perinecrotic area (penumbra of the infarct wavefront) continues for days after onset of reperfusion (Fig. 4.3). A temporal progression of necrosis after reperfusion underpins the efficacy of modified reperfusion protocols or cardioprotective drugs administered at reperfusion to salvage myocardium at risk of postischemic injury. As will become more apparent below, the first few moments of reperfusion are critical to the initiation of the "reperfusion injury cascade"—those series of events that are set in motion during the opening moments of reperfusion, and which propagate and/or initiate other later events. The duration of this critical time of early reperfusion has not been established completely, but the initial studies of Zhao et al. [15] and Kin et al. [45] using the brief (seconds to minutes) intervention termed postconditioning (multiple cycles of brief periods of reperfusion followed by brief ischemia applied immediately at the onset of reperfusion, also called "stutter" reperfusion [46]) suggest that this window is very short indeed.

No-Reflow in Reperfused Myocardium

The adherence of neutrophils and platelet aggregates to dysfunctional endothelium, combined with increased extravascular compression secondary to interstitial edema, and plugging of small vessels with microthrombi and intravascular debris cause maldistribution of blood flow to the affected myocardium distal to the arterial injury. The impairment of blood flow may be so severe that there is no measurable perfusion to some regions of myocardium. Defects in myocardial blood flow after transient ischemia was first observed in the heart by Krug et al. [47] in 1966, and the moniker "no-reflow" was later coined by Ames et al. [48] in 1968 for this phenomenon in the brain. The no-reflow state in postischemic myocardium has been observed experimentally and clinically despite widely patent epicardial coronary

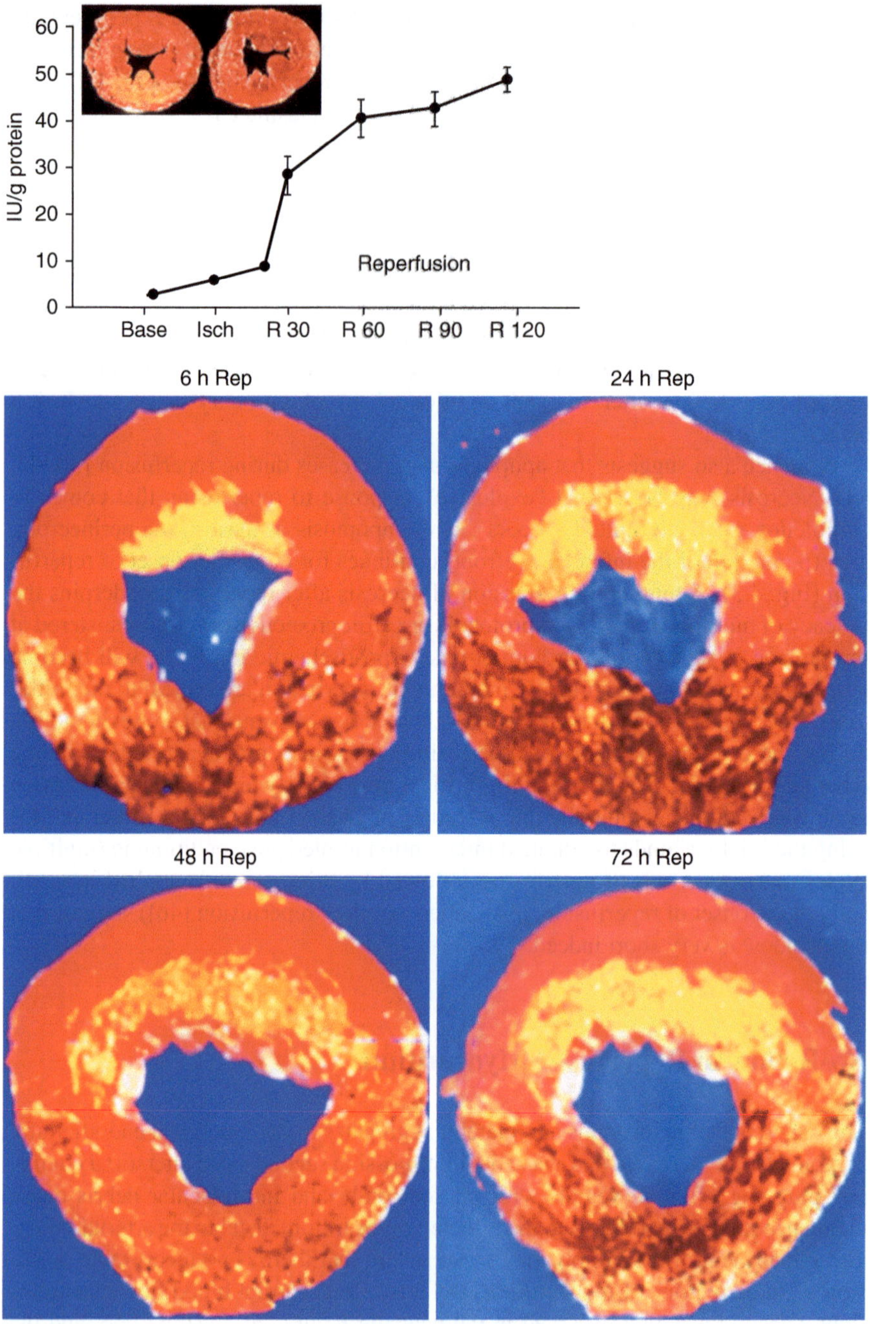
60
50
40
30
20
10
0
IU/g protein
Reperfusion
Base
Isch
R 30
R 60
R 90
R 120
6 h Rep
24 h Rep
48 h Rep
72 h Rep

Fig. 4.3 The time course of necrosis (TTC) and apoptosis (TUNEL staining of myocardial samples in the peri-infarcted region) in a canine model of 60 min LAD occlusion and 6, 24, 48, or 72 h of reperfusion [29]. *An* area of necrosis (TTC negative), *AAR* Area At Risk identified by in vivo distribution of unisperse blue dye after the LAD was relegated at the original occlusion site. *Determined by hematoxylin and eosin staining

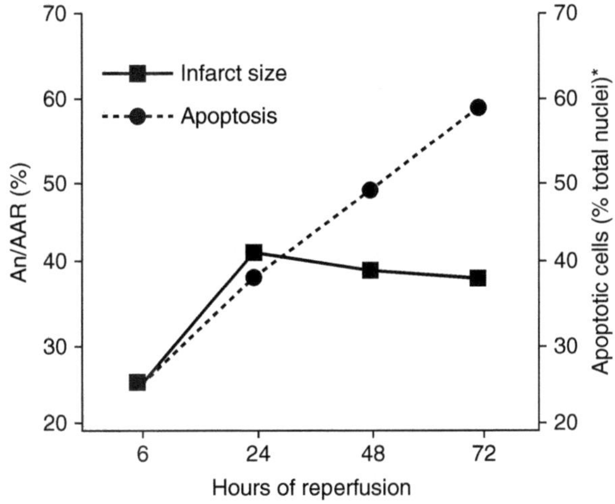

arteries [49–51]. This no-reflow zone is typically confined within the bounds of the infarct area. Recent evidence suggests that the no-reflow zone is dynamic and extends as the duration of reperfusion increases [52], implying that cells previously viable may die as the no-reflow zone extends outward toward the mid- and subepicardium, or that this mechanism of injury simply extends with time, hence its contribution of reperfusion injury. Clinically, the no-reflow observed after percutaneous coronary interventions (PCI, e.g., angioplasty) may present as continued chest pain and ST-segment elevation. The presence of no-reflow areas after

Fig. 4.2 The time course of infarct size estimated by appearance of plasma CK in a canine model of 60 min of LAD coronary artery occlusion followed by 2 h of reperfusion. The *color photograph* shows left ventricular slices from the same model of 60 min of LAD occlusion in which reperfusion was carried out for 6, 24, 48, or 72 h of reperfusion. After the prescribed period of reperfusion, the LAD was re-ligated, and unisperse blue dye was perfused in vivo by left atrial injection and allowed to circulate briefly. The left ventricle was excised and was then sliced transversely and incubated in 1% triphenyltetrazolium chloride (*TTC*) to differentiate the necrotic (*pale or yellow*) tissue from the nonnecrotic tissue in the area at risk. Note that the necrotic area extends toward the subepicardial region as the duration of reperfusion progresses. The infarct size was similar between 48 and 72 h of reperfusion. The *inset* shows transverse sections of porcine left ventricles treated with the double staining technique in which the LAD was occluded for 75 min by a fluoroscopically guided angioplasty balloon and reperfused for 4 h (*left*), or 4.25 h of occlusion without reperfusion (*right*). The two hearts had similar myocardial blood flow (microspheres) during baseline and at 60 min of ischemia (collateral blood flow). In the heart without reperfusion, blood flow in the area at risk was similar at 75 min of ischemia and 4.25 h of ischemia

reperfusion has been observed in about 30% of acute myocardial infarction cases and is associated with increased incidence of MI, complications, mortality, and heart failure [53, 54]. Accordingly, the presence of postreperfusion no-reflow is a predictor of adverse clinical events [51].

Mechanisms of Lethal Reperfusion Injury

Injury Induced by Reactive Oxygen Species (ROS)

Although oxygen was a waste product in a primordial world inhabited by plant life, it became essential for metabolism as animal cells evolved. Oxygen (O_2) is a terminal electron acceptor; the reduction of O_2 occurs normally in the mitochondrial electron transport chain to ultimately form H_2O. However, under certain conditions, O_2 forms free radicals, which are defined as atoms or small molecules that have one or more unpaired electrons. Unpaired electrons are unstable and highly reactive and seek a "partner" to achieve a more stable state. However, an incomplete reduction of O_2 forms the superoxide anion ($^-O^{\bullet}_2$), which has a half life of milliseconds at normal pH, is dismutated to hydrogen peroxide (H_2O_2) by superoxide dismutase (SOD), and finally is converted to the hydroxyl radical ($^{\bullet}OH$) (Fig. 4.4). Oxygen radicals are collectively included in the larger category of reactive oxygen species (ROS), while those radicals reacting with nitrogen are considered reactive nitrogen species (RNS). Although not fitting the definition of ROS, H_2O_2 is considered in the ROS category because of its intermediary position in the dismutation of $^-O^{\bullet}_2$ to $^{\bullet}OH$ and because of its high level of reactivity with biological molecules. Likewise, hypochlorous acid (HOCl) and chloramines are nonradical oxidants that contribute to injury of biological tissues.

As shown in Fig. 4.4, ROS are generated by many mechanisms, and cardiomyocytes and neutrophils (PMNs) are involved in this process. A predominant source of $^-O^{\bullet}_2$ is the PMN, which forms $^-O^{\bullet}_2$ from the NADPH oxidase that, under resting conditions, is relatively inactive because its subunits are separated in membrane and cytoplasmic compartments. In response to various soluble proinflammatory mediators such as TNFα(alpha), interkeukin-6 (IL-6) and −8 (IL-8), and complement fragments, the cytosolic and membrane-bound components assemble at the membrane and convert molecular oxygen to $^-O^{\bullet}_2$, which is released into the extracellular environment (or into the phagosome of PMNs). The $^-O^{\bullet}_2$ is further converted to H_2O_2 and subsequently to the hydroxyl radical ($^{\bullet}OH$), or HOCl- by myeloperoxidase, which can go on to form other oxidants (i.e., chloramines). The vascular endothelium also has a similar NAD(P)H oxidase (Nox) that can generate abundant $^-O^{\bullet}_2$ after activation by soluble mediators, ischemia-reperfusion, and PMNs.

Xanthine dehydrogenase is converted to the oxidant generating xanthine oxidase (XO) during ischemia, which forms $^-O^{\bullet}_2$ and H_2O_2 from the substrates hypoxanthine and xanthine derived from dephosphorylation of high energy

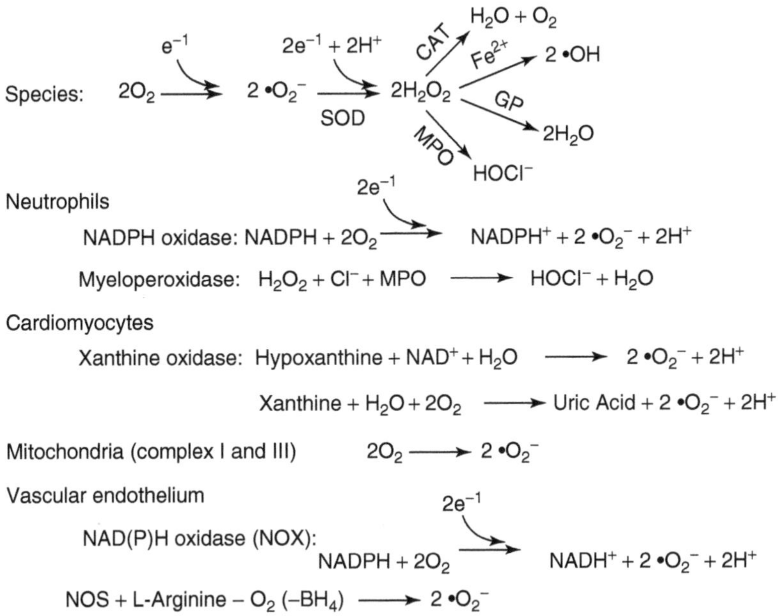

Fig. 4.4 The pathways and sources of ROS generation. *GP* glutathione peroxidase, *MPO* myeloperoxidase, *HOCl* hypochlorous acid, *SOD* superoxide dismutase, *CAT* catalase, *BH_4* tetrahydrobiopterin

phosphates (ATP, ADP, AMP) and breakdown of adenosine by adenosine deaminase. Hypoxanthine and xanthine accumulate during ischemia. Although the contribution of XO to overall ROS generation in humans has been questioned in the past, XO is reported to be localized to the vascular endothelium in substantial quantities [55, 56]. However, the importance of XO to the overall generation of ROS in humans is still controversial [57]. Other sources of ROS include the mitochondrial electron transport chain (at complexes I and III), oxidation of unsaturated free fatty acids involving cyclooxygenase, oxidation of catecholamines and P450, monoamine oxidase that transfers electrons from amines to oxygen, and p66Shc which oxidizes cytochrome c to form hydrogen peroxide. In addition, nitric oxide synthase will generate $^{-}O^{\bullet}_2$ under anoxic conditions or in the absence of the cofactor tetrahydrobiopterin (BH_4) [58].

The actions of ROS are thought to be concentration-dependent. At very low concentrations, i.e., the ROS generated normally by mitochondria (1–2%), ROS participates in signaling and may be part of the mechanisms by which the cell senses its redox status. However, larger amounts of ROS generated by activated PMNs, as a respiratory burst by NADPH oxidase from activated endothelium, or from the cardiomyocytes are cytotoxic. Mitochondria participate in this large-scale explosion of ROS generation by a process called ROS-triggered ROS release.

ROS in Ischemia and Reperfusion

By their destructive mechanisms, ROS play an important part in biological processes. Under normal conditions, $^{\bullet}OH$ generated by neutrophils kills bacteria. However, an overabundance of ROS can damage or destroy organelles, cells, and tissues, leading to an array of pathologies including DNA mutations possibly underlying cancer, Parkinson's disease, aging, and atherosclerosis. There is an abundance of evidence that overproduction of ROS is also involved in the pathophysiology of myocardial necrosis and apoptosis during reperfusion. In 1973 [12], Hearse and colleagues reported that reoxygenation of globally arrested (hyperkalemia), anoxic hearts for 100 min was accompanied by a release of creatine phosphokinase indicative of cell death, a phenomenon later called the "oxygen paradox." The exogenous administration of oxygen radical generators replicated the myocardial morphological damage and contractile dysfunctional observed after ischemia-reperfusion [59, 60]. Subsequent studies using oxygen radical scavengers confirmed that this explosive cell necrosis was caused by reactive oxygen species [61–65].

The temporal appearance of this massive generation of ROS is important. The release of ROS increases 1–2 orders of magnitude (relative to nonischemic myocardium) during the first minutes of reperfusion as measured directly using electron spin resonance techniques [66]. The rapid production of oxygen radicals has been reported in the in vivo rabbit model of ischemia-reperfusion by Grill et al. [67] using EPR (electron paramagnetc resonance) of biopsies taken during ischemia and periods of reperfusion. In addition, infusion of superoxide dismutase reduced the generation of oxygen-centered radicals during reperfusion. Ferrari et al. [68] reported in patients undergoing cardioplegic arrest and global ischemia during cardiac surgery that oxygen radicals estimated by release of oxidized glutathione (GSSG) sampled from coronary sinus blood were generated at reperfusion after longer ischemic times (>30 min), and the degree of GSSG formation was correlated with postoperative outcomes.

Mechanisms of Injury Induced by ROS

The formation of ROS from whatever source will cause damage to cardiomyocytes and vascular tissue, especially the coronary vascular endothelium which is the "front line" of defense against destructive processes or cells derived from the intravascular space. Their generation overwhelms the endogenous scavengers' superoxide dismutase, catalase, glutathione-glutathione peroxidase, and uric acid. The deleterious actions of ROS on cells and tissues includes: damage to DNA; lipid peroxidation leading to membrane damage and calcium (Ca^{2+}) overload; damage to the sarcoplasmic reticulum (SR) leading to Ca^{2+} dyshomeostasis and contractile dysfunction; denaturation of proteins that form enzymes and ion channels; impairment of metabolism, i.e., glycolysis; and activation of adhesion molecules on vascular endothelium, thereby stimulating an increase in PMN adhesion [69]. Importantly, ROS reduces the bioavailability of nitric oxide (NO˙) by a biradical reaction that proceeds at diffusion-limited speeds forming the potent oxidant peroxynitrite ($ONOO^-$). This reduction in NO˙ has far-reaching effects on the myocardium. The mitochondrial signaling functions of NO˙ may be impaired. The potent anti-inflammatory effects of endogenous NO˙ released by coronary vascular endothelium are diminished, thereby increasing its proinflammatory (and procoagulative) state. ROS may be responsible for causing damage to the NO˙ synthase enzyme or its regulation, which further limits both its capability of generating NO˙ and inhibiting inflammatory-mediated damage in a vicious cycle [70, 71]. The reduction in availability of endogenous NO˙ may contribute to the pathogenesis of infarction since inhibiting NO˙ or its production is associated with larger infarct sizes [72–74] while administration of authentic NO˙, the eNOS substrate L-arginine [75–77], or NO˙ donors at reperfusion reduce infarct size and global contractile dysfunction [78].

Calcium-Related Reperfusion Injury (Calcium Paradox)

Intracellular calcium is the most rigidly controlled constituent in the cell. Shen and Jennings [79] first reported that reperfusion following brief coronary occlusion was associated with accelerated accumulation of intracellular Ca^{2+}. After relatively short periods of ischemia, reperfusion is accompanied by a rapid increase in intracellular and mitochondrial Ca^{2+}. The loss of Ca^{2+} homeostasis has a number of causes: (1) the loss of membrane integrity may allow rapid entry of Ca^{2+} into the cell; (2) Ca^{2+} entry through the L-type channels, which may be facilitated by Ca^{2+} released by the glycocalyx; (3) impaired Ca^{2+} sequestration by the SR, leading to higher levels of cytosolic Ca^{2+}; and (4) reversal of the Na^+/Ca^{2+} exchanger favoring intracellular accumulation of Ca^{2+}. The physiological consequences of this Ca^{2+} accumulation are arrhythmias, hypercontracture of the cardiomyocytes causing cell death, and/or opening of the mitochondrial transition pores also leading to pursuit of cell death by necrotic or apoptotic pathways. In addition, the contractile apparatus becomes desensitized to Ca^{2+}, thereby impairing the contractile function of the myofibrils.

The conditions for intracellular accumulation of Ca^{2+} begin during ischemia with depletion of ATP with subsequent inhibition of the energy-dependent sarcolemmal Na^+/K^+ ATPase (extrudes Na^+ in exchange for K^+ influx) and the simultaneous build-up of H^+ secondary to anaerobic metabolism. In addition to a lack of ATP, the calpain-mediated degradation of ankyrin (anchors the ATPase molecule to the sarcolemmal membrane) at early reperfusion further impairs Na^+/K^+ ATPase pump function and Na^+ extrusion from the cell [80]. The intracellular accumulation of Na^+ stimulates reversal of the Na^+/Ca^{2+} antiporter, which normally extrudes intracellular Ca^{2+} in exchange for extracellular Na^+. The forward direction of the Na^+/H^+ exchanger can further increase Na^+ accumulation, but its activity is attenuated by the concomitant increase in extracellular H^+ which reduces the H^+ transsarcolemmal gradient fueling Na^+ influx. However, H^+ is washed out at reperfusion which reestablishes this gradient favoring Ca^{2+} efflux, leading to further increase in the intracellular Na^+ concentration, which in turn, promotes further Ca^{2+} accumulation through the Na^+/Ca^{2+} exchanger operating in the reverse mode.

The importance of intracellular Ca^{2+} accumulation via sarcolemmal channels or the coordinated actions of the Na^+/H^+ and Na^+/Ca^{2+} exchangers during reperfusion are not consistently supported by experimental evidence. Inhibitors of coronary blood Ca^{2+} during early reperfusion have shown an inconsistent reduction in infarct size [81, 82] as have Ca^{2+} channel blockers [81]. While administration of Na^+/H^+ exchange inhibitors before ischemia has been shown to be cardioprotective, administration specifically at reperfusion has not shown a consistent cardioprotection, with some studies showing benefit (contractile function [83]; infarct size [84]) and others no benefit (infarct size [85]). Accordingly, clinical trials in which inhibitors of the Na^+/H^+ exchanger (cariporide [86]; eniporide [87]; MCC-135 [88]) were administered at reperfusion to acute STEMI patients undergoing primary PCI or cardiac surgery requiring cardioplegic arrest have not shown benefit (reduced infarct size). MCC-135 is a new class of drug that both inhibits the Na^+/Ca^{2+} exchanger [83] and increases uptake of intracellular Ca^{2+} by sarcoplasmic reticulum. The failure of Na^+/H^+ exchange inhibitors to reduce infarct size when administered at reperfusion may not be related to the functioning of the exchanger itself but to the intact ability of the cardiomyocyte to rapidly normalize intracellular pH through other mechanisms (see below), which then permits hypercontracture to occur.

pH Paradox

Ischemia reduces delivery of O_2 to a highly metabolic myocardium. As O_2 is depleted, aerobic metabolism is replaced by anaerobiosis, with a lower yield of ATP and an accumulation of hydrogen ions (H^+). Both interstitial and tissue pH rapidly decrease with onset of ischemia. During ischemia, tissue acidosis inhibits the potentially deleterious effects of hypercontracture, cell-cell communication by gap junctions, calpain activation and proteolytic activity, the Na^+/H^+ exchanger, and opening of the mPTP. However, reperfusion rapidly restores tissue pH by washout of H^+ from the interstitial space, which then unleashes the aforementioned mechanisms to cause cell injury. In support of this connection between rapid normalization of tissue pH and lethal reperfusion injury, reperfusion with acidic perfusates during the first minutes of reperfusion [89, 90], or a gradual restoration of tissue pH as occurs with postconditioning [90, 91], or gradual reperfusion [92–95] are mechanical interventions that reduce infarct size.

Hypercontracture

The contraction bands noted by Jennings et al. [11] in reperfused myocardium represent hypercontracted sarcomeres [96] that induce mechanical stress to the sarcolemmal, leading to its disruption and cell death. The sarcolemma's vulnerability to contracture-induced stress is further augmented by a cytoskeleton made more fragile by degradation of sarcolemmal and cytoskeletal proteins by Ca^{2+} activated calpains [90, 97]. This cytoskeletal fragility can be passed to adjacent cells via gap junctions, thereby spreading necrosis to potentially viable cells [98]. Hypercontracture has been observed to occur in the first minutes of in vitro reoxygenation or in vivo reperfusion [96, 99, 100] coincident with intracellular enzyme release and contraction band necrosis. Avoiding hypercontracture prevents cell death and reduces infarct size [101–103], thereby confirming a correlation between hypercontracture and lethal reperfusion injury. Hypercontracture occurs when mitochondrial ATP synthesis transiently resumes during the early moments of reperfusion in the presence of Ca^{2+} accumulation by mechanisms discussed above. The transient availability of ATP from still functioning mitochondria fuels the sequestration of Ca^{2+} by the energy-requiring sarcoplasmic reticulum (SR) Ca^{2+} pump (SERCA) and its subsequent release through ryanodine receptor release channel (RyR) in a repeating cycle that sets up oscillatory Ca^{2+} patterns that contribute to Ca^{2+}-dependent contracture. However, intracellular Ca^{2+} from transarcolemmal influx and SR oscillatory Ca^{2+} transients provides a gradient force driving Ca^{2+} flux through the mitochondrial Ca^{2+} uniporter, thereby leading to opening of the mPTP and a failure to produce ATP, and a release of proapoptotic factors (e.g., cytochrome c). The reduced ATP levels may also contribute to a Ca^{2+}-independent contracture (rigor associated) [104].

Endothelial Dysfunction and the Inflammatory Response to Reperfusion

The vascular endothelium has the surface area of $1-6\times10^{13}$ cells covering an area of 1–7 m^2. As one of the body's largest organs, it acts as a barrier against fluid extravasation from the vascular space and regulates the synthesis and release of factors acting in autocrine and paracrine fashion that participate in hemostasis (blood coagulation), the immune response (inflammation), and vasoregulation (blood pressure and blood flow). Far from being an inert "cellophane" cell layer [105], the normal functional state of the vascular system is maintained in a noncoagulative, noninflammatory, and autoregulated state by the balanced release of factors that constrict (endothelin-1, thromboxane A2, leukotrienes) or dilate ($NO^{\bullet}$, cyclooxygenase derived prostanoids, and adenosine) vascular smooth muscle, promote (leukotrienes, platelet-activating factor) or inhibit (nitric oxide, adenosine) inflammation, and promote (von Willebrand Factor, platelet-activating factor) or inhibit (heparin, plasminogen activating factor) blood coagulation (Fig. 4.5) [106]. Stresses such as ischemia-reperfusion and oxidants will cause dysfunction, and shift the balance of release of these factors to a proconstrictive, procoagulant, and proinflammatory phenotype.

Ku et al. [107] first reported that ischemia was associated with a loss of endothelial-specific vasorelaxation responses to incremental concentrations of the endothelium-specific stimulator of $NO^{\bullet}$ synthase (eNOS) acetylcholine. This has

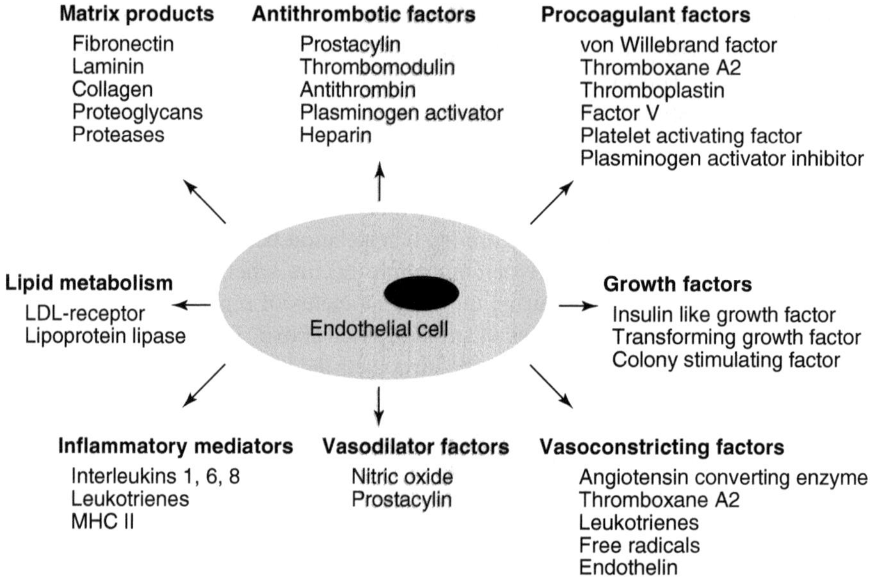

Fig. 4.5 Illustration of substances synthesized and released from the vascular endothelium. Both vasoconstrictors and vasodilators are produced to balance the regulation of vascular resistance. Likewise, both proinflammatory and anti-inflammatory factors are released. Ischemia-reperfusion upregulates the release of proinflammatory, procoagulant, and vasoconstrictive factors to change the postischemic phenotype from one that is homeostatic to one that is hostile [106]

been confirmed in numerous studies [72, 108–112] (reviewed in [113–117]); the microvessels may be more susceptible to this endothelial injury than the large epicardial vessels [118]. Subsequent experiments have shown the loss of vasoreactivity to be due to an impaired release of $NO^{\bullet}$ [71] and an overproduction of $^{-}O_2^{\bullet}$ which annihilates $NO^{\bullet}$ and forms the potent oxidant $ONOO^-$. The impaired synthesis and release of $NO^{\bullet}$ are important not only for loss of vascular tone regulation but also for presenting a procoagulant and proinflammatory surface that initiates microthrombi and neutrophil-mediated proinflammatory events (adherence, activation, diapedesis). Endothelial dysfunction and the resultant shift from the normal to a hostile state occur in the early moments of reperfusion [119] and can persist for days, weeks, or months [111, 120]. Zhao et al. [42], in the canine model of 60 min of coronary artery occlusion and up to 72 h of reperfusion, reported that endothelial dysfunction quantified by vasorelaxation responses to acetylcholine was blunted most after 6 h of reperfusion (the earliest observation point) and normalized over the next 3 days. The adherence of PMNs to the endothelial surface, however, continued to increase over that time period (Fig. 4.6). Indeed, endothelial dysfunction can occur in the absence of morphological injury and may precede morphological injury to cardiomyocytes; the endothelium can die by an apoptotic pathway that precedes cardiomyocyte apoptosis [121].

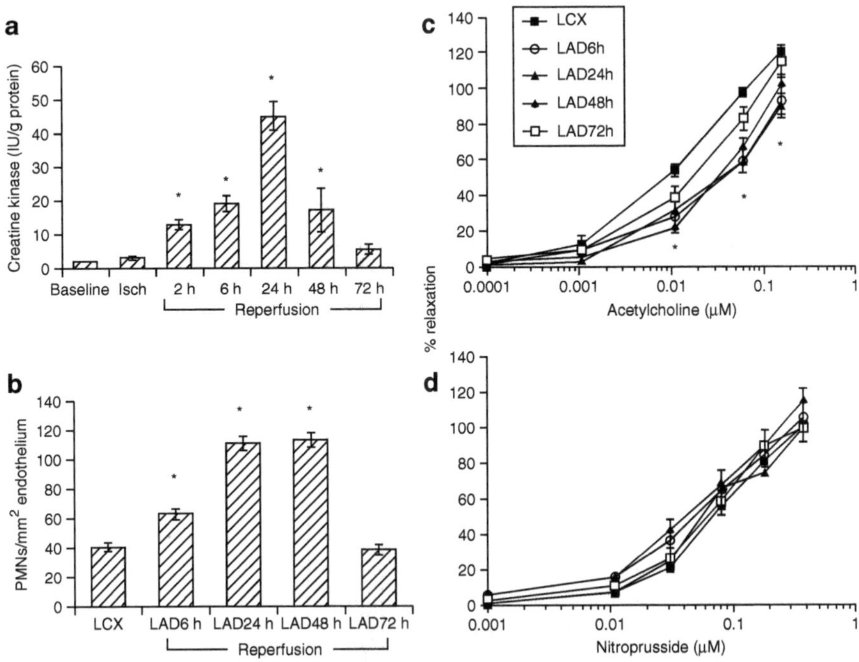

Fig. 4.6 (**a**) The time course of necrosis (plasma CK), (**b**) neutrophil adherence to ischemic-reperfused LAD coronary artery after coincubation of postischemic arterial segments with unstimulated PMNs, (**c**) endothelial dysfunction (vasorelaxation responses to incremental concentrations of acetylcholine in organ chambers), in comparison to(**d**) smooth muscle relaxation stimulated by incremental concentrations of sodium nitroprusside. (Modified from Zhao et al. [42], with kind permission from Elsevier Limited)

The studies by Lefer's group have shown that endothelial dysfunction after ischemia occurs rapidly after onset of reperfusion. The release of histamine, cytokines, and thrombin and the generation of $^{-}O_2^{\bullet}$ during the early moments of reperfusion activate the coronary vascular endothelium by expressing the early adhesion molecule P-selectin [122]. P-selectin expression reaches a peak within the first 20 min in experimental models and is subsequently shed in the form of soluble fragments. P-selectin binds to P-selectin glycoprotein-1 on PMNs, and this promotes the rolling of PMNs along the endothelial surface, which is a critical stage of the adhesion process and subsequent PMN transmigration into the myocardial parenchyma. Firm adherence to the endothelium occurs later with the upregulation of the β(beta)2 integrin CD11/CD18 on the PMN and its counter ligand, the immunoglobulin intercellular adhesion molecule type 1 (ICAM-1) on the endothelium, which is upregulated by ROS, IL-1, and TNFα(alpha), but the time course of expression is slower (~4 h) than that of P-selectin. Reperfusion therefore stimulates PMN adherence to the coronary vascular endothelial surface [42, 123, 124].

The study by Zhao et al. [42] shows that the accumulation of PMNs is primarily in the vascular space for the first 6 h of reperfusion and involves transmigration to the extravascular spaces thereafter. Indeed, there is an association between the accumulation of PMNs on the vascular endothelium, loss of endothelial function, and infarct size that suggests an interrelationship. Shandelya et al. [125] showed that PMNs contributed to postischemic injury in the isolated perfused rat heart preparation caused by ROS generation. Activation of PMNs requires the presence of plasma lipids [125] and complement [126]. (See the review by Vinten-Johansen [127] for a detailed description of the potential role of PMNs in reperfusion injury.) Such an interrelationship between endothelial cells and PMNs is supported by clinical data showing that activated PMNs and PMN-platelet aggregates sampled from coronary artery aspirates in patients undergoing primary PCI are more prominent locally in the culprit artery than in peripheral blood [128]. Plasma from MI patients has chemotactic activity and stimulates PMN adherence to endothelium and production of ROS [129, 130]. Patients with acute myocardial infarction also have increased plasma PMN elastase activity or myeloperoxidase activity [131], suggesting an increased level of activation and degranulation [132]; increased plasma myeloperoxidase was also associated with increased creatine kinase—MB enzyme release [131]. PMNs are observed to accumulate in the early rather than later phases of ischemia-reperfusion in patients with acute myocardial infarction [133]. In addition, elevated PMN counts and activators such as IL-6 after acute myocardial infarction and reperfusion are associated with diminished long-term survival [134].

Some studies support a functional role of PMNs and the inflammatory response to reperfusion on the pathogenesis of infarction. Infarct size has been reduced in experimental models of ischemia-reperfusion using PMN depletion by antiserum (34% reduction [135]; 37% reduction [136]; 77% reduction [137]; 35% reduction [138]), leukocyte filters (47% [139]), and immunoneutralization by administration at reperfusion of antibodies to adhesion molecules involved in early PMN—endothelial cell interactions (i.e., P-selectin on endothelium) [140, 141]. In addition, infarct size and PMN accumulation are decreased in mice deficient of CD18 on the PMN, and ICAM-1 [142, 143] or P-selectin [144] on the vascular endothelium. But not all studies on adhesion molecule depletion show infarct reduction [145]. Therefore, evidence strongly supports that inhibition of the early neutrophil—endothelial interactions that initiate the PMN-mediated inflammatory cascade at the onset of reperfusion reduces infarct size, as well as other forms of reperfusion injury. However, some studies do not strongly suggest a link between PMN-endothelial cell-mediated responses and lethal reperfusion injury [146, 147], and like many interventions, PMN inhibition may not effectively reduce infarct size after prolonged ischemic times exceeding 3–4 h [136].

From a broader perspective, not all experimental studies on various anti-inflammatory agents in the setting of postischemic injury have been positive [148]. (See Baxter [149] and Lefer [150] for an interesting point–counterpoint discussion). In studies using antibodies, it is important that the antibody cross-react with the specific target antigen, and as we now know, the treatments need to be administered within the short time window presented to attenuate the early moments of reperfusion injury. In addition, doses of any given anti-inflammatory agent vary widely among studies, and questions are raised about reaching effective plasma concentrations. Perhaps not surprisingly, clinical studies on anti-inflammatory agents have not shown a consistent reduction in infarct size [151, 152] although some agents (the protease inhibitor aprotinin [153]) have demonstrated benefit as an anti-inflammatory agent. The incongruity between largely positive preclinical and negative clinical studies is multifactorial and may relate to (1) the advanced age and presence of coronary artery disease and other risk factors of the patients versus the generally young healthy state of the experimental animal, (2) use of medications (aspirin, IIb/IIa inhibitors, heparin, and derivatives) that may interfere with the pharmacological agent under investigation, (3) inability of a medication with a singular and specific target (i.e., TNFα(alpha0)) to impact a very complex process with redundant mechanisms, (4) delayed or inconsistent application of the drug which misses the window of opportunity presented by the early moments of reperfusion, and (5) the timing of the drug administration in the experimental versus clinical situation plus the presence of a dynamic obstruction with occlusion and partial resolution of thrombus in the clinical milieu.

Activation of Toll-like receptors (TLR) has recently been implicated in the pathogenesis of reperfusion injury [154, 155]. TLRs are transmembrane receptors expressed on cardiomyocytes, endothelial cells, and PMNs. They recognize pathogen-associated molecular patterns on invading pathogens for host defense, and endogenous ligands (danger-associated molecular patterns (DAMPS)) released during stress such as heat shock proteins, high mobility group box (HMGB-1), and degradation products of heparan sulfate, fibronectin and hyaluronic acid (specifically for TLR2 and TLR4). They also take part in the innate immune response by recognizing molecules released by cells undergoing death processes. Recent data suggest that the TLR2 located on PMNs is involved in the inflammatory response to reperfusion, while parenchymal (cardiomyocyte and endothelium) TLR2 is not involved in lethal injury. Infarct size secondary to regional ischemia was reduced in TLR2-deficient mice. Chimeric $TLR2^{-/-}$ mice with wild type (positive for TLR2) bone marrow and negative for TLR2 in parenchymal tissue were found not to have infarct sizes different from wild type mice; wild type mice with $TLR2^{-/-}$ bone marrow had smaller infarct size comparable to that of TLR2 knockout mice. These data suggested that TLR2 signaling via circulating cells (e.g., inflammatory cells) is important in the pathogenesis of reperfusion injury. In addition, administration of a TLR2 antagonist at reperfusion reduced infarct size [155]. The TLR pathway may be a newly identified contributor to reperfusion injury and may therefore present a novel therapeutic target.

Soluble proinflammatory mediators such as complement (e.g., C5a) and cytokines such as TNFα(alpha) may contribute to the inflammatory response to irreversible ischemia-reperfusion injury. TNFα(alpha) is part of the signaling pathway of ROS generation by endothelial cells [156]. These mediators are increased during ischemia-reperfusion [157], agonists or mimetics replicate the lethal injury of the endogenous molecules, and antagonists reduce infarct size. The complement cascade is also involved in lethal reperfusion injury. Complement is activated during ischemia-reperfusion and ultimately forms the membrane attack complex, which forms transsarcolemmal pores and causes the transmembrane movement of water

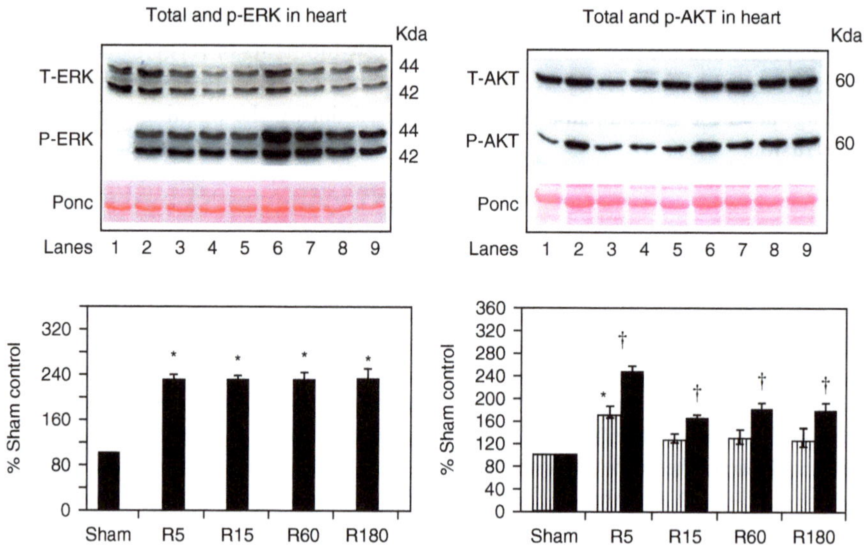

Fig. 4.7 The time course of phosphorylation of the antiapoptotic kinases ERK1/2 and Akt in the area at risk myocardium after 5, 15, 60, and 180 min of reperfusion following 30 min of left coronary artery occlusion in in vivo rats. Reperfusion was associated with an increased phosphorylation of ERK1/2 and Akt compared to sham, which remained stable over the period of reperfusion for phosphor-ERK1/2 but declined for phosphor-Akt after 15 min of reperfusion. Levels of kinases were not determined after ischemia only (Unpublished data by permission of Zhi-Qing Zhao)

increased the phosphorylation of ERK1/2. Darling et al. [46] also reported increased phosphorylation of ERK1/2 but not Akt, but this is controversial [180]. The endogenous "conditioning" strategies of preconditioning, perconditioning, and postconditioning [181] are associated with increased phosphorylation of RISK pathway components. The involvement of the RISK pathway in postconditioning has been shown in human atrial muscle subjected to simulated ischemia and reperfusion [182]. The RISK pathway may exert cardioprotection by inhibiting mPTP opening [183], which can inhibit both necrosis and apoptosis, and by improving Ca^{2+} handling by the sarcoplasmic reticulum [184]. The list of cardioprotective kinases that inhibit reperfusion injury is evolving to include JAK-STAT [118] PKCε(epsilon), PKC, PKG, and sphingosine kinase [185].

Effects of Age and Comorbidities on Reperfusion Injury

Cardiovascular disease is affected by various comorbidities, age, and gender that contribute to the pathology of reperfusion injury. Hypercholesterolemia, diabetes, and hypertension, for example, are associated with endothelial dysfunction and loss of NO• bioavailability that mitigates the anti-inflammatory effects of NO•. These comorbidities also reduce the resistance of oxidative stress.

Age

There is a generalized decrease in the tolerance to ischemia in experimental models [186–188] and in human myocardium [189] with aging involving many mechanisms.

1. ROS plays a central role in the aging process [190], and therefore ROS-related mechanisms to decreased tolerance to ischemia are likely. Therefore, there may be a compromise in the innate tolerance to stress at a time when aging increases the physiological and biochemical effects of stress [191] and the myocardium suffers greater damage from oxidative stress. Mitochondria from aged myocardium are larger and generate excessive ROS, while extramitochondrial enzymes (NADPH oxidase, monoamine oxidase) contribute to the overproduction of ROS, which may unfavorably alter the precarious balance between the signaling functions of ROS generated by mitochondria and deleterious ROS generated in substantially greater amounts from all sources. In addition, there is a decrease in the endogenous antioxidant capacity. Excessive levels of ROS may cause direct damage to cardiomyocytes and endothelial cells, may activate the coronary vascular endothelium and PMNs, and can stimulate mPTP opening during the reenergizing and realkalinization environment produced by reperfusion.
2. Ca^{2+} handling may be decreased in aged myocardium.
3. Loss of cardioprotective NO• secondary to increased endothelial dysfunction with age [192].
4. Compromised molecular signaling pathways (RISK) or levels of ligands, their cognate receptors, or signal transduction pathways operative in endogenous cardioprotection.

In the case of adenosine, the signal transduction pathways are impaired with age rather than the levels of adenosine or receptor expression being reduced (reviewed in Willems et al. [193]).

Comorbidities

Comorbidities represent significant risk factors for cardiovascular disease [194] and they contribute to the extent of lethal ischemia-reperfusion injury, mortality, morbidity, and heart failure [195, 196]. Some evidence suggests that the presence of comorbidities increases infarct size [197]. The mechanisms underlying this amplified response to ischemia-reperfusion include: (1) increased oxidant stress that poses the risk of serious tissue damage similar to that described above for oxidant-mediated injury in aged myocardium; (2) endothelial cell dysfunction and an increase in the activation state of endothelium to adopt a procoagulative, proinflammatory, and proconstrictive phenotype by limiting the bioavailability of $NO^{\bullet}$ at the level of precursor availability, impaired $NO^{\bullet}$ synthesis apparatus, increased degradation by $^{-}O_2^{\bullet}$ [198–201]; or (3) downregulation of the endogenous cardioprotective signaling pathways. In addition, diabetes is associated with a reduced phosphorylation of Akt that is increased by three cycles of ischemic preconditioning and abrogated by an Akt phosphorylation inhibitor [202]. There were parallel changes in infarct size, which suggested an association between the level of Akt phosphorylation and cardioprotection.

Clinical Implications of Reperfusion Injury and Concluding Remarks

Reperfusion injury contributes to fatal arrhythmias, to lethal injury (necrosis and apoptosis) that determines infarct size, and to post-MI remodeling leading ultimately to heart failure. This postischemic injury is encountered in settings where reperfusion is established, including PCI, cardiac surgery or organ transplantation, and resuscitation from sudden cardiac arrest and shock. Reperfusion injury decreases the salvage potential of reperfusion by transitioning potentially viable cells to irreversible injury. Attempts to reduce lethal injury and its survival consequences by reducing the ischemic time, a primary determinant of infarct size and myocardial injury, have been successful, but further efforts at improving response procedures by improved EMS alert and transport mechanisms or foreshortening in-hospital responses leading to reduced door-to-balloon time bring diminishing returns. The lessons learned from experience with postconditioning have taught us that reperfusion injury is initiated quickly after the onset of reperfusion and progresses quickly during the first few minutes of reperfusion possibly in a "wavefront" pattern. The progression of injury involves endothelial dysfunction and death, apoptosis, and necrosis, as well as nonlethal injury (Fig. 4.8). The early moments of reperfusion represent a high-risk, high-gain situation; the risk is that cardioprotective interventions will salvage less tissue if application immediately before or at reperfusion is delayed. The gain is that more tissue will be salvaged by modified reperfusion than heretofore appreciated. The understanding of the rapid time course of reperfusion injury will give new urgency to the clinical delivery of reperfusion therapies before or at the onset of reflow without delay. Indeed, the delay in applying reperfusion therapies may be only one reason that clinical trials of pharmacological agents targeting reperfusion injury have failed [204]. Further, more accurate identification of the mechanisms involved in reperfusion injury will open avenues for both new therapeutic options and new targets for pharmacological

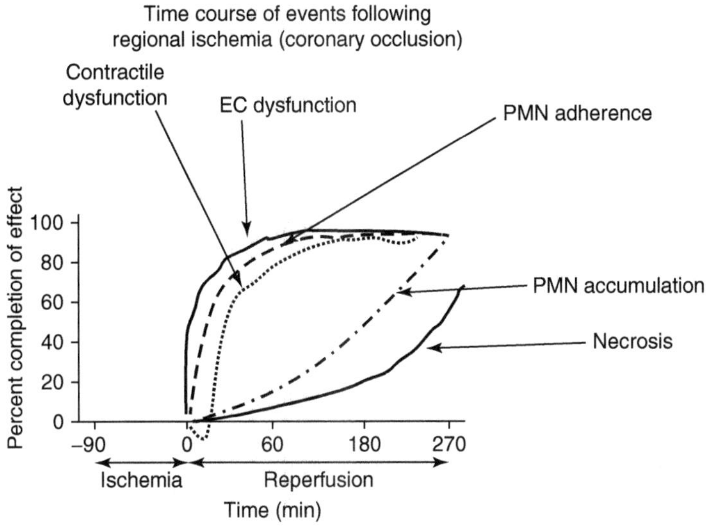

Fig. 4.8 The comparative time course of injury or dysfunction of regional contractility, endothelial vasoreactivity, PMN adherence to the ischemic-reperfused coronary artery endothelium, PMN transmigration and accumulation in the parenchyma, and necrosis. Each physiological effect is presented as a percentage of the total degree of dysfunction seen at the end of the reperfusion period (Adapted from Lefer et al. [203] with kind permission from FASEB)

and mechanical adjunctive therapies. In particular, those that can harness or enhance endogenous protective mechanisms that will "recapture" myocardium lost in the reperfusion process itself. Attenuating reperfusion injury has the potential to increase myocardial salvage and perhaps extend the salvage time, as suggested by preclinical studies.

References

1. Okrainec K, Banerjee DK, Eisenberg MJ. Coronary artery disease in the developing world. Am Heart J. 2004;148(1):7–15.
2. Patel B, Kloner RA. Analysis of reported randomized trials of streptokinase therapy for acute myocardial-infarction in the 1980s. Am J Cardiol. 1987;59(6):501–4.
3. Kloner RA, Forman MB, Gibbons RJ, et al. Impact of time to therapy and reperfusion modality on the efficacy of adenosine in acute myocardial infarction: the AMISTAD-2 trial. Eur Heart J. 2006;27(20):2400–5.
4. Anderson JL, Marshall HW, Bray BE, et al. A randomized trial of intracoronary streptokinase in the treatment of acute myocardial infarction. N Engl J Med. 1983;308(22):1312–8.
5. Markis JE, Malagold M, Parker JA, et al. Myocardial salvage after intracoronary thrombolysis with streptokinase in acute myocardial infarction. N Engl J Med. 1981;305(14):777–82.
6. Kennedy JW, Ritchie JL, Davis KB, et al. The western Washington randomized trial of intracoronary streptokinase in acute myocardial infarction. N Engl J Med. 1985;312(17):1073–8.

7. Braunwald E, Kloner RA. The stunned myocardium: prolonged, post-ischemic ventricular dysfunction. Circulation. 1982;66:1146–9.
8. Kim YD, Fomsgaard JS, Heim KF, et al. Brief ischemia-reperfusion induces stunning of endothelium in canine coronary artery. Circulation. 1992;85:1473–82.
9. DeFily DV, Chilian WM. Preconditioning protects coronary arteriolar endothelium from ischemia-reperfusion injury. Am J Physiol. 1993;265:H700–6.
10. Tennant R, Wiggers C. The effect of coronary occlusion on myocardial contraction. Am J Physiol. 1935;112:351–61.
11. Jennings RB, Sommers HM, Smyth GA, et al. Myocardial necrosis induced by temporary occlusion of a coronary artery in the dog. Arch Pathol Lab Med. 1960;70:68–78.
12. Hearse DJ, Humphrey SM, Chain EB. Abrupt reoxygenation of the anoxic potassium-arrested perfused rat heart: a study of myocardial enzyme release. J Mol Cell Cardiol. 1973;5(4): 395–407.
13. Cooley DA, Ruel GJ, Wukasch DC. Ischemic contracture of the heart: "stone heart". Am J Cardiol. 1972;29:575–7.
14. Gross GJ, Auchampach JA. Reperfusion injury: does it exist? J Mol Cell Cardiol. 2007; 42(1):12–8.
15. Zhao ZQ, Corvera JS, Halkos ME, et al. Inhibition of myocardial injury by ischemic postconditioning during reperfusion: comparison with ischemic preconditioning. Am J Physiol Heart Circ Physiol. 2003;285(2):H579–88.
16. Staat P, Rioufol G, Piot C, et al. Postconditioning the human heart. Circulation. 2005;112: 2143–8.
17. Jordan JE, Zhao ZQ, Sato H, et al. Adenosine A2 receptor activation attenuates reperfusion injury by inhibiting neutrophil accumulation, superoxide generation and coronary endothelial adherence. J Pharmacol Exp Ther. 1997;280(1):301–9.
18. Budde JM, Velez DA, Zhao Z, et al. Comparative study of AMP579 and adenosine in inhibition of neutrophil-mediated vascular and myocardial injury during 24 h of reperfusion. Cardiovasc Res. 2000;47(2):294–305.
19. Gomez L, Thibault H, Gharib A, et al. Inhibition of mitochondrial permeability transition improves functional recovery and reduces mortality following acute myocardial infarction in mice. Am J Physiol Heart Circ Physiol. 2007;293(3):H1654–61.
20. Piot C, Croisille P, Staat P, et al. Effect of cyclosporine on reperfusion injury in acute myocardial infarction. N Engl J Med. 2008;359(5):473–81.
21. Vinten-Johansen J, Rosenkranz ER, Buckberg GD, et al. Metabolic and histochemical benefits of regional blood cardioplegic reperfusion without cardiopulmonary bypass. J Thorac Cardiovasc Surg. 1986;92(3 Pt 2):535–42.
22. Yellon DM, Hausenloy DJ. Myocardial reperfusion injury. N Engl J Med. 2007;357(11): 1121–35.
23. Buckberg GD. Studies of controlled reperfusion after ischemia: I. when is cardiac muscle damaged irreversibly? J Thorac Cardiovasc Surg. 1986;92:483–7.
24. Buckberg GD. Myocardial protection: an overview. Semin Thorac Cardiovasc Surg. 1993;5:98–106.
25. Schlack W, Uebing A, Schafer M, et al. Regional contractile blockade at the onset of reperfusion reduces infarct size in the dog heart. Pflugers Archiv – Eur J Physiol. 1994;428: 134–41.
26. Piper HM, Kasseckert S, Abdallah Y. The sarcoplasmic reticulum as the primary target of reperfusion protection. Cardiovasc Res. 2006;70(2):170–3.
27. Ruiz-Meana M, Garcia-Dorado D. Translational cardiovascular medicine (II). Pathophysiology of ischemia-reperfusion injury: new therapeutic options for acute myocardial infarction. Rev Esp Cardiol. 2009;62(2):199–209.
28. Zhao ZQ, Morris CD, Budde JM, et al. Inhibition of myocardial apoptosis reduces infarct size and improves regional contractile dysfunction during reperfusion. Cardiovasc Res. 2003;59:132–42.

29. Zhao ZQ, Velez DA, Wang NP, et al. Progressively developed myocardial apoptotic cell death during late phase of reperfusion. Apoptosis. 2001;6(4):279–90.
30. Freude B, Masters TN, Robicsek F, et al. Apoptosis is initiated by myocardial ischemia and executed during reperfusion. J Mol Cell Cardiol. 2000;32(2):197–208.
31. Zhao ZQ, Morris CD, Budde JM, Wang NP, Muraki S, Sun HY, Guyton RA. Inhibition of myocardial apoptosis reduces infarct size and improves regional contractile dysfunction during reperfusion. Cardiovasc Res. 2003;59:132–142.
32. Reimer KA, Lowe JE, Rasmussen MM, et al. The wavefront phenomenon of ischemic cell death. 1. Myocardial infarct size vs duration of coronary occlusion in dogs. Circulation. 1977;56(5):786–94.
33. Reimer KA, Jennings RB. The "wavefront phenomenon" of myocardial ischemic cell death. II. Transmural progression of necrosis within the framework of ischemic bed size (myocardial at risk) and collateral flow. Lab Invest. 1979;40(6):633–44.
34. Backstrom T, Lockowandt U, Liska J, et al. Monitoring of porcine myocardial ischemia and reperfusion by intravasal microdialysis. Scand Cardiovasc J. 2002;36(1):27–34.
35. Klein HH, Schubothe M, Nebendahl K, et al. Temporal and spatial development of myocardial infarcts in porcine hearts without significant collateral blood flow. Tex Heart Inst J. 1984; 11(2):154–9.
36. Ganz W, Watanabe I, Kanamasa K, et al. Does reperfusion extend necrosis? A study in a single territory of myocardial ischemia: half reperfused and half not reperfused. Circulation. 1990;82: 1020–33.
37. Miura T. Does reperfusion induce myocardial necrosis? Circulation. 1990;82:1070–2.
38. Przyklenk K. Lethal myocardial "reperfusion injury": the opinions of good men. J Thromb Thrombolysis. 1997;4:5–6.
39. Vinten-Johansen J, Johnston WE, Mills SA, et al. Reperfusion injury after temporary coronary occlusion. J Thorac Cardiovasc Surg. 1988;95(6):960–8.
40. Van den Hoek TL, Shao Z, Li C, et al. Reperfusion injury on cardiac myocytes after simulated ischemia. Am J Physiol. 1996;270(4 Pt 2):H1334–41.
41. Matsumura K, Jeremy RW, Schaper J, et al. Progression of myocardial necrosis during reperfusion of ischemic myocardium. Circulation. 1998;97(795):804.
42. Zhao ZQ, Nakamura M, Wang NP, et al. Dynamic progression of contractile and endothelial dysfunction and infarct extension in the late phase of reperfusion. J Surg Res. 2000; 94(2):133–44.
43. Fliss H, Gattinger D. Apoptosis in ischemic and reperfused rat myocardium. Circ Res. 1996; 79:949–56.
44. Zhao ZQ, Nakamura M, Wang NP, et al. Reperfusion induces myocardial apoptotic cell death. Cardiovasc Res. 2000;45(3):651–60.
45. Kin H, Zhao ZQ, Sun HY, et al. Postconditioning attenuates myocardial ischemia-reperfusion injury by inhibiting events in the early minutes of reperfusion. Cardiovasc Res. 2004; 62(1):74–85.
46. Darling CE, Jiang R, Maynard M, et al. Postconditioning via stuttering reperfusion limits myocardial infarct size in rabbit hearts: role of ERK1/2. Am J Physiol Heart Circ Physiol. 2005;289(4):H1618–26.
47. Krug A, Du Mesnil de Rochemont Du, Korb G. Blood supply of the myocardium after temporary coronary occlusion. Circ Res. 1966;19(1):57–62.
48. Ames 3rd A, Wright RL, Kowada M, et al. Cerebral ischemia. II. The no-reflow phenomenon. Am J Pathol. 1968;52(2):437–53.
49. Kloner RA, Ganote CE, Jennings RB. The "no-reflow" phenomenon after temporary coronary occlusion in the dog. J Clin Invest. 1974;54:1496–508.
50. Dillon WC, Hadian D, Ritchie ME. Refractory no-reflow successfully treated with local infusion of high-dose adenosine and verapamil – a case report. Angiology. 2001;52(2):137–41.
51. Jaffe R, Charron T, Puley G, et al. Microvascular obstruction and the no-reflow phenomenon after percutaneous coronary intervention. Circulation. 2008;117(24):3152–6.

52. Reffelmann T, Kloner RA. The no-reflow phenomenon: a basic mechanism of myocardial ischemia and reperfusion. Basic Res Cardiol. 2006;101(5):359–72.
53. Abbo KM, Dooris M, Glazier S, et al. Features and outcome of no-reflow after percutaneous coronary intervention. Am J Cardiol. 1995;75(12):778–82.
54. Morishima I, Sone T, Okumura K, et al. Angiographic no-reflow phenomenon as a predictor of adverse long-term outcome in patients treated with percutaneous transluminal coronary angioplasty for first acute myocardial infarction. J Am Coll Cardiol. 2000;36(4):1202–9.
55. Zweier JL, Kuppusamy P, Lutty GA. Measurement of endothelial cell free radical generation: evidence for a central mechanism of free radical injury in postischemic tissues. Proc Natl Acad Sci USA. 1988;85(11):4046–50.
56. Zweier JL, Broderick R, Kuppusamy P, et al. Determination of the mechanism of free radical generation in human aortic endothelial cells exposed to anoxia and reoxygenation. J Biol Chem. 1994;269(39):24156–62.
57. Berry CE, Hare JM. Xanthine oxidoreductase and cardiovascular disease: molecular mechanisms and pathophysiological implications. J Physiol. 2004;555(Pt 3):589–606.
58. Xia Y, Dawson VL, Dawson TM, et al. Nitric oxide synthase generates superoxide and nitric oxide in arginine-depleted cells leading to peroxynitrite-mediated cellular injury. Proc Natl Acad Sci USA. 1996;93(13):6770–4.
59. Ytrehus K, Myklebust R, Mjos OD. Influence of oxygen radicals generated by xanthine oxidase in the isolated perfused rat heart. Cardiovasc Res. 1986;20(8):597–603.
60. Corretti MC, Koretsune Y, Kusuoka H, et al. Glycolytic inhibition and calcium overload as consequences of exogenously generated free radicals in rabbit hearts. J Clin Invest. 1991;88(3): 1014–25.
61. Lucas SK, Gardner TJ, Flaherty JT, et al. Beneficial effects of mannitol administration during reperfusion after ischemic arrest. Circulation. 1980;62:I-34–41.
62. Stewart JR, Blackwell WH, Crute SL, et al. Inhibition of surgically induced ischemia/reperfusion injury by oxygen free radical scavengers. J Thorac Cardiovasc Surg. 1983;86(2): 262–72.
63. Jolly SR, Kane WJ, Bailie MB, et al. Canine myocardial reperfusion injury: its reduction by the combined administration of superoxide dismutase and catalase. Circ Res. 1984;54: 277–85.
64. Mitsos SE, Fantone JC, Gallagher KP, et al. Canine myocardial reperfusion injury: protection by a free radical scavenger, N-2-Mercaptopropionyl glycine. J Cardiovasc Pharmacol. 1986;8: 978–88.
65. Ambrosio G, Flaherty JT, Duilio C, et al. Oxygen radicals generated at reflow induce peroxidation of membrane lipids in reperfused hearts. J Clin Invest. 1991;87(6):2056–66.
66. Zweier JL, Flaherty JT, Weisfeldt ML. Direct measurement of free radical generation following reperfusion of ischemic myocardium. Proc Natl Acad Sci USA. 1987;84(5):1404–7.
67. Grill HP, Zweier JL, Kuppusamy P, et al. Direct measurement of myocardial free radical generation in an in vivo model: effects of postischemic reperfusion and treatment with human recombinant superoxide dismutase. J Am Coll Cardiol. 1992;20:1604–11.
68. Ferrari R, Alfieri O, Curello S, et al. Occurrence of oxidative stress during reperfusion of the human heart. Circulation. 1990;81(1):201–11.
69. Serrano Jr CV, Mikhail EA, Wang P, et al. Superoxide and hydrogen peroxide induce CD18-mediated adhesion in the postischemic heart. Biochim Biophys Acta. 1996;1316(3): 191–202.
70. Ma XL, Tsao PS, Viehman GE, et al. Neutrophil-mediated vasoconstriction and endothelial dysfunction in low-flow perfusion-reperfused cat coronary artery. Circ Res. 1991;69: 95–106.
71. Ma XL, Weyrich AS, Lefer DJ, et al. Diminished basal nitric oxide release after myocardial ischemia and reperfusion promotes neutrophil adherence to coronary endothelium. Circ Res. 1993;72(2):403–12.
72. Johnson III G, Tsao PS, Lefer AM. Cardioprotective effects of authentic nitric oxide in myocardial ischemia with reperfusion. Crit Care Med. 1991;19:244–52.

73. Jones SP, Girod WG, Palazzo AJ, et al. Myocardial ischemia-reperfusion injury is exacerbated in absence of endothelial cell nitric oxide synthase. Am J Physiol. 1999;276(5 Pt 2): H1567–73.
74. Williams MW, Taft CS, Ramnauth S, et al. Endogenous nitric oxide (NO) protects against ischaemia-reperfusion injury in the rabbit. Cardiovasc Res. 1995;30(1):79–86.
75. Nakanishi K, Vinten-Johansen J, Lefer DJ, et al. Intracoronary L-arginine during reperfusion improves endothelial function and reduces infarct size. Am J Physiol. 1992;263(6 Pt 2): H1650–8.
76. Pernow J, Uriuda Y, Wang QD, et al. The protective effect of L-arginine on myocardial injury and endothelial function following ischaemia and reperfusion in the pig. Eur Heart J. 1994; 15:1712–9.
77. Lefer AM. Attenuation of myocardial ischemia-reperfusion injury with nitric oxide replacement therapy (Review). Ann Thorac Surg. 1995;60:847–51.
78. Draper NJ, Shah AM. Beneficial effects of a nitric oxide donor on recovery of contractile function following brief hypoxia in isolated rat heart. J Mol Cell Cardiol. 1997;29:1195–203.
79. Shen AC, Jennings RB. Kinetics of calcium accumulation in acute myocardial ischemic injury. Am J Pathol. 1972;67:441–52.
80. Inserte J, Garcia-Dorado D, Hernando V, et al. Calpain-mediated impairment of Na^+/K^+ – ATPase activity during early reperfusion contributes to cell death after myocardial ischemia. Circ Res. 2005;97(5):465–73.
81. Klein HH, Pich S, Lindert S, et al. Treatment of reperfusion injury with intracoronary calcium channel antagonists and reduced coronary free calcium concentration in regionally ischemic, reperfused porcine hearts. J Am Coll Cardiol. 1989;13(6):1395–401.
82. Nakanishi K, Lefer DJ, Johnston WE, et al. Transient hypocalcemia during the initial phase of reperfusion extends myocardial necrosis after 2 hours of coronary occlusion. Coron Artery Dis. 1991;2:1009–21.
83. Satoh N, Kitada Y. Cardioprotective effect of MCC-135 is associated with inhibition of Ca^{2+} overload in ischemic/reperfused hearts. Eur J Pharmacol. 2004;499(1–2):179–87.
84. Gumina RJ, Mizumura T, Beier N, et al. A new sodium/hydrogen exchange inhibitor, EMD 85131, limits infarct size in dogs when administered before or after coronary artery occlusion. J Pharmacol Exp Ther. 1998;286(1):175–83.
85. Klein HH, Pich S, Bohle RM, et al. Myocardial protection by Na^+–H^+ exchange inhibition in ischemic, reperfused porcine hearts. Circulation. 1995;92:912–7.
86. Theroux P, Chaitman BR, Danchin D, et al. Inhibition of the sodium-hydrogen exchanger with cariporide to prevent myocardial infarction in high-risk ischemic situations. Circulation. 2000;102:3032–8.
87. Zeymer U, Suryapranata H, Monassier JP, et al. The Na^+/H^+ exchange inhibitor eniporide as an adjunct to early reperfusion therapy for acute myocardial infarction – results of the evaluation of the safety and cardioprotective effects of eniporide in acute myocardial infarction (ESCAMI) trial. J Am Coll Cardiol. 2001;38(6):1644–50.
88. Jang IK, Weissman NJ, Picard MH, et al. A randomized, double-blind, placebo-controlled study of the safety and efficacy of intravenous MCC-135 as an adjunct to primary percutaneous coronary intervention in patients with acute myocardial infarction: evaluation of MCC-135 for left ventricular salvage in acute myocardial infarction (EVOLVE). Am Heart J. 2008; 155(1):113.e1–e8.
89. Cohen MV, Yang XM, Downey JM. The pH hypothesis of postconditioning: staccato reperfusion reintroduces oxygen and perpetuates myocardial acidosis. Circulation. 2007;115(14):1895–903.
90. Inserte J, Barba I, Hernando V, et al. Delayed recovery of intracellular acidosis during reperfusion prevents calpain activation and determines protection in postconditioned myocardium. Cardiovasc Res. 2009;81(1):116–22.
91. Vinten-Johansen J, Zhao ZQ, Jiang R, et al. Preconditioning and postconditioning: innate cardioprotection from ischemia-reperfusion injury. J Appl Physiol. 2007;103(4):1441–8.
92. Vinten-Johansen J, Lefer DJ, Nakanishi K, et al. Controlled coronary hydrodynamics at the time of reperfusion reduces postischemic injury. Coron Artery Dis. 1992;3:1081–93.

93. Sato H, Jordan JE, Zhao ZQ, et al. Gradual reperfusion reduces infarct size and endothelial injury but augments neutrophil accumulation. Ann Thorac Surg. 1997;64(4):1099–107.
94. Musiolik J, van Caster P, Skyschally A, et al. Reduction of infarct size by gentle reperfusion without activation of reperfusion injury salvage kinases in pigs. Cardiovasc Res. 2010;85: 110–7.
95. Okamoto F, Allen BS, Buckberg GD, et al. Studies of controlled reperfusion after ischemia. XIV. Reperfusion conditions: importance of ensuring gentle versus sudden reperfusion during relief of coronary occlusion. J Thorac Cardiovasc Surg. 1986;92:613–20.
96. Barrabes JA, Garcia-Dorado D, Ruiz-Meana M, et al. Myocardial segment shrinkage during coronary reperfusion in situ. Relation to hypercontracture and myocardial necrosis. Pflugers Arch. 1996;431(4):519–26.
97. Inserte J, Garcia-Dorado D, Ruiz-Meana M, et al. Ischemic preconditioning attenuates calpain-mediated degradation of structural proteins through a protein kinase A-dependent mechanism. Cardiovasc Res. 2004;64(1):105–14.
98. Ruiz-Meana M, Garcia-Dorado D, Hofstaetter B, et al. Propagation of cardiomyocyte hypercontracture by passage of Na(+) through gap junctions. Circ Res. 1999;85(3):280–7.
99. Garcia-Dorado D, Gonzalez MA, Barrabes JA, et al. Prevention of ischemic rigor contracture during coronary occlusion by inhibition of Na^+–H^+ exchange. Cardiovasc Res. 1997;35: 80–9.
100. Inserte J, Garcia-Dorado D, Ruiz-Meana M, et al. Effect of inhibition of Na^+/Ca^{2+} exchanger at the time of myocardial reperfusion on hypercontracture and cell death. Cardiovasc Res. 2002;55:739–48.
101. Garcia-Dorado D, Theroux P, Duran JM, et al. Selective inhibition of the contractile apparatus. A new approach to modification of infarct size, infarct composition, and infarct geometry during coronary artery occlusion and reperfusion. Circulation. 1992;85:1160–74.
102. Siegmund B, Klietz T, Schwartz P, et al. Temporary contractile blockade prevents hypercontracture in anoxic-reoxygenated cardiomyocytes. Am J Physiol. 1991;260(2 Pt 2):H426–35.
103. Sebbag L, Verbinski SG, Reimer KA, et al. Protection of ischemic myocardium in dogs using intracoronary 2,3-butanedione monoxime (BDM). J Mol Cell Cardiol. 2003; 35(2):165–76.
104. Ladilov Y, Efe O, Schafer C, et al. Reoxygenation-induced rigor-type contracture. J Mol Cell Cardiol. 2003;35(12):1481–90.
105. Kaiser L, Sparks Jr HV. Endothelial cells: not just a cellophane wrapper. Arch Intern Med. 1987;147:569–73.
106. Galley HF, Webster NR. Physiology of the endothelium. Br J Anaesth. 2004;93(1):105–13.
107. Ku DD. Coronary vascular reactivity after acute myocardial ischemia. Science. 1982;218:576–8.
108. Dignan RJ, Kadletz M, Dyke CM, et al. Microvascular dysfunction after myocardial ischemia. J Thorac Cardiovasc Surg. 1995;109(5):892–7.
109. Dignan RJ, Dyke CM, Abd-Elfattah AS, et al. Coronary artery endothelial cell and smooth muscle dysfunction after global myocardial ischemia. Ann Thorac Surg. 1992;53:311–7.
110. Pearson PJ, Schaff HV, Vanhoutte PM. Acute impairment of endothelium-dependent relaxations to aggregating platelets following reperfusion injury in canine coronary arteries. Circ Res. 1990;67(2):385–93.
111. Pearson PJ, Schaff HV, Vanhoutte PM. Long-term impairment of endothelium-dependent relaxations to aggregating platelets after reperfusion injury in canine coronary arteries. Circulation. 1990;81(6):1921–7.
112. Sobey CG, Dusting GJ, Grossman HJ, et al. Impaired vasodilation of epicardial coronary arteries and resistance vessels following myocardial ischemia and reperfusion in anesthetized dogs. Coron Artery Dis. 1990;1:363–74.
113. Boyle EM, Pohlman TH, Cornejo CJ, et al. Endothelial cell injury in cardiovascular surgery: ischemia-reperfusion. Ann Thorac Surg. 1996;62:1868–75.

114. Boyle EM, Verrier ED, Spiess BD. Endothelial cell injury in cardiovascular surgery: the procoagulant response. Ann Thorac Surg. 1996;62:1549–57.
115. Sellke FW, Boyle EM, Verrier ED. Endothelial cell injury in cardiovascular surgery: the pathophysiology of vasomotor dysfunction. Ann Thorac Surg. 1996;62:1222–8.
116. Verrier E. The microvascular cell and ischemia-reperfusion injury. J Cardiovasc Pharmacol. 1996;27 suppl 1:S26–30.
117. Boyle EM, Pohlman TH, Johnson MC, et al. Endothelial cell injury in cardiovascular surgery: the systemic inflammatory response. Ann Thorac Surg. 1997;63:277–84.
118. Lacerda L, Somers S, Opie LH, et al. Ischaemic postconditioning protects against reperfusion injury via the SAFE pathway. Cardiovasc Res. 2009;84(2):201–8.
119. Tsao PS, Aoki N, Lefer DJ, et al. Time course of endothelial dysfunction and myocardial injury during myocardial ischemia and reperfusion in the cat. Circulation. 1990;82:1402–12.
120. Kaeffer N, Richard V, Francois A, et al. Preconditioning prevents chronic reperfusion-induced coronary endothelial dysfunction in rats. Am J Physiol. 1996;271:H842–9.
121. Scarabelli T, Stephanou A, Rayment N, et al. Apoptosis of endothelial cells precedes myocyte cell apoptosis in ischemia/reperfusion injury. Circulation. 2001;104(3):253–6.
122. Weyrich AS, Buerke M, Albertine KH, et al. Time course of coronary vascular endothelial adhesion molecule expression during reperfusion of the ischemic feline myocardium. J Leukoc Biol. 1995;57:45–55.
123. Chatelain P, Latour JG, Tran D, et al. Neutrophil accumulation in experimental myocardial infarcts: relation with extent of injury and effect of reperfusion. Circulation. 1987;75(5):1083–90.
124. Sheridan FM, Cole PG, Ramage D. Leukocyte adhesion to the coronary microvasculature during ischemia and reperfusion in an in vivo canine model. Circulation. 1996;93(10):1784–7.
125. Shandelya SM, Kuppusamy P, Weisfeldt ML, et al. Evaluation of the role of polymorphonuclear leukocytes on contractile function in myocardial reperfusion injury. Evidence for plasma-mediated leukocyte activation. Circulation. 1993;87:536–46.
126. Shandelya SM, Kuppusamy P, Herskowitz A, et al. Soluble complement receptor type 1 inhibits the complement pathway and prevents contractile failure in the postischemic heart. Evidence that complement activation is required for neutrophil-mediated reperfusion injury. Circulation. 1993;88:2812–26.
127. Vinten-Johansen J. Involvement of neutrophils in the pathogenesis of lethal myocardial reperfusion injury. Cardiovasc Res. 2004;61(3):481–97.
128. Botto N, Sbrana S, Trianni G, et al. An increased platelet-leukocytes interaction at the culprit site of coronary artery occlusion in acute myocardial infarction: a pathogenic role for "no-reflow" phenomenon? Int J Cardiol. 2007;117(1):123–30.
129. Siminiak T, Egdell RM, O'Gorman DJ, et al. Plasma-mediated neutrophil activation during acute myocardial infarction: role of platelet-activating factor. Clin Sci (Lond). 1995;89(2):171–6.
130. Siminiak T, Zozulinska D, Zeromska M, et al. Evidence for plasma-mediated neutrophil superoxide anion production during myocardial infarction. Cardiology. 1993;82(6):377–82.
131. Chang LT, Chua S, Sheu JJ, et al. Level and prognostic value of serum myeloperoxidase in patients with acute myocardial infarction undergoing primary percutaneous coronary intervention. Circ J. 2009;73(4):726–31.
132. Dinerman JL, Mehta JL, Saldeen TGP, et al. Increased neutrophil elastase release in unstable angina pectoris and acute myocardial infarction. J Am Coll Cardiol. 1990;15(7):1559–63.
133. Bell D, Jackson M, Millar AM, et al. The acute inflammatory response to myocardial infarction: imaging with indium-111 labelled autologous neutrophils. Br Heart J. 1987;57(1):23–7.
134. Jaremo P, Nilsson O. Interleukin-6 and neutrophils are associated with long-term survival after acute myocardial infarction. Eur J Intern Med. 2008;19(5):330–3.

135. Granfeldt A, Jiang R, Wang NP, et al. Inhibition of neutrophils is critical to the in vivo cardioprotection of postconditioning. Circulation. 2008;118(18 Meeting Abstracts):S292.
136. Jolly SR, Kane WJ, Hook BG, et al. Reduction of myocardial infarct size by neutrophil depletion: effect of duration of occlusion. Am Heart J. 1986;112(4):682–90.
137. Romson JL, Hook BG, Kunkel SL, et al. Reduction of the extent of ischemic myocardial injury by neutrophil depletion in the dog. Circulation. 1983;67(5):1016–23.
138. De Lorgeril M, Basmadjian A, Lavallee M, et al. Influence of leukopenia on collateral flow, reperfusion flow, reflow ventricular fibrillation, and infarct size in dogs. Am Heart J. 1989; 117(3):523–32.
139. Litt MR, Jeremy RW, Weisman HF, et al. Neutrophil depletion limited to reperfusion reduces myocardial infarct size after 90 minutes of ischemia: evidence for neutrophil-mediated reperfusion injury. Circulation. 1989;80:1816–27.
140. Lefer DJ, Flynn DM, Buda AJ. Effects of a monoclonal antibody directed against P-selectin after myocardial ischemia and reperfusion. Am J Physiol. 1996;270(1 Pt 2):H88–98.
141. Weyrich AS, Ma XY, Lefer DJ, et al. In vivo neutralization of P-selectin protects feline heart and endothelium in myocardial ischemia and reperfusion injury. J Clin Invest. 1993;91(6):2620–9.
142. Palazzo AJ, Jones SP, Girod WG, et al. Myocardial ischemia-reperfusion injury in CD18- and ICAM-1-deficient mice. Am J Physiol. 1998;275(6 Pt 2):H2300–7.
143. Zhao ZQ, Lefer DJ, Sato H, et al. Monoclonal antibody to ICAM-1 preserves postischemic blood flow and reduces infarct size after ischemia-reperfusion in rabbit. J Leukoc Biol. 1997;62(3):292–300.
144. Palazzo AJ, Jones SP, Anderson DC, et al. Coronary endothelial P-selectin in pathogenesis of myocardial ischemia-reperfusion injury. Am J Physiol. 1998;275(5 Pt 2):H1865–72.
145. Briaud SA, Ding ZM, Michael LH, et al. Leukocyte trafficking and myocardial reperfusion injury in ICAM-1/P-selectin-knockout mice. Am J Physiol Heart Circ Physiol. 2001;280(1): H60–7.
146. Arai M, Masui Y, Goldschmidt-Clermont P, et al. P-selectin inhibition prevents early neutrophil activation but provides only modest protection against myocardial injury in dogs with ischemia and forty-eight hours reperfusion. J Am Coll Cardiol. 1999;34(1):280–8.
147. Jones SP, Girod WG, Granger DN, et al. Reperfusion injury is not affected by blockade of P-selectin in the diabetic mouse heart. Am J Physiol. 1999;277(2 Pt 2):H763–9.
148. Tanaka M, Brooks SE, Richard VJ, et al. Effect of anti-CD18 antibody on myocardial neutrophil accumulation and infarct size after ischemia and reperfusion in dogs. Circulation. 1993; 87:526–35.
149. Baxter GF. The neutrophil as a mediator of myocardial ischemia-reperfusion injury: time to move on. Basic Res Cardiol. 2002;97(4):268–75.
150. Lefer DJ. Do neutrophils contribute to myocardial reperfusion injury? Basic Res Cardiol. 2002;97(4):263–7.
151. Harlan JM, Winn RK. Leukocyte-endothelial interactions: clinical trials of anti-adhesion therapy. Crit Care Med. 2002;30(5):S214–9.
152. Baran KW, Nguyen M, McKendall GR, et al. Double-blind, randomized trial of an anti-CD18 antibody in conjunction with recombinant tissue plasminogen activator for acute myocardial infarction. Limitation of myocardial infarction following thrombolysis in acute myocardial infarction (LIMIT AMI) study. Circulation. 2001;104:2778–83.
153. Buerke M, Pruefer D, Dahm M, et al. Serine protease inhibitor (Aprotinin) attenuates myocardial necrosis and apoptosis following ischaemia and long-term reperfusion in rats. Eur Heart J. 1999;20(P996):163.
154. Arslan F, Keogh B, McGuirk P, et al. TLR2 and TLR4 in ischemia reperfusion injury. Mediators Inflamm. 2010;2010:704202.
155. Arslan F, Smeets MB, O'Neill LA, et al. Myocardial ischemia/reperfusion injury is mediated by leukocytic toll-like receptor-2 and reduced by systemic administration of a novel anti-toll-like receptor-2 antibody. Circulation. 2010;121(1):80–90.

156. Zhang C, Xu X, Potter BJ, et al. TNF-alpha contributes to endothelial dysfunction in ischemia/reperfusion injury. Arterioscler Thromb Vasc Biol. 2006;26(3):475–80.
157. Vakeva A, Morgan BP, Tikkanen I, et al. Time course of complement activation and inhibitor expression after ischemic injury of rat myocardium. Am J Pathol. 1994;144:1357–68.
158. Meldrum DR. Tumor necrosis factor in the heart. Am J Physiol. 1998;274(3 Pt 2): R577–95.
159. Di Lisa F, Bernardi P. Mitochondria and ischemia-reperfusion injury of the heart: fixing a hole. Cardiovasc Res. 2006;70(2):191–9.
160. Griffiths EJ, Halestrap AP. Mitochondrial non-specific pores remain closed during cardiac ischaemia, but open upon reperfusion. Biochem J. 1995;307:93–8.
161. Griffiths EJ, Halestrap AP. Protection by Cyclosporin A of ischemia/reperfusion-induced damage in isolated rat hearts. J Mol Cell Cardiol. 1993;25:1461–9.
162. Halestrap AP, Kerr PM, Javadov S, et al. Elucidating the molecular mechanism of the permeability transition pore and its role in reperfusion injury of the heart. Biochim Biophys Acta. 1998;1366(1–2):79–94.
163. Argaud L, Gateau-Roesch O, Muntean D, et al. Specific inhibition of the mitochondrial permeability transition prevents lethal reperfusion injury. J Mol Cell Cardiol. 2005;38(2): 367–74.
164. Ge ZD, Pravdic D, Bienengraeber M, et al. Isoflurane postconditioning protects against reperfusion injury by preventing mitochondrial permeability transition by an endothelial nitric oxide synthase-dependent mechanism. Anesthesiology. 2010;112(1):73–85.
165. Yao Y, Li L, Gao C, et al. Sevoflurane postconditioning protects chronically-infarcted rat hearts against ischemia-reperfusion injury by activation of pro-survival kinases and inhibition of mitochondrial permeability transition pore opening upon reperfusion. Biol Pharm Bull. 2009;32(11):1854–61.
166. Hausenloy DJ, Yellon DM, Mani-Babu S, et al. Preconditioning protects by inhibiting the mitochondrial permeability transition. Am J Physiol Heart Circ Physiol. 2004;287(2):H841–9.
167. Argaud L, Gateau-Roesch O, Raisky O, et al. Post-conditioning inhibits mitochondrial permeability transition. Circulation. 2005;111:194–7.
168. Argaud L, Gateau-Roesch O, Augeul L, et al. Increased mitochondrial calcium coexists with decreased reperfusion injury in postconditioned (but not preconditioned) hearts. Am J Physiol Heart Circ Physiol. 2008;294(1):H386–91.
169. Hausenloy DJ, Tsang A, Yellon DM. The reperfusion injury salvage kinase pathway: a common target for both ischemic preconditioning and postconditioning. Trends Cardiovasc Med. 2005;15(2):69–75.
170. Schulman D, Latchman DS, Yellon DM. Urocortin protects the heart from reperfusion injury via upregulation of p42/p44 MAPK signaling pathway. Am J Physiol Heart Circ Physiol. 2002;283(4):H1481–8.
171. Zhao ZQ, McGee S, Nakanishi K, et al. Receptor-mediated cardioprotective effects of endogenous adenosine are exerted primarily during reperfusion after coronary occlusion in the rabbit. Circulation. 1993;88(2):709–19.
172. Gross ER, Gross GJ. Ligand triggers of classical preconditioning and postconditioning. Cardiovasc Res. 2006;70(2):212–21.
173. Kin H, Zatta AJ, Lofye MT, et al. Postconditioning reduces infarct size via adenosine receptor activation by endogenous adenosine. Cardiovasc Res. 2005;67(1):124–33.
174. Zatta AJ, Kin H, Yoshishige D, et al. Evidence that cardioprotection by postconditioning involves preservation of myocardial opioid content and selective opioid receptor activation. Am J Physiol Heart Circ Physiol. 2008;294:H1444–51.
175. Marzilli M, Orsini E, Marraccini P, et al. Beneficial effects of intracoronary adenosine as an adjunct to primary angioplasty in acute myocardial infarction. Circulation. 2000;101(18): 2154–9.

176. Assali AR, Sdringola S, Ghani M, et al. Intracoronary adenosine administered during percutaneous intervention in acute myocardial infarction and reduction in the incidence of "no reflow" phenomenon. Catheter Cardiovasc Interv. 2000;51(1):27–31.
177. Yellon DM, Baxter GF. Reperfusion injury revisited: is there a role for growth factor signaling in limiting lethal reperfusion injury? Trends Cardiovasc Med. 1999;9(8):245–9.
178. Hausenloy DJ, Mocanu MM, Yellon DM. Ischemic preconditioning protects by activating pro-survival kinases at reperfusion. Am J Physiol Heart Circ Physiol. 2005;288:H971–6.
179. Yang XM, Proctor JB, Cui L, et al. Multiple, brief coronary occlusions during early reperfusion protect rabbit hearts by targeting cell signaling pathways. J Am Coll Cardiol. 2004; 44(5):1103–10.
180. Ovize M, Baxter GF, Di Lisa F, et al. Postconditioning and protection from reperfusion injury: where do we stand? Position paper from the Working Group of Cellular Biology of the Heart of the European Society of Cardiology. Cardiovasc Res. 2010;87(3):406–23.
181. Xin P, Zhu W, Li J, et al. Combined local ischemic postconditioning and remote preconditioning recapitulate the cardioprotective effects of local ischemic preconditioning. Am J Physiol Heart Circ Physiol. 2010;298:H1819–31.
182. Sivaraman V, Mudalagiri NR, Di Salvo C, et al. Postconditioning protects human atrial muscle through the activation of the RISK pathway. Basic Res Cardiol. 2007;102(5):453–9.
183. Davidson SM, Hausenloy D, Duchen MR, et al. Signalling via the reperfusion injury signalling kinase (RISK) pathway links closure of the mitochondrial permeability transition pore to cardioprotection. Int J Biochem Cell Biol. 2006;38(3):414–9.
184. Abdallah Y, Gkatzoflia A, Gligorievski D, et al. Insulin protects cardiomyocytes against reoxygenation-induced hypercontracture by a survival pathway targeting SR Ca^{2+} storage. Cardiovasc Res. 2006;70(2):346–53.
185. Vessey DA, Li L, Honbo N, et al. Sphingosine 1-phosphate is an important endogenous cardioprotectant released by ischemic pre- and postconditioning. Am J Physiol Heart Circ Physiol. 2009;297(4):H1429–35.
186. Boengler K, Konietzka I, Buechert A, et al. Loss of ischemic preconditioning's cardioprotection in aged mouse hearts is associated with reduced gap junctional and mitochondrial levels of connexin 43. Am J Physiol Heart Circ Physiol. 2007;292(4):H1764–9.
187. Willems L, Zatta A, Holmgren K, et al. Age-related changes in ischemic tolerance in male and female mouse hearts. J Mol Cell Cardiol. 2005;38(2):245–56.
188. O'Brien JD, Ferguson JH, Howlett SE. Effects of ischemia and reperfusion on isolated ventricular myocytes from young adult and aged Fischer 344 rat hearts. Am J Physiol Heart Circ Physiol. 2008;294(5):H2174–83.
189. Mariani J, Ou R, Bailey M, et al. Tolerance to ischemia and hypoxia is reduced in aged human myocardium. J Thorac Cardiovasc Surg. 2000;120(4):660–7.
190. Harman D. Free radical theory of aging: an update: increasing the functional life span. Ann N Y Acad Sci. 2006;1067:10–21.
191. Boucher F, Tanguy S, Besse S, et al. Age-dependent changes in myocardial susceptibility to zero flow ischemia and reperfusion in isolated perfused rat hearts: relation to antioxidant status. Mech Ageing Dev. 1998;103(3):301–16.
192. Amrani M, Goodwin AT, Gray CC, et al. Ageing is associated with reduced basal and stimulated release of nitric oxide by the coronary endothelium. Acta Physiol Scand. 1996;157(1): 79–84.
193. Willems L, Ashton KJ, Headrick JP. Adenosine-mediated cardioprotection in the aging myocardium. Cardiovasc Res. 2005;66(2):245–55.
194. Houterman S, Verschuren WM, Hofman A, et al. Serum cholesterol is a risk factor for myocardial infarction in elderly men and women: the Rotterdam Study. J Intern Med. 1999;246(1): 25–33.
195. De Luca G, Gibson CM, Bellandi F, et al. Diabetes mellitus is associated with distal embolization, impaired myocardial perfusion, and higher mortality in patients with ST-segment elevation myocardial infarction treated with primary angioplasty and glycoprotein IIb-IIIa inhibitors. Atherosclerosis. 2009;207:181–5.

196. Abbott RD, Donahue RP, Kannel WB, et al. The impact of diabetes on survival following myocardial infarction in men vs women. The Framingham Study. JAMA. 1988;260(23): 3456–60.
197. Girod WG, Jones SP, Sieber N, et al. Effects of hypercholesterolemia on myocardial ischemia-reperfusion injury in LDL receptor-deficient mice. Arterioscler Thromb Vasc Biol. 1999;19(11):2776–81.
198. Cerwinka WH, Granger DN. Influence of hypercholesterolemia and hypertension on ischemia-reperfusion induced P-selectin expression. Atherosclerosis. 2001;154:337–44.
199. Cooper A, Heagerty AM. Endothelial dysfunction in human intramyocardial small arteries in atherosclerosis and hypercholesterolemia. Am J Physiol. 1998;275(Heart Circ Physiol 44): H1482–8.
200. Dandona P, Aljada A. Advances in diabetes for the millennium: diabetes and the endothelium. MedGenMed. 2004;6(3 Suppl):6.
201. Harrison DG. Endothelial dysfunction in atherosclerosis (Review). Basic Res Cardiol. 1994; 89 Suppl 1:87–102.
202. Tsang A, Hausenloy DJ, Mocanu MM, et al. Preconditioning the diabetic heart: the importance of Akt phosphorylation. Diabetes. 2005;54(8):2360–4.
203. Lefer AM, Tsao PS, Lefer DJ, et al. Role of endothelial dysfunction in the pathogenesis of reperfusion injury after myocardial ischemia. FASEB J. 1991;5(7):2029–34.
204. Bolli R, Becker L, Gross G, et al. Myocardial protection at a crossroads: the need for translation into clinical therapy. Circ Res. 2004;95:125–34.

Chapter 5
Translating Cardioprotective Strategies into Clinical Settings

Nathan Mewton, François Roubille, Olivier Lairez, Gilles Rioufol, Meyer Elbaz, Christophe Piot, and Michel Ovize

Abstract The major objective of the treatment of ST elevation myocardial infarction (STEMI) patients is to reduce infarct size, which is the major prognostic factor in this population. Most of the progress has consisted in improving reperfusion therapy, both by opening as quickly as possible and by preventing reocclusion of the culprit coronary artery. Basic science research used in well-described animal models allowed to clearly establish the major determinants of infarct size, i.e., area at risk, collateral flow, duration of ischemia, and timing of the protective intervention with

N. Mewton, M.D., Ph.D.
Department of Cardiology and Clinical Research, Inserm U 1060 (CARMEN), Lyon, France

Service d'Exploration Fonctionnelles Cardiovasculaires,
Hospices Civils de Lyon, Université Claude Bernard Lyon1, Lyon, France

F. Roubille, M.D., Ph.D. • C. Piot, M.D., Ph.D.
Department of Cardiology, Inserm U661, Montpellier, France

Hopital Arnaud de Villeneuve, Université de Montpellier I and II, Montpellier, France

O. Lairez, M.D., Ph.D. • M. Elbaz, M.D., Ph.D.
Department of Cardiology, Service de Cardiologie, Hôpital Rangueuil,
University Paul Sabatier, Toulouse, France

G. Rioufol, M.D., Ph.D.
Department of Cardiology, Inserm U 1060 (CARMEN), Lyon, France

Interventional Cardiology, Hospices Civils de Lyon, Université Claude Bernard Lyon1,
Lyon, France

M. Ovize, M.D., Ph.D. (✉)
Department of Cardiology and Clinical Research, Inserm U 1060 (CARMEN), Lyon, France

Service d'Exploration Fonctionnelles Cardiovasculaires, Hospices Civils de Lyon,
Université Claude Bernard Lyon1, Lyon, France

Hôpital Louis Pradel, 59 Bd Pinel, 69394 Lyon, France

University of Lyon, Lyon, France
e-mail: michel.ovize@chu-lyon.fr

J.C. Kaski et al. (eds.), *Management of Myocardial Reperfusion Injury*,
DOI 10.1007/978-1-84996-019-9_5, © Springer-Verlag London 2012

respect to reflow. Recent reports have proven that lethal reperfusion injury exists, that it is of significant importance, and that it can be prevented by protective interventions applied immediately before reflow. Therefore, after taking care of the vessel, it is now time to better protect the muscle against lethal reperfusion injury. In spite of several past negative infarct size reduction studies, recent proof-of-concept studies have shown that infarct size reduction is possible in STEMI patients, at least in part because the major determinants of infarct size have been taken into account. Increased understanding of underlying mechanisms from animal models together with encouraging results from phase II infarct size reduction clinical trials should help us improve the design of future studies aimed at reducing infarct size in STEMI patients.

Keywords Ischemia • Reperfusion injury • Stemi • Cardioprotection • Animal models • Proof-of-concept trials

Although major progress has been made, cardiovascular diseases remain a major threat to the health worldwide [1]. The epidemiology of diabetes, obesity, the failure to significantly reduce smoking, specifically in teenagers, the lack of physical exercise, all contribute to the upcoming "global tsunami" of cardiovascular diseases [2]. The decline observed in the incidence of cardiovascular disease in Western countries has been counterbalanced by an alarming epidemic of cardiovascular disease in "emergent countries" [3]. Estimates are that the number one and two causes of death worldwide will remain ischemic heart and cerebrovascular diseases in the next decade.

Many efforts have been made during the last three decades to improve reperfusion therapy, with impressive advances in the treatment of acute coronary syndromes and more specifically reperfusion therapy. Most progress comes from technical and pharmacological innovation which have allowed optimal treatment, in acute clinical settings, both unstable/ruptured atherosclerotic plaque and thrombotic events. In contrast, while experimental results have been very encouraging, little, if any, improvement has been made in protecting the myocardium against ischemia-reperfusion injury in acute coronary syndromes, including ST-segment elevation myocardial infarction (STEMI). We propose to analyze in this chapter some aspects of this issue of the failure to translate protective strategies into clinical practice.

Failure to Translate "Cardioprotective" Strategies

Definition and Scope

The term "cardioprotection" (in the field of ischemia-reperfusion injury, i.e., ischemic cardiomyopathies) should be defined. For basic scientists, it refers to the reduction of myocardial infarct size in most cases. For a clinician, it is less clear and probably corresponds to an intervention that ultimately prevents heart failure. Although there are indisputable links between these two views, practical aspects when coming to design of experimental or clinical trials are somewhat different.

For the sake of clarity, we will consider here that the term "cardioprotection" refers to "any intervention that eventually improves functional recovery of the heart following a prolonged ischemia-reperfusion injury." This (unfortunately) encompasses not only treatments that might reduce infarct size, but also all interventions that attenuate adverse LV remodeling way after the acute phase, including, for example, the well-recognized beneficial effects of ACE inhibitors and statins. In fact, using such a vague definition does not help basic scientists and clinicians to understand each other and to better translate therapeutic advances to the patient. In contrast, "infarct size reduction" is a more precise concept. It does belong to the "cardioprotection" field, since reducing infarct size results in attenuation of adverse remodeling, improvement of functional recovery, and amelioration of outcome, both in experimental preparations and in clinical settings. In this chapter, we will then focus our attention on infarct size reduction studies. Obviously, since STEMI patients are the highest-risk population requiring infarct size reduction, we will further focus our attention on this subset of the acute coronary syndromes.

Negative Infarct Size Reduction Trials

Despite thousands of experimental reports showing a significant infarct size reduction by ischemia- or pharmacological pre- and postconditioning over the last 25 years, there is still a major doubt among clinicians and the pharmaceutical industry regarding the reality and clinical benefit of therapies aimed at reducing infarct size in STEMI patients. Indeed, several large-scale clinical trials have failed to show a significant infarct size reduction with any drug during the past years, even though some of these agents had been convincing in animal models [4–6]. This has been true for antioxidants, Na^+/H^+ exchanger inhibitors, or anti-inflammatory agents, among other types of drugs. For example, although numerous reports had shown that cariporide could significantly reduce infarct size and improve postischemic functional recovery in animal models and encouraging data had been obtained from the Guardian study, the Expedition trial failed to show a significant benefit in 5,761 patients undergoing coronary artery bypass graft surgery; in fact, there was the possibility of harmful effects [7, 8]. The K_{ATP}^+ channel opener nicorandil could reduce infarct size and improve contractile function in most animal models, yet the J-WIND trial failed to show any significant benefit when administered to STEMI patients [5]. Erythropoïetin successfully limited myocardial ischemia-reperfusion injury using in vitro or in vivo experimental preparations but has now been reported as inefficient in several clinical studies (e.g., [9]). Many other examples could be mentioned.

What is wrong with the process of translation to clinical practice? Is it because the experimental models are not relevant and that differences among species play an important role? Is it because the clinical settings of acute myocardial infarction which is a dynamic and evolving process does not fit the animal models with ischemia and abrupt reperfusion? A better understanding of this failure to translate most of these studies requires that we thoroughly analyze the specificities of experimental preparations on one hand and the design of clinical studies on the other.

Current Care of Ischemia-Reperfusion Injury in STEMI Patients

Reperfusion therapy is the first therapeutic objective when treating STEMI patients [10]. This statement arises from the classical concept that the duration of ischemia is a major determinant of infarct size and that the larger the infarct size, the greater the risk of adverse LV remodeling and the worse the clinical outcome [11, 12]. Reduction of infarct size therefore represents the primary goal of the treatment of STEMI patients.

Based on the idea that ischemia is the primary cause of irreversible tissue damage in acute myocardial infarction, major efforts have been made over the last three decades to develop tools and strategies to reopen the occluded culprit coronary artery as quickly as possible. The "time to reperfusion" has been significantly reduced by improving prehospital care (time to onset of chest pain to first medical care and transfer to cardiology center) and hospital admission (door to balloon time) in most STEMI patients. Revascularization techniques (thrombolysis, angioplasty, stenting, thromboaspiration) have dramatically improved over the years to reach a high level of safety and efficacy, allowing optimal reperfusion reperfusion in more than 90% of cases. Several treatments have now been developed and are combined to prevent coronary artery reocclusion acutely and improve plaque stabilization and persistent coronary patency in STEMI patients. As a consequence, several studies have confirmed that reperfusion therapy can limit infarct size and improve functional recovery in humans [1, 13–17]. One can now consider that reperfusion therapy has clearly improved the prognosis of STEMI patients and is very likely close to its optimal efficiency [18].

It is however important to acknowledge that all these efforts made to reduce infarct size in STEMI patients have focused on the coronary vessel patency. Ischemic injury has been carefully looked at, but reperfusion injury has been neglected. Time has come to focus upon cardiac muscle, which largely impacts the patient's prognosis. Indeed, none of the drugs currently recommended for treating STEMI patients during the acute phase targets the jeopardized myocardium. This is in sharp contrast with major steps forward that have been made recently from experimental preparations as well as from phase II clinical trials regarding our understanding of the physiology of lethal ischemia and reperfusion injury. We will review here some aspects of these recent advances that may help to better understand

Table 5.1 Improving "clinical models" for infarct size reduction phase II trials in STEMI patients

Endpoints: infarct size-related events
Determinants of infarct size:
Do not include patients with visible collaterals
Assess area at risk/include patients with large area at risk
Therapeutic window:
Do not include patients with TIMI flow grade > 1 before treatment
Administer study treatment before reperfusion

why we have so far failed to translate infarct size reduction from the experimental to clinical setting Table 5.1.

Considering "Reperfusion Injury" as a Major Component of Infarction

It has recently become clear through animal studies that reperfusion can per se irreversibly damage the previously ischemic myocardium: this has been termed "lethal reperfusion injury." This concept specifically refers to cell death associated with prolonged ischemia that can be prevented by an intervention applied at the time of reperfusion. Therefore, it is the component of cell death occurring as a consequence of reperfusion. The overall irreversible cardiac damage following a period of prolonged ischemia-reperfusion is thus the combination of two different types of insult: first the ischemia- and second the reperfusion-induced damage.

The clear-cut demonstration of the existence of lethal reperfusion injury came from the initial work of Vinten-Johansen's group [19]. Zhao et al. first reported in the dog heart that three episodes of 30 s of reperfusion/30 s of ischemia performed immediately after a prolonged 60-min ischemic insult dramatically attenuated irreversible myocardial injury: they named it "ischemic postconditioning" [19]. Several other investigators have now been able to reproduce this initial experiment and found that ischemic postconditioning is also efficient in the pig, rabbit, rat, and mouse hearts [20–23]. Experimental work has further shown that this infarct size reduction translates into an improved functional recovery and even decreased mortality in the vivo mouse model of acute myocardial infarction [24]. Importantly, the time window to trigger postconditioning protection is very narrow in animal models. In the rat, when the brief episodes of ischemia-reperfusion that trigger postconditioning are delayed by only 1 minute, the protection does not develop. In other words, most of the lethal reperfusion injury is triggered within the first minutes of reflow after a prolonged ischemia [25]. Whether a comparable time course applies to the human heart is currently unknown.

Overall, these important preclinical studies have proven that a large amount of myocardium is destroyed after the reopening of the culprit coronary artery and that this "reperfusion infarct" influences LV remodeling and functional recovery in animal models. In addition, the signaling pathways involved in postconditioning are being better understood, and recent reports suggest that mitochondrial permeability transition pore opening plays a major role in lethal reperfusion injury [26–32]. Recent studies have identified new molecular targets, and pharmacological postconditioning appears to be as efficient as ischemic postconditioning, creating new opportunities for protective therapy in STEMI patients.

Differences Between the Clinical Setting and Animal Models

The physiology of acute myocardial infarction, and then of infarct size reduction therapy, has been described long ago in animal models. Jennings' group and others have clearly established that the size of the infarct caused by a prolonged ischemic insult followed by reperfusion is determined by four critical factors: the duration of ischemia, the size of the area at risk, the amount of collateral circulation to the ischemic territory during coronary artery occlusion, and the timing of treatment administration with respect to reperfusion. Another factor has to be taken into account, specifically when it comes to clinical trials, i.e., the primary endpoint.

To understand why extrapolation from animal models to clinical settings of STEMI often failed, one might take the major common characteristics of all animal models of acute myocardial infarction and analyze how these correspond to the clinical setting of STEMI Table 5.1. The proposal would then be to build a reliable "human model" to perform infarct size reduction studies in patients and be able to test in STEMI patients the drugs that have passed the preclinical step successfully.

The Study Endpoint

In animal models, the study endpoint is, by definition, infarct size that can be accurately measured by histology. In clinical trials, infarct size can also be reasonably quantified and measured using surrogates like cardiac enzymes release or via imaging (single photon emission computed tomography (SPECT), magnetic resonance imaging (MRI)) techniques. However, in some "cardioprotection" clinical trials, there might be a misleading interpretation of clinical endpoints, which may not necessarily be related to infarct size per se. Some, including infarct size, LV remodeling, heart failure, or ventricular fibrillation, closely reflect the impact of ischemia and reperfusion injury on the myocardium. Others, however, including recurrent ischemia, reinfarction, unstable angina, or need for a new revascularization, are related to the vessel (coronary artery) patency and the ongoing atherothrombotic process and therefore should not be used for the evaluation of infarct size reduction therapy.

The Duration of Ischemia

In all animal models, the duration of ischemia is identical according to the study design [33]. It is even established in order to have the best chance to show a difference between the untreated and the treated group. For example, one knows that the optimal effect of a given protective drug can better be observed when the duration of ischemia is between 40 and 60 min in the pig model [34]. Unlike animal models, choosing the duration of ischemia is highly variable among patients. Including STEMI patients with the duration of ischemia (time between onset of chest pain to reperfusion by angioplasty) less than 12 h, as recommended by the current guidelines, increases the heterogeneity of the population when compared to animal models. The dynamic and evolving nature of occlusion due to thrombus and spontaneous lysis may also introduce considerable heterogeneity. In addition, it remains to be determined (both in animal models and humans) whether the extent of myocardial reperfusion injury is proportional to the duration of ischemia. In other words, it is not known whether postconditioning may be as efficient when the duration of ischemia is short compared to when it is long. In fact, one report in the rat model would suggest the contrary [35].

The Size of the Area at Risk

Reimer et al. have clearly shown that the size of the area at risk can explain more than 60% of the final infarct size in the dog and therefore represents its major determinant [33]. In most clinical studies, the size of the area at risk is not even assessed. It should be acknowledged that the emergency situation of STEMI in humans makes it very difficult to obtain an area at risk measurement. However, at least for small-size trials, techniques like sestamibi-SPECT, LV angiography, or even the simple but reliable BARI score [36, 37] allow an estimate of this major determinant of infarct size for use as a covariate of infarct size when analyzing the data.

Furthermore, assessing area at risk is important since clinical studies have demonstrated that there is heterogeneity of the size of area at risk in STEMI patients, and only patients with a large risk region benefit from infarct size reduction therapy.

The Collateral Circulation

Eventually, many animal species, including man, display coronary collateral circulation that may bring some residual flow to the ischemic bed after a coronary artery occlusion. This is why in animal models, either collateral flow must be measured or species known to be devoid of native collaterals should be chosen for infarct size reduction studies. Collateral flow cannot be reliably measured in emergency clinical settings of acute myocardial infarction. At least, eliminating patients with overt collateral circulation to the ischemic territory at admission coronary angiography (approximately 15% of all STEMI patients) will avoid inclusion of patients already protected against ischemia and reperfusion injury and may partly prevent statistical dilution of the data.

The Timing of Treatment

The fourth major determinant of infarct size is the timing of administration of the protective treatment with respect to reperfusion. The postconditioning studies performed in animal preparations have clearly established that protective interventions must be applied before the onset of reperfusion. When delayed by only a few minutes after reflow, no protection can be expected. For infarct size reduction clinical studies to comply with the concept of prevention of lethal reperfusion injury, the culprit coronary artery must be occluded (i.e., TIMI flow grade at the time of treatment administration must be 0 or 1) at the time of study treatment administration. Thus, patients with TIMI flow grade of 2 or 3 should not be eligible for infarct size reduction trials, since it is very likely that they had undergone reperfusion injury before the treatment was administered.

One has, however, to acknowledge that other factors may have some influence on ischemia and reperfusion injury. Experimental models generally use healthy, young and male animals, which does not fit with the classical profile seen in study populations of infarct size reduction trials. In addition, unlike patients, animals do not display the comorbidities (e.g., diabetes or hypertension) that, according to preclinical studies, may influence resistance to ischemia and reperfusion [32, 38]. Laboratory animals do not receive treatments (e.g., antiplatelet agents, heparin, ACE inhibitors, statins) that might modify the tolerance to ischemia and reperfusion. Yet, in clinical trials, it is expected that the randomization process would balance most of the impact of these confounding factors upon the potential beneficial effect of a given intervention.

In other words, in vivo animal models of acute myocardial infarction are very well controlled and have largely contributed to our understanding of the physiology of acute myocardial infarction. These models are robust, provided the determinants are appropriately assessed. Efforts must be made to design infarct size reduction clinical studies by complying as much as possible to the animal model fundamentals, i.e. assessment of these major determinants of infarct size.

Toward a "Human Model" for Infarct Size Reduction Trials

Aside from the reported negative trials, recent small-size clinical studies have proven that infarct size reduction is feasible in STEMI patients provided care is taken to consider the major determinants of ischemia-reperfusion injury.

In a proof-of-concept trial, Staat et al. aimed to determine whether postconditioning might be protective in patients with ongoing acute myocardial infarction [39]. They included patients with a first STEMI, chest pain for less than 6 h, and a need for angioplasty revascularization in a multicenter, controlled, randomized study. Following direct stenting, control patients underwent no additional intervention. In postconditioned patients, the angioplasty balloon was first deflated immediately after stent implantation and then reinflated for 1 min at low pressure. This deflation/inflation cycle was repeated four times before final reperfusion was allowed. Area under the curve of creatine kinase (CK) release, a surrogate for infarct size, was significantly reduced by 36% in postconditioned versus control group. This study demonstrated for the first time that angioplasty postconditioning protects the human heart. Furthermore, it showed that lethal reperfusion injury does exist in STEMI patients, that it causes significant myocardial damage, and that it can be prevented by a timely intervention. Thibault et al. and Mewton et al. further demonstrated that infarct size reduction persisted at 6–12 months after acute myocardial infarction and was associated with an improved functional recovery at 1 year [40, 41]. In another study, Piot et al. administered cyclosporine, a potent inhibitor of the opening of the mitochondrial permeability transition pore, immediately prior to reperfusion in STEMI patients [42]. In this randomized, controlled, proof-of-concept trial, they showed that cyclosporine reduced CK release (and MRI infarct size) by near 30%. More recently, Bötker et al. reported that remote conditioning by repeated cuff inflation on the arm was able to increase myocardial salvage in STEMI patients [43]. These carefully designed small-size studies have demonstrated that infarct size can be further reduced in STEMI patients by attenuating lethal reperfusion injury in a safe and simple manner.

Importantly, these small-size studies may have been positive mostly because of the attempt to control the determinants of infarct size in STEMI patients. In the Staat, Thibault, and Piot studies, patients with overt collateral circulation to the ischemic bed were not included [39, 40, 42]. In these studies, as well as in the Botker study, the size of the area at risk was assessed before reperfusion, either using LV angiography or by SPECT. Interestingly, all four studies found a significant correlation between infarct size and the size of the risk region, very similar to that observed in animal models (Fig. 5.1). This analysis brought major information, primarily confirming that patients who benefit the most from protective intervention are those who display large areas at risk, i.e., mostly patients with LAD coronary artery occlusion. These studies confirmed that patients with a small area at risk develop small infarcts, then have a good prognosis, and may not therefore expect a major benefit from any adjunctive therapy against lethal reperfusion injury. Eventually, in all four studies reporting an infarct size reduction effect of postconditioning, the timing of treatment was very precise and always fully applied before reopening of the culprit coronary artery.

In order to understand why previously published infarct size reduction studies performed in STEMI patients have been negative, one may verify whether the major determinants of infarct size have been determined by the investigators and taken into consideration for analyzing the data. As for most of them, the four major

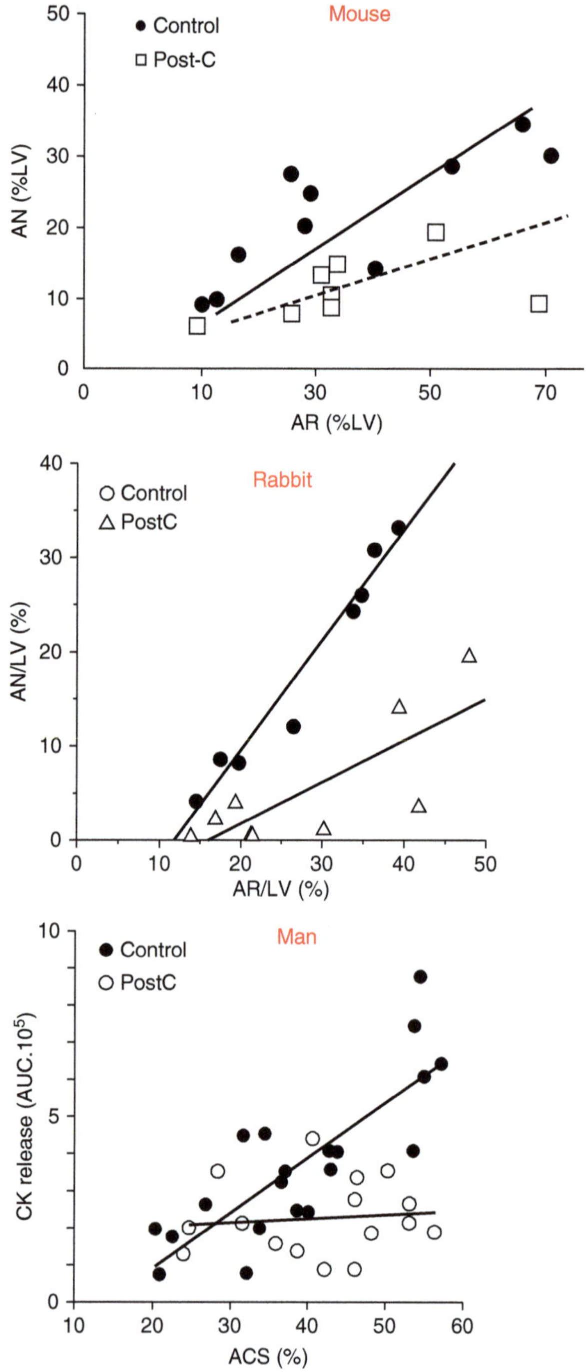

Fig. 5.1 Infarct size as a function of area at risk in the mouse, rabbit and human heart

determinants of infarct size have not been evaluated. In all cases, patients with visible collaterals at admission coronary angiography were included, and area at risk was not assessed. This likely increased the heterogeneity of the study population and dramatically decreased the statistical power of the study, likely contributing to mask a potential positive effect. Noteworthy, an infarct size-reducing effect of the treatment is sometimes found in the high-risk subpopulation of patients when heterogeneity is reduced [4].

After having made so much effort and being successful in reperfusion therapy for STEMI patients, time has come to pay attention at the muscle downstream the vessel. Accumulating evidence from basic and proof-of-concept clinical trials clearly indicates that there is a major opportunity to prevent lethal myocardial reperfusion injury and hopefully improve clinical outcome. We must not miss the opportunity to better protect STEMI patients by improving the design of both phase II and phase III infarct size reduction clinical trials. In terms of demonstrating changes in mortality and heart failure as a function of a reduction in infarct size, there are some formidable hurdles to be overcome. The majority of patients seek medical care after 90 minutes to 2 h of symptoms, and at this time "it might be too late to make a difference." On the other hand, among patients presenting within 70 minutes of symptoms, the mortality and infarct size after prompt reperfusion therapy are so low that it would be difficult "to demonstrate a difference" [44].

Nonetheless, this remains one of the last frontiers of reperfusion therapy and it certainly deserves further investigations.

References

1. Sans S, Kesteloot H, Kromhout D. The burden of cardiovascular diseases mortality in Europe. Task force of the European society of cardiology on cardiovascular mortality and morbidity statistics in Europe. Eur Heart J. 1997;18:1231–48.
2. Anand SS, Yusuf S. Stemming the global tsunami of cardiovascular disease. Lancet. 2011;377(9765):529–32.
3. Tunstall-Pedoe H, Kuulasmaa K, Mähönen M, Tolonen H, Ruokokoski E, Amouyel P. Contribution of trends in survival and coronary-event rates to changes in coronary heart disease mortality: 10-year results from 37 WHO MONICA project populations. Monitoring trends and determinants in cardiovascular disease. Lancet. 1999;353:1547–57.
4. Mahaffey KW, Puma JA, Barbagelata NA, et al. Adenosine as an adjunct to thrombolytic therapy for acute myocardial infarction: results of a multicenter, randomized, placebo-controlled trial: the Acute Myocardial Infarction STudy of ADenosine (AMISTAD) trial. J Am Coll Cardiol. 1999;34:1711–20.
5. Kitakaze M, Asakura M, Kim J, J-WIND investigators, et al. Human atrial natriuretic peptide and nicorandil as adjuncts to reperfusion treatment for acute myocardial infarction (J-WIND): two randomised trials. Lancet. 2007;370:1483–93.
6. Lincoff AM. Presentation of PROTECTION-AMI trial. American College of Cardiology. Scientific Services, New Orleans, Apr 2011.
7. Theroux P, Chaitman BR, Danchin N, et al. Inhibition of the sodium-hydrogen exchanger with cariporide to prevent myocardial infarction in high-risk ischemic situations. Main results of the GUARDIAN trial. Guard during ischemia against necrosis (GUARDIAN) investigators. Circulation. 2000;102:3032–8.

8. Mentzer Jr MR, Bartels C, Bolli R, on behalf of the EXPEDITION Study Investigators, et al. Sodium-hydrogen exchange inhibition by cariporide to reduce the risk of ischemic cardiac events in patients undergoing coronary artery bypass grafting: results of the EXPEDITION Study. Ann Thorac Surg. 2008;85:1261–70.
9. Najjar SS, Rao SV, Melloni C, for the REVEAL Investigators, et al. Intravenous erythropoietin in patients with ST-segment elevation myocardial infarction REVEAL: a randomized controlled trial. JAMA. 2011;305:1863–72.
10. Wijns W, Kolh P, Danchin N, et al. Guidelines on myocardial revascularization. Eur Heart J. 2010;31:2501–55.
11. Gibbons RJ, Valeti US, Aaroz PA, Jaffe AS. The quantification of infarct size. J Am Coll Cardiol. 2004;44:1533–42.
12. Miller TD, Christian TF, Hopfenspirger MR, Hodge DO, Gersh BJ, Gibbons RJ. Infarct size after acute myocardial infarction measured by quantitative tomographic 99mTc sestamibi imaging predicts subsequent mortality. Circulation. 1995;92:334–41.
13. Anderson GF, Chu E. Expanding priorities – confronting chronic disease in countries with low income. N Engl J Med. 2007;356:209–11.
14. Randomised trial of intravenous streptokinase, oral aspirin, both, or neither among 17,187 cases of suspected acute myocardial infarction: ISIS-2. ISIS-2 (Second International Study of Infarct Survival) Collaborative Group. ISIS-2 Lancet. 1988;2:349–60.
15. Gruppo Italiano per lo Studio della Streptochinasi nell'Infarto Miocardico (GISSI). Effectiveness of intravenous thrombolytic treatment in acute myocardial infarction. Lancet. 1986;1(8478):397–402.
16. White HD, Chew DP. Acute myocardial infarction. Lancet. 2008;372:570–84.
17. Gelfand EV, Cannon CP. Myocardial infarction: contemporary management strategies. J Intern Med. 2007;262:59–77.
18. Jernberg T, Johanson P, Held C, Svennblad B, Lindbäck J, Wallentin L, SWEDEHEART/RIKS-HIA. Association between adoption of evidence-based treatment and survival for patients with ST-elevation myocardial infarction. JAMA. 2011;305:1677–84.
19. Zhao Z-Q, Corvera JS, Halkos ME, et al. Inhibition of myocardial injury by ischemic postconditioning during reperfusion: comparison with ischemic preconditioning. Am J Physiol. 2003;285:H579–88.
20. Argaud L, Gateau-Roesch O, Raisky O, Loufouat J, Robert D, Ovize M. Postconditioning inhibits mitochondrial permeability transition. Circulation. 2005;111:194–7.
21. Yang X-M, Proctor JB, Cui L, Krieg T, Downey JM, Cohen MV. Multiple, brief coronary occlusions during early reperfusion protect hearts by targeting cell signaling pathways. J Am Coll Cardiol. 2004;44:1103–10.
22. Tsang A, Hausenloy DJ, Mocanu MM, Yellon DM. Postconditioning: a form of "modified reperfusion" protects the myocardium by activating the phosphatidylinositol 3-kinase-Akt pathway. Circ Res. 2004;95:230–2.
23. Argaud L, Prigent AF, Chalabreysse L, Loufouat J, Lagarde M, Ovize M. Ceramide in the antiapoptotic effect of ischemic preconditioning. Am J Physiol. 2004;286:H246–51.
24. Gomez L, Thibault H, Gharib A, et al. Inhibition of mitochondrial permeability transition improves functional recovery and reduces mortality following acute myocardial infarction in mice. Am J Physiol. 2007;293:H1654–61.
25. Kin H, Zhao ZQ, Sun HY, et al. Postconditioning attenuates myocardial ischemia-reperfusion injury by inhibiting events in the early minutes of reperfusion. Cardiovasc Res. 2004;62:74–85.
26. Crompton M. The mitochondrial permeability transition pore and its role in cell death. Biochem J. 1999;341:233–49.
27. Halestrap AP, Clarke SJ, Javadov SA. Mitochondrial permeability transition pore opening during myocardial reperfusion – a target for cardioprotection. Cardiovasc Res. 2004;61:372–85.
28. Nakagawa T, Shimizu S, Watanabe T, et al. Cyclophilin D-dependent mitochondrial permeability transition regulates some necrotic but not apoptotic cell death. Nature. 2005;434:652–7.

29. Baines CP, Kaiser RA, Purcell NH, et al. Loss of cyclophilin D reveals a critical role for mitochondrial permeability transition in cell death. Nature. 2005;434:658–62.
30. Hausenloy DJ, Maddock HL, Baxter GF, Yellon DM. Inhibiting mitochondrial permeability transition pore opening: a new paradigm for myocardial preconditioning? Cardiovasc Res. 2002;55:534–43.
31. Argaud L, Gateau-Roesch O, Muntean D, et al. Specific inhibition of the mitochondrial permeability transition prevents lethal reperfusion injury. J Mol Cell Cardiol. 2005;38:367–74.
32. Ovize M, Baxter GF, Di Lisa F, Working Group of Cellular Biology of Heart of European Society of Cardiology, et al. Postconditioning and protection from reperfusion injury: where do we stand? Position paper from the working group of cellular biology of the heart of the European Society of Cardiology. Cardiovasc Res. 2010;87:406–23.
33. Reimer KA, Lowe JE, Rasmussen MM, Jennings RB. The wavefront phenomenon of ischemic cell death. 1. Myocardial infarct size vs duration of coronary occlusion in dogs. Circulation. 1977;56:786–94.
34. Ovize M, Aupetit JF, Rioufol G, et al. Preconditioning reduces infarct size but accelerates time to ventricular fibrillation in the pig heart. Am J Physiol. 1995;269:H72–9.
35. Mannintveld OC, Te Lintel HM, van den Bos EJ, et al. Cardiac effects of postconditioning depend critically on the duration of index ischemia. Am J Physiol. 2007;292:H1551–60.
36. Ortiz-Pérez JT, Lee DC, Meyers SN, Davidson CJ, Bonow RO, Wu E. Determinants of myocardial salvage during acute myocardial infarction: evaluation with a combined angiographic and CMR myocardial salvage index. JACC Cardiovasc Imaging. 2010;3:491–500.
37. Graham MM, Faris PD, Ghali WA, Galbraith PD, Norris CM, Badry JT, Mitchell LB, Curtis MJ, Knudtson ML, APPROACH Investigators (Alberta Provincial Project for Outcome Assessment in Coronary Heart Disease). Validation of three myocardial jeopardy scores in a population-based cardiac catheterization cohort. Am Heart J. 2001;142:254–61.
38. Ferdinandy P, Schulz R, Baxter GF. Interaction of cardiovascular risk factors with myocardial ischemia/reperfusion injury, preconditioning, and postconditioning. Pharmacol Rev. 2007; 76:142–54.
39. Staat P, Rioufol G, Piot C, et al. Postconditioning the human heart. Circulation. 2005;112: 2143–8.
40. Thibault H, Piot C, Staat P, et al. Long-term benefit of postconditioning. Circulation. 2008;117:1037–44.
41. Mewton N, Croisille P, Gahide G, et al. Effect of cyclosporine on left ventricular remodeling after reperfused myocardial infarction. J Am Coll Cardiol. 2010;55:1200–5.
42. Piot C, Croisille C, Staat P, et al. Effect of cyclosporine on reperfusion injury in acute myocardial infarction. N Engl J Med. 2008;359:473–81.
43. Bøtker HE, Kharbanda R, Schmidt MR, et al. Remote ischaemic conditioning before hospital admission, as a complement to angioplasty, and effect on myocardial salvage in patients with acute myocardial infarction: a randomised trial. Lancet. 2010;375:727–34.
44. Weaver WD, Cerqueira M, Hallstrom AP, Litwin PE, Martin JS, Kudenchuk PJ, Eisenberg M. Prehospital-initiated vs hospital-initiated thrombolytic therapy. The Myocardial Infarction Triage and Intervention Trial. JAMA. 1993;270:1211–6.

Part III
Diagnosis of Myocardial Reperfusion Injury: Assessment and Quantification

Chapter 6
Cardiac Catheter Laboratory

Eva von Schmilowski and Howard Swanton

Abstract Successful reperfusion in acute myocardial infarction by either thrombolysis or angioplasty results in early ST segment resolution which is a marker of prognostic benefit. A combination of ST resolution and myocardial blush grade is a useful predictor of survival. Microvascular obstruction can be assessed by cardiovascular magnetic resonance (CMR) and/or myocardial contrast echocardiography. Incomplete ST resolution indicates incomplete vessel reopening with the risks of reperfusion ventricular tachyarrhythmias. If these occur late they carry a worse prognosis. Optimal anti-platelet and antithrombotic pharmacotherapy is vital in successful primary percutaneous coronary angioplasty (PPCI) coupled with aspiration thrombectomy. The no-reflow phenomenon is a complex multifactorial problem with numerous techniques and drugs aimed at its prevention. There are several angiographic scoring systems for assessing reperfusion, but grading this often requires the combination of more than one variable.

Keywords Reperfusion injury • PCI pharmacotherapy • No-reflow phenomenon ST segment resolution • Imaging area at risk • Angiographic scores • Microvascular perfusion

---

E. von Schmilowski, M.D., Ph.D.
Department of Cardiology, The Royal Brompton Hospital,
Sydney street, London SW3 6NP, UK
e-mail: ecardiodoc@gmail.com

H. Swanton, M.A., M.D., FRCP, FESC, FACC (✉)
Cardiology Department, The Heart Hospital, University College London Hospitals,
16-18 Westmoreland Street, London W1G 8PH, UK
e-mail: howard.swanton@uclh.org

J.C. Kaski et al. (eds.), *Management of Myocardial Reperfusion Injury*,
DOI 10.1007/978-1-84996-019-9_6,

The Electrocardiogram: Introduction

The ECG remains the first investigation used in the assessment of a patient with a history suggestive of a myocardial infarction. Although it has considerable diagnostic and prognostic value, the ECG has its limitations. Information on the site and extent of the infarct may be available, as well as the speed and extent of reperfusion following primary coronary angioplasty (PPCI) or thrombolysis. The ST segment recovery following reperfusion has prognostic value.

However, the ECG is an isolated test in a moment in time of an event which extends over several hours. It needs to be repeated at regular intervals to identify changes and to provide the most information. In addition, the conventional 12-lead ECG is not an ideal investigation for patients with posterior infarction or pre-existing LBBB. Provided the operator interpreting the ECG is aware of its limitations, it still remains an investigation of fundamental importance against which all other measures of reperfusion are still compared.

ST Elevation: Area at Risk

Evidence of dynamic ECG change is important in confirming the diagnosis of an ST elevation myocardial infarction (STEMI). An ECG should be always recorded during chest pain and compared with an ECG from an asymptomatic period if possible. Dynamic ST segment changes such as ST elevation and depression or dynamic T wave inversion indicate an ongoing process in the coronary artery and, consequently, a higher risk of myocardial infarction.

The number of ECG leads showing evidence of ischaemic change is an important prognostic factor. In general, the greater the number of involved leads, the larger is the ischaemic area and the higher the risk. Although a lower amount of ST elevation and a higher incidence of pre-infarct angina are independent predictors of an aborted myocardial infarction, the amount of ST elevation is not a very sensitive predictor of the area at risk. It is likely, however, that opening an occluded coronary artery results in preservation of myocardial tissue if the area at risk is not too extensive.

Unfortunately, the ECG does not provide conclusive and consistent information for all STEMI patients. Whereas it is reliable in the assessment of the anterior wall, posterior ischaemia in the region of the left circumflex coronary artery is often not visible on a normal standard 12-lead ECG and the patient needs to be monitored for a few hours in order to observe potential ST-T segment changes. If a posterior infarct is suspected (plane ST depression in leads V1–V3), extending the chest leads round the back of the chest (V7–9) should show mirror image ST elevation.

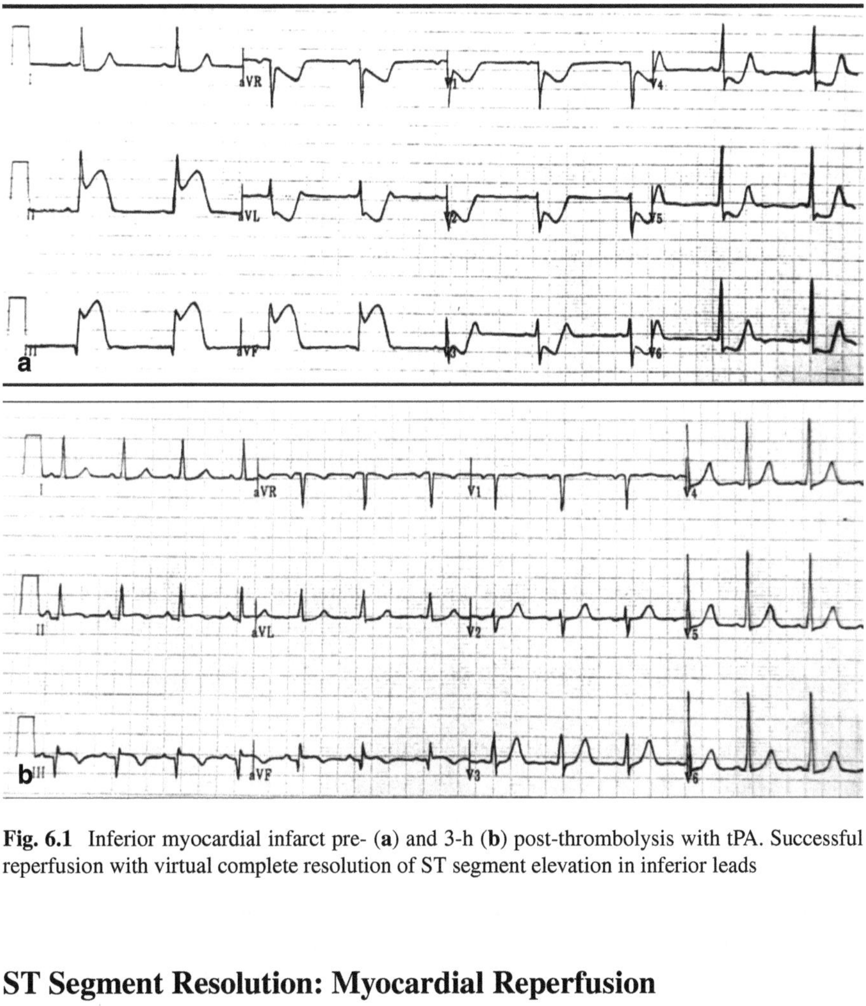

Fig. 6.1 Inferior myocardial infarct pre- (**a**) and 3-h (**b**) post-thrombolysis with tPA. Successful reperfusion with virtual complete resolution of ST segment elevation in inferior leads

ST Segment Resolution: Myocardial Reperfusion

Successful reperfusion occurs at both the epicardial and microvascular level, when complete ST resolution is seen 90 min after fibrinolysis. Patients with rapid ST resolution have a smaller infarct area than those with persistent ST elevation. Immediate ST resolution is the gold standard in patients having PPCI as the outcome in this group is optimal (see below). Successful reperfusion in a patient with an inferior infarct following tPA is shown in Fig. 6.1.

If ST elevation persists, it usually indicates an occluded infarct-related artery (IRA). Incomplete ST resolution suggests a failure of myocardial and microvascular reperfusion. The value of ST resolution in both diagnostic and prognostic terms has been reviewed by De Lemos et al. [1].

Patients with anterior infarction show significantly less ST resolution than those with inferior infarction, despite minor differences in epicardial blood flow. This may suggest that ST resolution is a less precise predictor of epicardial reperfusion in patients with anterior MI than in those with inferior MI. Unfortunately, ST resolution after successful recanalization does not consistently predict myocardial salvage in patients with anterior acute MI.

Several techniques have been used to determine successful myocardial reperfusion following either thrombolysis or primary PCI. ST segment resolution (STR) has long been the standard benchmark even though it is a surrogate end point. TIMI flow and myocardial blush grade (MBG) at angiography, gadolinium-enhanced cardiovascular magnetic resonance (CMR), and myocardial contrast echocardiography (MCE) all have their proponents often studied in conjunction with ST resolution.

A recent study from patients undergoing primary PCI (PPCI) has shown that immediate ST resolution following PPCI carries a better outcome than resolution delayed to 90 min, which itself was superior to incomplete resolution. Thus the major adverse cardiac event (MACE) rate at 1 year was 7.6% in 217 patients whose ST segments resolved immediately and completely at PPCI, 17.1% in 188 patients whose ST resolution was delayed to 90 min post-PPCI, and 20.2% in those 217 patients whose ST segments did not resolve completely by 90 min. The LV ejection fraction was higher and the incidence of heart failure and all cause mortality lowest in patients whose ST segments resolved immediately [2]. It appears that the extent and timing of ST resolution has important prognostic value and is an indicator of microvascular reperfusion and hence left ventricular function.

It is possible that ST resolution may be of more prognostic benefit after fibrinolysis than after PPCI. Data from the DANAMI-2 sub-study is available in 1,421 patients [3]. This showed that ST segment resolution after 4 h following fibrinolysis was associated with a decreased mortality but increased reinfarction rates. However ST resolution was not predictive of 30-day mortality in the 602 patients receiving PPCI. The authors felt that lack of ST segment resolution following PPCI in patients receiving optimal medical therapy may have been of little consequence.

Their conclusion is disputed however by Buller et al. [4] who noted that if both strategies were combined, then ST resolution had definite prognostic benefit, and previous larger studies have confirmed that early ST segment resolution after primary PCI was associated with better 90-day outcomes [5].

A combination of ST segment resolution (STR) and myocardial blush grade improves risk stratification, although neither is a direct measurement of myocardial perfusion. Sorajja et al. [6] noted that although the results of the two are often discordant after PPCI, the combination was a powerful predictor of survival post-PPCI. In patients who had >70% STR plus a myocardial blush grade of 2/3, 30-day mortality was 0.6% and 1-year mortality was 1.2%. In patients who had incomplete STR < 70% and an MBG 0/1, mortality was 8.3% at 30 days and 10.1% at 1 year. Of the two variables, ST segment change was the stronger prognostically on multivariate analysis.

Microvascular obstruction (MVO) identified by cardiovascular magnetic resonance (CMR) may be a more powerful predictor of functional recovery than ST resolution or TIMI flow grading. Nijveldt et al. [7] studied 60 patients between

2 and 9 days following PPCI determining MVO by first pass perfusion imaging. They found that microvascular obstruction was related to incomplete ST resolution but not to TIMI flow grade or myocardial blush grade. MVO was the strongest predictor of changes in ventricular volumes or ejection fraction at follow-up. Other workers [8] had found CMR of value in studying no reflow (see below).

Finally, myocardial contrast echocardiography has been used to assess the degree of microvascular damage in the AMICI study [9]. Using a continuous infusion of SonoVue, they calculated the length of the endocardial contrast defect (CD) 1-day post-PPCI, comparing this with the TIMI flow, myocardial blush grade, ST resolution, peak CK release and wall motion scores. In patients with TIMI 3 flow, the only independent variable of LV remodelling was the endocardial contrast defect. This was superior to ST resolution and myocardial blush grade in patients with TIMI 3 flow. Although LV remodelling was less frequent in patients with established TIMI 3 flow, it still occurred, and TIMI 3 flow should not give the interventionist a false sense of security.

Unfortunately, we still do not have the ideal tool for investigating microvascular obstruction, and of all the techniques described above, CMR is probably the best, but at the same time the least available. Myocardial contrast echocardiography remains underused in acute MI patients. The interventionist will continue to rely on ST resolution, TIMI flow, and myocardial blush grade as surrogate markers of a process which remains tantalizingly difficult to measure.

Reperfusion Arrhythmias

This is one of the four types of myocardial dysfunction resulting from reperfusion. No reflow is discussed below. Myocardial stunning and lethal reperfusion injury are covered in other chapters.

Reperfusion is often associated with an increase in the number of episodes of arrhythmia. Accelerated idioventricular rhythm during thrombolysis in patients with STEMI indicates successful reperfusion. Other important evidence of successful thrombolysis is relief of pain and more than 50% resolution of ST segment elevation within 90 min.

The risk of accelerated idioventricular rhythm during thrombolysis is low as this is generally well tolerated and does require specific treatment. A bradycardia-hypotension syndrome, most frequently observed in inferior wall myocardial infarction, normally resolves spontaneously or following atropine and volume administration.

Ventricular arrhythmias (VT/VF) and myocardial stunning in patients with STEMI may occur either during primary PCI or more commonly immediately after primary PCI as a response to reperfusion caused by TIMI 3 flow restoration. Ninety per cent of these malignant ventricular arrhythmias occur within 48 h of the procedure. Factors associated with an increased risk for early VT/VF on multivariate analysis are the following [10]:

- Pre-PCI TIMI flow grade 0
- Inferior infarction
- Higher total baseline ST deviation

- Lower creatinine clearance
- Killip class > I
- Lower systolic blood pressure
- Greater body weight
- Baseline heart rate > 70/min

The main purpose of primary PCI is to achieve complete reperfusion. When reperfusion is good and the vessel has opened up completely, the arrhythmia risk is small, but incomplete reopening is associated with an increased risk of an arrhythmia (see below). Ventricular tachyarrhythmias are associated with worse outcomes and a higher risk of early death [10]. Therefore, any ventricular arrhythmias particularly after PCI should not be ignored.

In Mehta's study of 5,745 patients in 296 hospitals undergoing primary PCI for ST elevation MI 329 (5.7%) developed VT/VF either early (during the procedure) or late (after the procedure). Overall, 90-day mortality was 3.6% in patients with no ventricular arrhythmias and 23.2% in patients with VT/VF. Ninety-day mortality in patients with late VT/VF was greater than in patients who developed it during the procedure: 33.3% versus 17.2% [10].

The risk of late VT/VF is increased among patients with:

- Lower systolic blood pressure
- ST resolution < 70%
- Baseline heart rate > 70/min
- Higher total baseline ST deviation
- Pre-PCI TIMI flow grade 0
- Post-PCI TIMI flow grade < 3
- Lack of beta blocker use on admission

It will be seen that these factors are similar to those in the early VT/VF group, but include poor TIMI flow and incomplete ST resolution post-PCI. This group needs careful monitoring post-procedure.

Coronary Angiography

Reperfusion in Acute ST Elevation Myocardial Infarction

Pharmaco-Invasive Reperfusion Therapy

Keeley, Boura, and Grines' [11] meta-analysis compared primary angioplasty with thrombolytic therapy. They showed a significant reduction in death, recurrent nonfatal infarction and recurrent ischaemia with primary angioplasty compared with thrombolysis. This study has resulted in a change in strategy with all patients where possible being transferred to interventional cardiac centres for primary percutaneous coronary intervention. Where geographical considerations make this impossible, then prehospital thrombolysis is followed by transfer to the centre for elective angiography and possible angioplasty.

PCI After Failed Thrombolysis (Formerly Rescue PCI)

Failure of thrombolytic therapy to relieve pain or reduce the ST segment elevation <50% after 90 min of thrombolytic administration is considered to be failed thrombolysis. In failed reperfusion, all high-risk patients treated primarily with thrombolytics, abciximab, heparin and aspirin have better outcomes when transferred immediately for PCI rather than continuing medical therapy or attempting repeat thrombolysis without intervention [12, 13].

Early PCI After Successful Thrombolysis (Formerly Known as Facilitated PCI)

Theoretically, a combination of prehospital thrombolysis followed by primary PCI should be superior to either intervention alone. Thrombolysis would offer the best choice for immediate myocardial salvage, and angioplasty would subsequently deal with the stenosis preventing reocclusion and reinfarction. It was therefore hoped that facilitation with early 'upstream' administration of these agents would reduce mortality and reinfarction in STEMI patients. The administration of a thrombolytic (full or half dose) and/or a glycoprotein IIb/IIIa inhibitor prior to early primary PCI described previously as facilitated PCI has not proved beneficial, and it may be harmful. The lack of benefit with facilitated PCI was also shown in the On-TIME trial [14], TITAN-TIMI 34 trial [15], ASSENT-4 trial [16] and FINESSE trial [17]. The only facilitation recommended is the use of aspirin and full-dose clopidogrel (600 mg) prior to the catheter lab, and the use of abciximab once in the catheter lab (0.25-mg/kg bolus plus 0.125-ug/kg/min infusion up to 10 ug/min for 12 h).

The On-TIME trial [14] randomized 507 STEMI patients to upstream tirofiban or its use only in the catheter laboratory. Although early tirofiban administration resulted in a better TIMI 2–3 flow and myocardial perfusion (blush grade), there were no benefits in death or reinfarction at 1 year. The use of early or late eptifibatide was studied in the TITAN-TIMI 34 trial [15]. Once again, early eptifibatide was associated with better reperfusion (TIMI 3 flow and lower TIMI frame counts at the time of the procedure), but there were no differences in post-procedural ST resolution or myocardial perfusion. The ASSENT-4 trial [16] failed to show a benefit of pretreatment with tenecteplase and had to be terminated early because of an increased stroke risk in the facilitated group (particularly in those patients aged >75 years). The FINESSE trial [17] failed to show a benefit with half-dose reteplase plus abciximab or abciximab alone over the simple use of abciximab in the catheter laboratory. Although studies suggest facilitation improves immediate perfusion, unfortunately, this does not translate into improved long-term outcomes, and it merely increases the subsequent bleeding risk.

Primary Percutaneous Coronary Intervention

This is now established worldwide as the optimum treatment for acute myocardial infarction. In England, approximately 75% of patients received primary PCI, and the percentage rises annually. Hospital mortality rates are now 4.5% with primary PCI compared with thrombolysis mortality running at 9.5%. Optimal reperfusion therapy for myocardial infarction has been reviewed [18, 19].

All patients with STEMI should be taken directly to a PCI centre. Trained paramedics in the ambulance interpret the ECG, give loading doses of clopidogrel 600 mg, aspirin 500-mg iv bolus (or 300 mg orally), heparin 5,000-IU iv bolus and warn the cardiothoracic centre of their arrival. Telemetry of difficult ECGs to a local cardiologist may help. Direct transfer of the patient on arrival in the hospital to the catheter laboratory is important. Admission via A&E has been shown to prolong the delay and increase mortality. Primary PCI should be considered in all patients with STEMI, particularly high-risk patients in cardiogenic shock <18 h from symptoms, <75 years old and in whom fibrinolytic therapy is contraindicated or who have already received thrombolytics.

It is still important that the PCI-related delay is as short as possible, and primary PCI is not time independent. Primary PCI is the preferred reperfusion treatment at any time delay, even with early presenters. Time to reperfusion is as important with primary PCI as it is with thrombolysis. Delay from symptom onset to balloon inflation must be as short as possible (see no-reflow section below).

Procedural Factors in Primary PCI

Several procedural factors influence the outcomes of primary angioplasty in acute MI. These are:

- Adjunctive therapy
- Thrombus aspiration
- Choice of stent: bare metal stent versus drug-eluting stent

Adjunctive Therapy During Primary PCI

Major bleeding is a powerful predictor of mortality in patients undergoing primary PCI for STEMI. In high-risk patients, treatment with bivalirudin rather than a combination of heparin and glycoprotein IIb/IIIa inhibitors (GPI) results in a significant reduction in bleeding, thrombocytopenia and transfusions and, consequently, a lower mortality.

Glycoprotein IIb/IIIa Inhibitors (GPI) (See Also No-Reflow Section)

Abciximab may now be administered once the wire is across the stenosis/occlusion and in the true lumen. Abciximab should be avoided if there is any history of a bleeding tendency, peptic ulceration, gastrointestinal bleeding, epistaxes or bleeding haemorrhoids. If there has been difficulty with femoral artery access requiring multiple punctures, its use should be reconsidered. Patients should receive both the bolus dose in the lab (via the intracoronary route if possible) and start the 12-h infusion iv when back on the cardiac care ward.

Thrombus Aspiration (See Also No-Reflow Section)

Intracoronary thrombus increases the risk of no-reflow, distal embolization, abrupt closure and major adverse cardiovascular events (MACE). Thrombus should be removed either mechanically or pharmacologically in order to improve the safety of primary PCI. Thrombectomy improves perfusion and should be performed as the first therapeutic procedure, before any balloon dilatation. Thrombus aspiration helps avoid thrombus propagation down the culprit vessel following balloon dilatation and also migration of thrombus down a side branch or large adjacent vessel when the balloon catheter is removed. The aspiration catheter should be passed if possible to the distal part of the coronary artery also as thrombus may propagate distally. Usually, this manoeuvre is highly successful with both red and white thrombus seen. Several passes of the catheter are made. Angiography should then show a distal vessel and the length of the lesion causing the original occlusion. In young patients where the thrombus is the main lesion, thrombus aspiration alone may be enough to create an excellent result. Thrombus aspiration has been shown to improve clinical outcomes at 1 year in the TAPAS trial [20].

Choice of Stent

Drug-eluting stents (DES) are now used. Bare metal stents (BMS) were initially recommended because of the slightly lower stent-thrombosis risk, but the TYPHOON trial has shown better outcomes with DES up to 4 years with significant reduction in restenosis and the need for repeat revascularization [21]. The choice of DES necessitates good patient compliance with long-term dual anti-platelet therapy. If the patient has a bleeding risk, or is on long-term anticoagulation, or is likely to need surgery within the year, then a BMS should be considered.

Prevention of Complications During Primary PCI

There are several studies on the prevention of overall complications during and following primary PCI. Of particular relevance are studies in adjunctive anti-platelet pharmacology. Increasingly potent and faster-acting anti-platelet drugs are available, but with this potency come increased bleeding risks.

Platelet Inhibition Pre-primary PCI Treatment

Four drugs are at present in use which inhibit the platelet P_2Y_{12} receptor: clopidogrel, prasugrel, cangrelor and ticagrelor.

Clopidogrel

This prodrug which inhibits the P_2Y_{12} receptor on platelets has been in standard use prior to PCI for many years. The HORIZONS-AMI trial [22] has confirmed that patients treated with a 600-mg loading dose of clopidogrel prior to PCI have a better outcome than patients receiving 300 mg. The incidence of stent thrombosis was lower with a 600-mg dose, and there was no increased stroke risk or risk of thrombocytopenia regardless of what antithrombotic treatment the patient received.

Three concerns have been expressed with regard to the use of clopidogrel. First is the delayed onset of action, second the variation in response to clopidogrel due to genetic polymorphisms and third possible problems in co-administration with proton pump inhibitors.

Some patients have shown a lack of response to therapy in spite of good compliance. A genetic variation in metabolism has been found [23]. Two-step clopidogrel activation occurs via the CYP-450 cytochrome isoenzymes. Carriers of two specific alleles of CYP2C19 and CYP3A4 isoenzymes have a reduced response to clopidogrel.

The TRITON-TIMI 38 trial suggested that patients with the loss of function CYP2C19 allele had an increased risk of cardiovascular events post-PCI [24].

Proton pump inhibitors (PPI) are metabolized by the CYP2C19 isoenzyme, and co-treatment with omeprazole has been shown to reduce the platelet inhibitory effect of clopidogrel. A large retrospective study of 8,025 patients being discharged from Veterans Affairs hospitals following acute coronary syndromes showed that of the 63.9% patients who were taking a proton pump inhibitor with clopidogrel on multivariate analysis, there was a significantly increased risk of recurrent ACS and rehospitalization [25]. However, the COGENT study which was stopped early found no increase in cardiac events in those patients who received omeprazole in addition to clopidogrel over a 12-month period [26]. Further studies are needed, but the need for a PPI must be considered carefully in patients undergoing a primary PCI for ST elevation MI.

Prasugrel

This acts directly and irreversibly on the P_2Y_{12} receptor with a faster onset of platelet inhibition than clopidogrel. It undergoes a one-step CYP oxidation in the liver but seems not to be influenced by variability in CYP2CI9 isoenzymes and has a lower variability of platelet response.

A comparison of the use of prasugrel (loading dose 60 mg, maintenance dose 10 mg) and clopidogrel (loading dose 300 mg, maintenance dose 75 mg) in acute coronary syndromes was made in the TRITON-TIMI 38 study [24] and a sub-study of 3,534 ST elevation MI patients undergoing primary PCI reported by Montalescot et al. [27]. This confirmed the earlier larger study in patients with acute coronary syndromes: showing a small benefit for prasugrel over clopidogrel. At 30 days, the primary end point in this sub-study (cardiovascular death, nonfatal MI or nonfatal stroke) was 6.5% in the prasugrel group and 9.5% in the clopidogrel group ($p = 0.0017$), with the benefit still apparent at 15 months.

However:

- There was no difference in the cardiovascular death rate.
- The trial was underpowered for a single end point.
- Only 300 mg clopidogrel was used as the loading dose.
- There was more major and minor bleeding in the prasugrel group, particularly in those patients who needed CABG.

The small benefit with prasugrel over clopidogrel must be weighed against the increased bleeding risk. It should be avoided in patients over 75 years (CVA risk), patients who have a history of CVA or TIA, and a dose reduction is necessary in patients <60 kg. Diabetic patients should receive prasugrel rather than clopidogrel (TRITON-TIMI 38 sub-study).

Cangrelor

This is a rapidly acting reversible P_2Y_{12} receptor inhibitor which is given parenterally. It is an ATP analogue with and immediate onset of action following a bolus dose. It was studied in the CHAMPION and CHAMPION PLATFORM trials [28]. Both of these trials included patients who have primarily acute coronary syndromes, and cangrelor was given in a double-blind fashion to half the patients prior to 600 mg clopidogrel. Both trials failed to show an advantage for cangrelor in spite of its earlier onset of action.

Ticagrelor

This drug is an oral reversible P_2Y_{12} receptor inhibitor which does not require in vivo metabolism. It is an active drug and has a stronger and faster onset of action than clopidogrel. It was compared with clopidogrel in 18,624 patients with acute coronary syndromes (with or without ST elevation MI) in the PLATO trial [29]. At 12 months, the primary end point of death from vascular causes, myocardial infarction or stroke was reduced in the ticagrelor group to 9.8% compared with 11.7% in the clopidogrel group ($p=0.001$). There was no significant increase in major bleeding. There was a significant reduction in death from any cause with ticagrelor (4.5% vs. 5.9% for clopidogrel), although the trial was not powered to detect a mortality difference. In addition, a significant number of patients in the clopidogrel group did not receive optimum dosing.

However, ticagrelor had new side effects such as dyspnoea, bradyarrhythmias and a rise in serum uric acid and creatinine. Part of the ticagrelor molecule is similar to adenosine which might account for these side effects.

No-Reflow Phenomenon

Following balloon inflation and/or stent deployment, the vessel is widely patent at the lesion site, but following injection, dye is still held up and does not flow briskly down the artery: creeping down the vessel if at all. Dye in the artery just proximal to the lesion site may appear to oscillate slightly with each systole, but simply fails to progress distally in spite of an apparently satisfactory angioplasty procedure. There is abnormal and inadequate tissue perfusion in the segment of the target vessel with no evidence of spasm, dissection, thrombus or obvious embolic obstruction. The result is a myocardial blush grade (MBG) of 0–1, with poor TIMI flow grade 0–1. This is the no-reflow phenomenon: disturbed and reduced myocardial perfusion in the absence of visible vessel obstruction.

It is a frustrating condition for the interventionist who having deployed a stent is faced with a patient who may still have chest pain and ST elevation. It is more common in primary PCI (up to 50% cases) and saphenous vein graft PCI than in elective native vessel PCI. This is thought to be due to the thrombus burden of acute myocardial infarction or the bulky atheroma of vein grafts. Thrombogenic factors are generated from activated platelets, traumatized endothelium and denuded intimal cells. The mechanism is poorly understood but is thought to be due to obstruction at microvascular level. Animal experiments suggest multiple factors contributing to both ischaemic and reperfusion injury.

The subject has been extensively reviewed [30–32], and the mechanisms thought responsible for the phenomenon are summarized below:

- Coronary spasm. This may be provoked by the guide wire, or by the tip of the guiding catheter, or is the direct result of trauma at the site of dilatation. Thromboxane A2 (TXA2) and endothelin-1 (ET-1) release from cell damage will contribute to this. Pre-intervention plasma levels of thromboxane and endothelin-1 are probably important, but there is little data on this.
- Microemboli migrating distally. This might be thrombus or plaque debris. It is a particular problem in cases involving rotablation where temporary pacing is advisable. Unfortunately, distal filter protection has not been successful in

improving outcomes in PPCI, but thrombus aspiration prior to dilatation has been shown to reduce mortality at 1 year [20].

- Endothelial cell swelling. Endothelial oedema with bleb or protrusion formation has been seen in experimental models and may be due to free-radical release. These protrusions contribute to microvascular obstruction. P-selectins are expressed causing monocyte adherence to the endothelial surface.
- Platelet activation with platelet microemboli. Thrombin is released from intraluminal and adherent thrombus driving a procoagulable state. Vigorous anti-platelet treatment is necessary. Pretreatment with the platelet P_2Y_{12} receptor inhibitor clopidogrel or prasugrel is standard therapy, together with the use of a glycoprotein IIb/IIIa receptor antagonist which blocks the final common pathway of platelet activation (see below).
- White cell adherence to the endothelium. Activated neutrophils are attracted to the infarct zone and contribute to vascular plugging with platelets and endothelial blebs. Expression of P-selectins and ICAM (cell adhesion molecules) on the endothelial cell surface ensures white cell adherence. The white cells release free radicals, proteolytic enzymes and pro-inflammatory cytokines.
- Collapse in the capillary bed due to a drop in capillary perfusion pressure. It is important to avoid hypotension and/or bradycardia, and volume loading is necessary especially if nitrates are used.
- Red cells becoming less deformable when hypoxic contribute to plugs in the distal capillaries.
- Possible irreversible myocyte injury. Intracellular acidosis, sodium and calcium overload with additional reactive oxygen species stimulate the opening of the mitochondrial permeability transition pore (mPTP) causing further calcium overload, mitochondrial and cell swelling with disruption and cell death. Cell swelling and oedema contribute to microvascular obstruction.

It will be seen that this is a highly complex phenomenon with multiple factors contributing to microvascular obstruction in variable amounts. In summary, the principle mechanisms are ischaemic injury caused by spasm, endothelial swelling and bleb formation, reperfusion injury caused largely by platelets and white cells and prolonged mechanical obstruction by distal embolization.

Prediction of the No-Reflow Phenomenon

The experienced operator in PPCI procedures will be aware of the factors increasing the likelihood of a no-reflow phenomenon:

- Long ischaemic time prior to coronary intervention. Prolonged ischaemia increases tissue oedema which will impede microvascular flow following PPCI.
- Large thrombotic burden visible on the first angiogram. This may be seen as adherent thrombus at the occlusion site or more free-floating thrombus proximal to it. Thrombus generates thrombin and increases platelet activation, as well as being an embolic risk.

- A large infarct-related vessel: >4.0 mm
- A vessel supplying a large segment of myocardium: commonly the LAD
- Persistent dye distal to the lesion site.
- Saphenous vein graft cases

Other contributing factors which may not be routinely considered in emergency PPCI cases but which are undoubtedly contributory are:

- Platelet reactivity and platelet volume
- Plasma thromboxane and endothelin-1 levels prior to intervention
- Intrinsic/natural antioxidant levels in the myocardium
- Acute hyperglycaemia
- Neutrophil count prior to the procedure
- Statin status

Prevention of the No-Reflow Phenomenon

From the above predictors, it will be seen that every effort must be made to reduce the pain to balloon time. This involves education of the general public, successful liaison with the ambulance service and a 24/7 PPCI service with an easily accessible and experienced on call team. The ambulance personnel must be instructed to deliver the patient straight to the catheter laboratory, bypassing the A&E department which has been shown to cause unnecessary delays. Anti-platelet agents can be given in the ambulance. Upstream IIb/IIIa antagonists however in STEMI are best reserved for the catheter laboratory.

Thrombus aspiration as the first part of the PPCI procedure should be attempted where possible. Thrombectomy has been shown to be associated with significant improvement in reperfusion as judged by ST resolution and myocardial blush grade [33]. A sub-study of the REMEDIA trial using myocardial contrast echocardiography showed thrombus aspiration improved microvascular obstruction [34].

The TAPAS trial [20] showed convincingly that thrombus aspiration using the Export catheter improved 30-day MACE, 1-year mortality and reinfarction in patients undergoing PPCI. Successful aspiration was achieved in 72.9% patients. Complete ST resolution was achieved in 56.6% patients treated with thrombus aspiration but only in 44.2% in patients treated without it. Thrombus aspiration improved the myocardial blush grade (MBG). In patients treated with aspiration, the MBG was 0/1 in 17% but 26.3% in those treated with conventional angioplasty. The MBG correlated closely with 1-year mortality. Mortality at 1-year was 3.7% in patients with an MBG of 3, 4.7% with an MBG of 2 and 11% if the MBG was 0 or 1.

Stenting itself will of course help reduce no reflow by trapping thrombus against the arterial wall and preventing distal embolization. The stent should if possible be long enough to achieve this. Optical coherence tomography (OCT) studies after stenting have shown microthrombi protruding through and between the stent struts, but there is no doubt that stenting is an effective stabilizer of thrombus.

Theoretically, distal protection should improve microvascular circulation by trapping and removing thrombus and atheromatous debris, reducing the embolic burden. Unfortunately, trials have shown that distal protection does not protect or improve outcomes in PPCI for ST elevation MI. In the EMERALD trial, visible debris was filtered in 73% of 252 patients, but there was no improvement in microvascular flow or event-free survival [35]. In fact, late 15-month follow-up in the DEDICATION trial showed an increase in late stent thrombosis in those patients treated with distal protection (2.9% in the distal protection group vs. 0.3% in the PCI alone group) [36]. It is clear that distal protection cannot be used as a routine strategy in PPCI for acute ST elevation MI as even in skilled hands (and it is not always an easy procedure) it conveys no benefit.

Treatment with glycoprotein IIb/IIIa inhibitors is both a theoretical and proven therapy in PPCI. These drugs block the final common pathway of platelet aggregation, preventing fibrinogen cross-binding to the IIb/IIIa receptors on the platelet surface. The evidence is strongest for abciximab which also blocks the vitronectin receptor and reduces white cell adherence to the endothelium. Abciximab has been shown to reduce remodelling at 6 months and improve myocardial perfusion with a substantial reduction in no reflow [37]. This group found adenosine improved perfusion but did not prevent remodelling. Intracoronary abciximab bolus may be preferable to the intravenous route [38] with the higher concentrations available at the site of the thrombus when delivered locally. This Leipzig study suggested a reduced infarct size and better myocardial perfusion with the intracoronary route. The TIMI flow grades were not different in the two groups.

Chronic statin therapy pre-PPCI appears to reduce the incidence of no reflow [39] with a 9.1% incidence in the statin-treated group versus 34.1% in the non-treated group.

Hyperglycaemia has been identified as a risk factor for no reflow [40], and treatment of hyperglycaemia in acute MI with insulin and glucose infusion followed by sc insulin carried a mortality benefit in the first DIGAMI trial [41].

Treatment of the No-Reflow Phenomenon

Unfortunately, many of the drugs tested in the treatment of the no-reflow phenomenon have been unsuccessful, and the preventive techniques described above will remain better than a cure which remains elusive. In some cases, the phenomenon is gradually reversible over a few minutes. Intracoronary drug therapy should be given as soon as possible together with volume loading to help avoid hypotension. Temporary pacing may be needed for resistant bradycardia. Nitrates and adenosine together may be enough to restore brisk flow. No single drug has proved superior to others, and the agents can be given in combination provided hypotension is avoided. The vasodilators have different additional metabolic effects. Commonly used agents are:

Nicorandil

This drug is a combination of nicotinamide nitrate and an ATP-sensitive K^+ channel opener. Animal work has shown reduced infarct size following coronary ligation. It is a vasodilator, inhibits free-radical production from white cells and stimulates preconditioning. Ito [42] studied a group of 81 patients with an anterior infarct using myocardial contrast echocardiography as a measure of myocardial perfusion following successful PPCI. Forty patients had an infusion of nicorandil. It reduced no reflow, improved LV wall motion scores and reduced the incidence of ventricular arrhythmias and congestive cardiac failure. A larger randomized double-blind trial of 368 patients with long-term follow-up [43] used 12 mg nicorandil given iv just prior to reperfusion. Nicorandil improved TIMI 3 flow and ST resolution and reduced TIMI frame counts. At a mean follow-up of 2.4 years, there was a substantial reduction in mortality and congestive cardiac failure in the nicorandil group. Suggested dose is 12 mg iv prior to reperfusion.

Sodium Nitroprusside

This is a nitric oxide donor independent of cell metabolism with anti-platelet and vasodilating properties. It is light sensitive.

A randomized trial of 60 ug intracoronary nitroprusside versus placebo given distal to the occlusion at PPCI failed to show any improvement in measures of myocardial perfusion. Corrected TIMI frame count, ST resolution and myocardial blush score were the same in both groups [44]. In spite of these findings, 6-month outcomes were better in the nitroprusside group. Other much smaller studies have confirmed nitroprusside can reverse no reflow but without long-term outcome data. Suggested dose is 60–120 ug.

Adenosine

This endogenous nucleoside vasodilator inhibits platelet and white cell aggregation and reduces calcium overload. It reduces no reflow and the level of incomplete ST resolution but has not been shown to effect long-term outcomes. Studies vary in their choice of dose from 4 mg i.c. [45] to 60 mg i.c. The drug is safe with such a short half-life. A small first trial with adenosine as an adjunct to thrombolysis [46] suggested it reduced infarct size as assessed by sestamibi scanning. A larger second study with thrombolysis or primary PCI [47] used a 50–70-ug/kg/min infusion for 3 h. Although infarct size was reduced at the higher dose, clinical outcomes were no different in the adenosine group. ST resolution appears to be faster with adenosine, but it does not influence overall long-term results. The ideal dose and regime have yet to be established.

Verapamil

In a study of 212 patients, Werner et al. [48] used intracoronary verapamil in 10.8% patients who developed no reflow after PPCI. Coronary flow was assessed by TIMI frame counts (see below). Verapamil 1 mg infused over 2 min reduced the TIMI frame count and reversed the no reflow possibly by reducing coronary spasm. The drug has not been widely tested. It certainly may improve coronary flow following PPCI but may induce bradycardia or AV block necessitating temporary pacing. Suggested dose is 0.5–2.5 mg over 2 min i.c.

Abciximab (See Above)

This effectively inhibits platelet activation, preventing the formation of microthrombi. Recently formed small thrombi visible on angiography can be seen to disappear after abciximab administration. It seems to be more effective with the bolus given directly via the intracoronary route and should be administered before balloon dilatation. Dose is 0.25-mg/kg iv bolus followed by infusion of 10 ugm/min for 12 h.

Other Drugs

Cyclosporine A

This drug inhibits the opening of the mitochondrial permeability transition pore, and a small study found that when given at the time of PPCI infarct size was reduced (as measured by CK release), but TIMI flow was similar in the two groups [49]. A CMR study at 6 months showed that the reduction in infarct size had persisted, the LV end-systolic volume remained attenuated and the LVEF remained better in the cyclosporine group [50].

Atrial Natriuretic Peptide (ANP)

The J-WIND trial [51] of a 3-day intravenous infusion of ANP in acute myocardial infarction showed a reduction in infarct size (total CK release) and an improved LV ejection fraction (angiographic assessment).

We still do not have the ideal drug to reverse no reflow and prevent reperfusion injury. The problem is compounded by the fact that measuring microvascular function remains a major challenge, and we still rely on surrogate markers such as ST resolution.

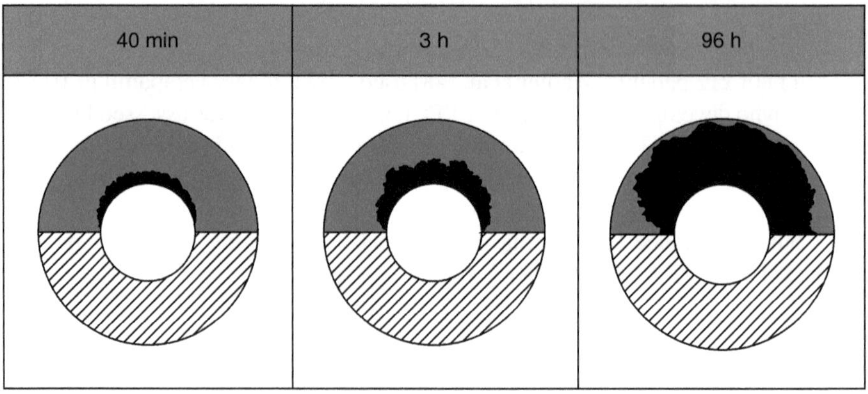

Fig. 6.2 Wavefront concept of myocardial infarction based on duration of coronary occlusion. *Grey area* – area at risk. *Black area* – final infarct. (Adapted from Reimer and Jennings [52])

Regional Wall Motion Abnormalities (RMWA): Area at Risk

Shortly after the onset of chest pain and long before evidence of ECG changes, myocardial ischaemia produces regional wall motion abnormalities (RWMA). The wavefront concept of myocardial infarction states that infarction increases in a transmural wavefront, starting from the endocardium moving out to the epicardium [52] without much lateral extension. The longer the duration of the occluded artery, the more severe is the ischaemia. Occlusion lasting longer than 1 h leads to subendocardial necrosis and subsequently increases the transmural extent of the infarct (transmurality) until infarct size covers the entire area at risk (Fig. 6.2). Based on this concept, the infarct-related artery should be opened as quickly as possible to limit the duration of ischaemia in the occluded area and protect viable myocardium in the area at risk. Reopening the artery late (e.g. 3–28 days after the infarction) is of no value as demonstrated by Hochman et al. [53] in the OAT study and may even increase the risk of late reinfarction. Infarct size is also dependent on haemodynamic factors such as blood pressure and heart rate, and residual flow in the area at risk is determined by the potential presence of collaterals and antegrade flow in the infarct-related artery.

Area at Risk: Definition and Assessment

The definition of the area at risk of infarction is the myocardial area located distal to and supplied by the acutely occluded infarct-related coronary artery. This is determined by summing the lengths of all distal coronary branches (see below). Precise assessment of the area at risk is clinically important as it allows estimation

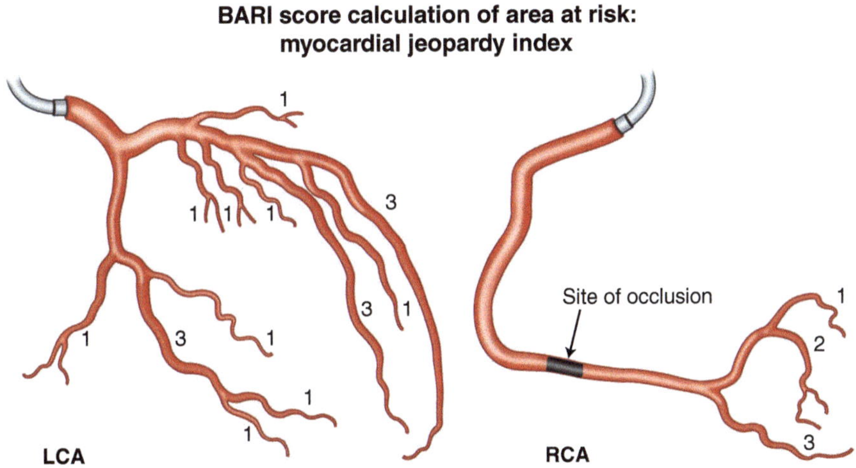

Fig. 6.3 Area at risk estimated according to BARI score. Area at risk = 6 points. Total LV = 24 points. BARI (%) LV = 25%

of potential infarct size, the effectiveness of reperfusion therapy and myocardial salvage. Myocardial salvage = area at risk – area of infarction.

Angiographic Scores

These have been designed for patients with STEMI to assess the anatomical area at risk and myocardial salvage. Both scores provide prognostic information based on the estimated proportion of the LV that is dependent on the size of the occluded coronary artery.

BARI Score (Bypass Angioplasty Revascularization Investigation Myocardial Jeopardy Index)

This score applies to patients with chronic coronary artery disease. It allows an estimation of the entire jeopardized myocardial area at risk based on detailed vascular anatomy – the length and diameter of the distal segments of all the main coronary arteries (LAD, LCx, RCA, diagonals, obtuse marginals, PDA and PLA branches). Each artery is graded from 0 – as an insignificant artery – to 3 as a large artery. Scores affected by the culprit lesion in the IRA are summed and divided by the total score supplying blood to the entire left ventricle. The result is the myocardial area at risk as percentage of left ventricle myocardial volume Fig. 6.3 [54].

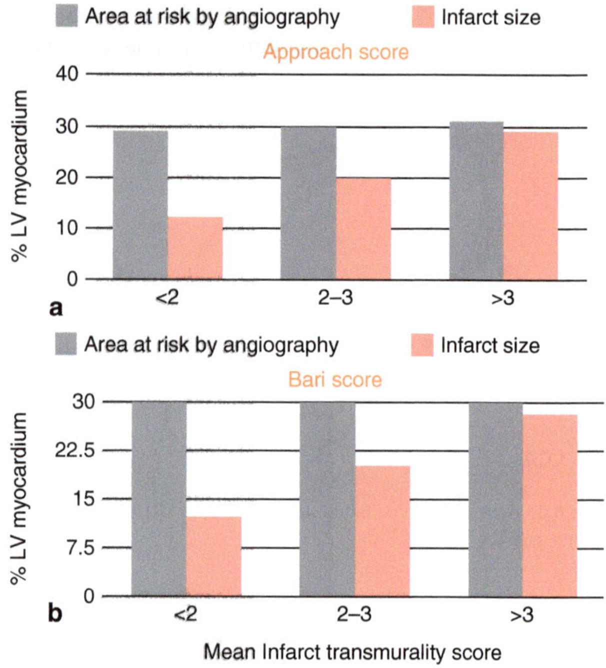

Fig. 6.4 Angiographic area at risk and infarct size related to mean infarct transmurality score: (**a**) using the APPROACH score, (**b**) using BARI score (Adapted from Ortiz-Perez et al. [56])

Modified APPROACH Score (Alberta Provincial Project for Outcome Assessment in Coronary Heart Disease)

The modified APPROACH score is simpler, based on dominance, location of occlusion and size of the coronary branches of the infarct-related artery [55]. These are related to the left ventricle and allow a calculation of the jeopardized myocardial area for a specific part of the occlusion. The area at risk is estimated as a percentage of the left ventricular myocardium.

Area at Risk and Infarct Size

In patients with an acute MI, early reperfusion benefits left ventricular function and remodelling and also reduces severity of RWMA and infarct size. Angiographic studies with CMR (cardiac magnetic resonance) assessment show that in cases of complete transmural myocardial infarction treated by reperfusion therapy with long periods of pre-intervention ischaemia, the anatomical area at risk visible at angiography calculated by the BARI and APPROACH scores is very similar to the infarct size calculated as the infarct-endocardial surface area at CMR [56]. In patients with prompt reperfusion therapy and only sub-endocardial infarction, the infarct size is smaller than the risk area (Fig. 6.4). In consequence, combining measurements of anatomical area at risk at angiography and infarct size assessed at CMR may help determine myocardial salvage achieved by reperfusion therapy. The other advantage of the use of an angiographic scoring system is that it can be used to assess risk area in patients investigated and

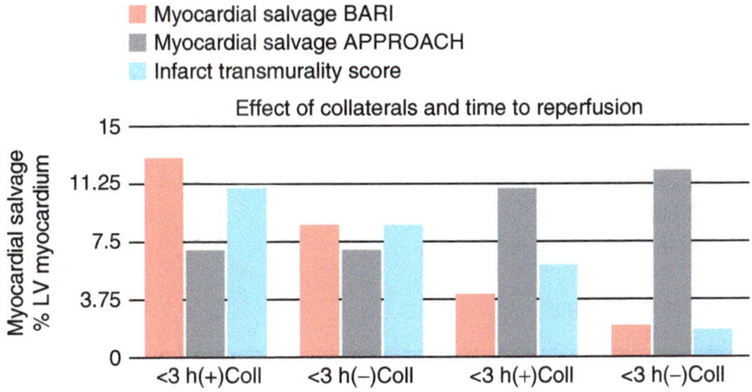

Fig. 6.5 Effect of collaterals and time to reperfusion on myocardial salvage (Adapted from Ortiz-Perez et al. [56])

treated out of hours in the middle of the night [57]. The use of Technetium-99-m sestamibi has long been used as an agent to define myocardium at risk and infarct size [58], and similar myocardial salvage has been proven with both primary PCI and thrombolysis. However, it is unlikely to be available on a 24-h basis.

Myocardial Salvage and Infarct Transmurality

There is a relation between myocardial salvage and infarct transmurality. Patients with developed collateral flow, or those who had early reperfusion, present a lower infarct transmurality score and consequently increased myocardial salvage defined as the difference between infarct size and initial area at risk. The presence of collateral flow does not decrease the lateral boundaries of the infarct that are established after the first hour of symptom onset. Collaterals however have been shown to reduce the infarct transmurality score (Fig. 6.5).

Imaging

RWMA can be precisely identified before angiography using two-dimensional echocardiography. A substantial reduction in regional blood flow associated with an MI presents as akinesis or dyskinesis. Hypokinesis is not reliable enough as too sensitive a marker for severe ischaemia. Hyperkinesis may be seen in the non-infarcted segments. Several modern imaging techniques such as CMR, SPECT and contrast CMRI are also of great value. These are described in detail in other chapters.

Coronary Angiography Jeopardy Scores: Area at Risk

The jeopardy score is a simple method for estimating the amount of myocardium at risk for ischaemia based on the coronary anatomy and particular location of the lesion. Coronary circulation is divided into six arterial segments:

- Left anterior descending coronary artery (LAD)
- Major anterolateral (diagonal) branch

Table 6.1 The jeopardy score for characterizing the area at risk

Arterial system supplying myocardial territory	Score	Comments
Left anterior descending	1	Maximum left anterior descending system score, including branches
Major anterolateral (diagonal) branch	1	
First major septal perforator	1	
Left circumflex	1	Maximum left circumflex system score, including branches
Major circumflex marginal branch	1	
Posterior descending	1	Maximum score for right coronary system

- First major septal perforator
- Left circumflex coronary artery (LCx)
- Major circumflex marginal branch
- Posterior descending artery

Each segment with a significant stenosis that is >75% lumen diameter is given one point. Also, each segment distal to a segment with a significant stenosis is given one point. The maximum number of points is six. To determine the amount of myocardium at risk or in other words the area of risk, it is necessary to score each angiogram by giving a point to segments that are distal to the infarct culprit segment. The maximum score, six points, indicates patients with the largest burden of ischaemia. The jeopardy score does not provide information about the number of significantly diseased arteries and is not being used in daily practice (Table 6.1).

Myocardial Perfusion (TIMI Flow, Myocardial Blush Grade)

The main purpose of primary angioplasty in acute myocardial infarction is to restore normal blood flow in the infarct-related coronary artery. This can be achieved in almost 90% of patients, and the result of reperfusion can be assessed during angioplasty using TIMI flow and blush grades. Whereas TIMI flow grade describes epicardial blood flow, myocardial blush grade refers to myocardial viability in the IRA. Both scores are simple to use and very helpful as prognostic tools in patients after primary PCI.

Sometimes, however, primary PCI is limited by suboptimal myocardial reperfusion (a failure of microvascular reperfusion). This is partly caused by microembolization of thrombus into the distal circulation (see no-reflow section above). In these situations TIMI flow in the IRA is impaired, and myocardial blush is lower (0 or 1). Distal microembolization during primary PCI may contribute to poor myocardial reperfusion, and the use of adjunctive aspiration thrombectomy, by removing thrombus prior to balloon inflation, has become a standard first-step procedure in primary PCI as mentioned above.

Table 6.2 TIMI flow grades

TIMI grade	Contrast penetration
TIMI 0	No flow
TIMI 1	Flow is minimal and there is no perfusion. Contrast passes beyond the lesion, but fails to opacify the entire coronary bed distal to the lesion for the duration of the cine sequence
TIMI 2	There is partial perfusion. Contrast passes across the lesion and opacifies the coronary bed distal to the lesion. However, the entry of contrast into the vessel distal to the lesion and its clearance from the distal bed, or both, are visibly slower than in non-occluded segments
TIMI 3	Perfusion is complete. Antegrade flow into the distal segment to the lesion and clearance from the distal bed are as rapid as in non-occluded segments

It has been reported that in more than 30% of patients, impaired myocardial perfusion persists with low blush grade in spite of successful angioplasty, a fully opened IRA and good TIMI 3 flow. Several mechanisms such as no-reflow or low-reflow phenomenon or distal embolization have been described as factors associated with this situation. Patients with suboptimal myocardial reperfusion have limited myocardial salvage and increased mortality.

TIMI (Thrombolysis in Myocardial Infarction) Flow Grade (Table 6.2)

TIMI grade describes the degree of epicardial blood flow after reperfusion therapy. Good flow (TIMI 3 flow) after primary PCI is associated with a lower risk of complications and an improvement in LV function. Generally, the higher TIMI grade, the lower mortality. If the artery is completely occluded and there is no flow beyond the point of occlusion, TIMI flow is 0. If there is minimal penetration across the lesion without perfusion, TIMI flow is described as grade 1. Grade TIMI 2 refers to partial perfusion with slow flow within a well-visualized artery. After successful reperfusion with completely restored perfusion, rapid TIMI 3 flow is achieved (Figs. 6.6 and 6.7).

Corrected TIMI Frame Count (CTFC)

This has been designed to estimate TIMI flow more precisely and objectively, particularly in high-risk patients. It is a more reproducible and accurate assessment of flow than the TIMI flow scoring system above which although quick and instantaneous is subjective [59]. The definition of CTFC is the time taken for contrast to

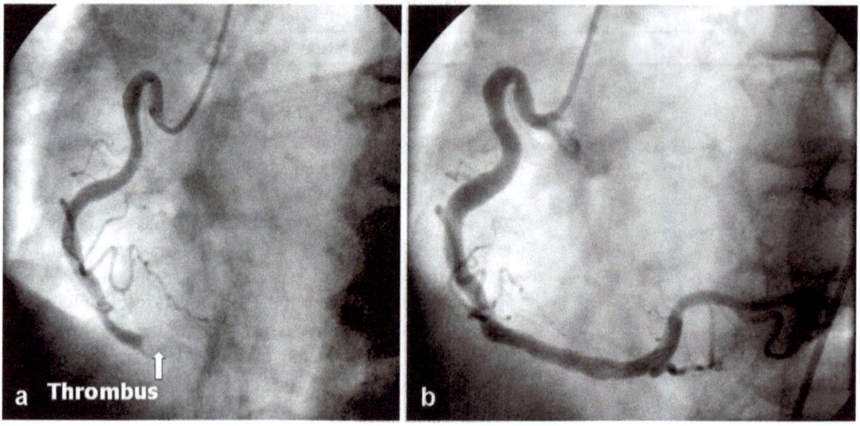

Fig. 6.6 Primary PCI of totally occluded right coronary artery (**a**) with thrombus visible (*arrowed*). Result after thrombus aspiration and stenting TIMI 3 flow achieved (**b**)

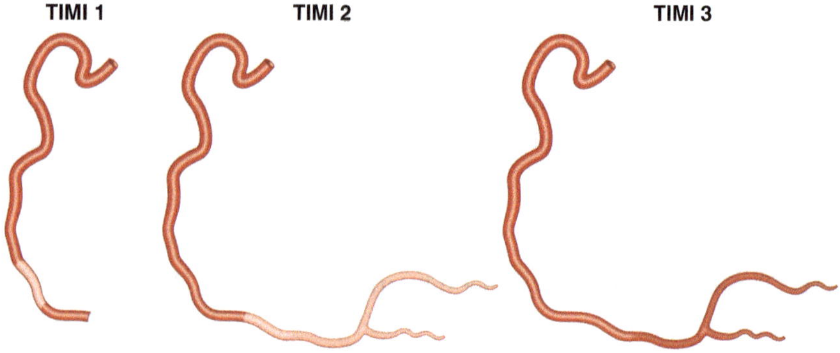

Fig. 6.7 Diagram of TIMI flow grades in the right coronary artery shown in Fig. 6.6

enter the distal part of the artery. Frame 0 is the starting frame, and this is the first frame in which contrast touches two borders of the proximal segment of the major coronary artery. Contrast moves forward in the following frames reaching the distal segment of the artery (frame 21). Standard distal landmarks are identified for each of the main coronary arteries and are as follows:

- In the LAD, the distal bifurcation – sometimes called the whale's tale
- In the LCx, the most distal branch of the obtuse marginal branch that includes the infarct-related artery
- In the RCA, the first branch of the posterolateral (LV branch) artery (Fig. 6.8).

In patients during primary PCI, flow rate in the IRA is important and associated with outcomes. The faster the flow, the lower is the mortality. Studies have shown that mortality increases by 0.7% for every ten frame rise. However, in patients with acute MI flow in the non-infarct-related arteries is also slower and can be restored

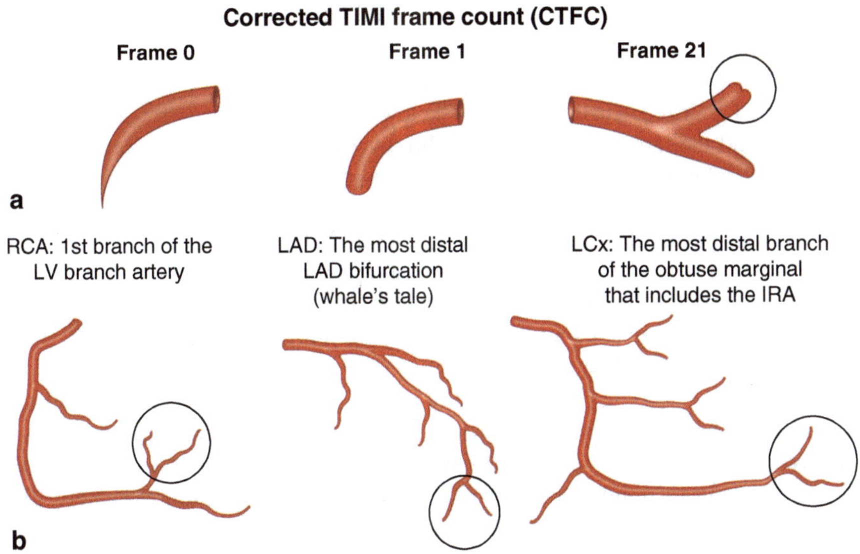

Fig. 6.8 (**a**) Corrected TIMI frame count (CTFC). (**b**) Standard distal landmarks describing main coronary arteries (*circles*)

Table 6.3 Blush score grade

Blush score grade	Blush (contrast opacification)
Blush score 0	No blush in the myocardial area
Blush score 1	Minimal blush or persistent stain without contrast clear-out
Blush score 2	Moderate blush, with slow contrast clear-out
Blush score 3	Normal blush with rapid contrast clear-out

to normal following successful reopening of the IRA. There are hypotheses that this impaired flow in the non-involved arteries may be caused by necrosis in shared microvasculature or vasoconstriction in the vascular bed. Residual stenoses will also play an important role in this mechanism.

Myocardial Blush Score (Grade) for Myocardial Perfusion (Table 6.3)

Normal epicardial blood flow achieved during primary PCI in acute MI is not always associated with restored microvascular perfusion. Myocardial perfusion can be assessed using the myocardial blush score (MBS). This is based on the presence of contrast density (described as blush) in the distal microvasculature of the downstream myocardium after passage through the epicardial coronary artery. To assess the MBS precisely, angiographic runs should be long enough to allow careful visualization of the contrast density within the infarct area. MBS also provides information about myocardial viability during angioplasty. The restoration of normal myocardial perfusion following PCI is associated with increased survival.

The presence of a blush is an independent predictor of infarct size, LV function and survival after reperfusion therapy. The lower the MBS (0 or 1), the higher is the mortality and the larger the infarct size. Multivessel disease or acute anterior wall myocardial infarction is generally associated with a larger myocardial infarction, and in these patients, MBG 0 or 1 is more common. Minimal or no blush indicates lack of tissue perfusion in the area at risk.

Blush score 0 is considered as the absence of contrast opacification in the myocardial area at risk. Contrast fails to enter the microvasculature; there is either minimal or no blush or opacification of the myocardium in the segment of the IRA, indicating a lack of perfusion.

Blush score 1 describes the presence of minimal contrast opacification. Contrast slowly enters but fails to exit the microvasculature; there is blush or opacification of the myocardium in the segment of the IRA that fails to clear from the microvasculature, and contrast staining is still visible on the next injection (approximately 30 s between injections).

Blush score 2 refers to moderate contrast opacification. Contrast entry and exit from the microvasculature is delayed; there is blush or opacification of the myocardium in the segment of the IRA that is strongly persistent at the end of the washout phase. Contrast is still clearly visible after a couple of cardiac cycles, and either does not diminish or only minimally diminishes intensity during washout.

Blush score 3 represents normal contrast opacification with adequate contrast entry and exit from the microvasculature. The opacification of the myocardium clears normally and is similar to that in the non-infarct-related coronary artery. Blush or opacification of the myocardium in the IRA clears normally. Blush that is of only mild intensity throughout the washout phase but fades minimally is also classified as grade 3 Fig. 6.9.

Angiographic Perfusion Score (APS) (Table 6.4) **[60]**

This is a simple angiographic score that combines both epicardial and myocardial perfusion. The score is the sum of TIMI flow graded from 0 to 3 and myocardial blush score graded from 0 to 3. Successful perfusion is describe as APS 10–12, whereas failed perfusion as APS 0–3. Angiographic perfusion score is clinically relevant and should be used before and after PCI. The results are associated with infarct size and mortality.

Conclusion

It will be seen that there is no ideal angiographic scoring system for assessing reperfusion. TIMI flow and myocardial blush grading have the advantage of being simple and instantaneous. Attempts to grade microvascular perfusion often involve combining more than one variable such as TIMI flow and myocardial blush grade possibly with the addition of ST resolution. Myocardial contrast echocardiography

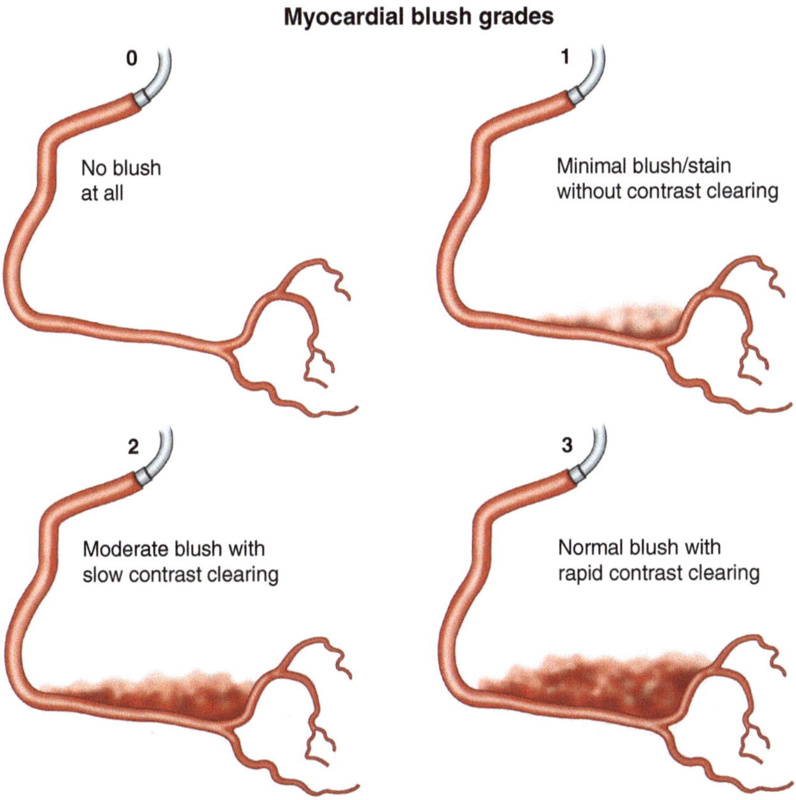

Fig. 6.9 Myocardial blush grade (MBG). MBG *0*: no blush. MBG *1*: minimal blush present or persistent contrast stain. MBG *2*: contrast persists but is gone by next injection. MBG *3*: normal appearance of blush. Rapid contrast clear-out

Table 6.4 Angiographic perfusion score [60]

APS grade	Perfusion
APS 0–3	No perfusion
APS 4–9	Partial perfusion
APS 10–12	Full perfusion

and CMR could be used more as they provide valuable information, but the logistics of providing CMR in the acute infarct setting are considerable.

As well as difficulties in quantitating reperfusion, there are additional difficulties in preventing and treating reperfusion injury. Research has confirmed that this is a complex multifactorial problem. The large number of drugs tried in this condition testifies to our very limited success in managing it. Although primary percutaneous coronary intervention has had a huge impact on infarct mortality, this could be reduced still further if no reflow and reperfusion injury could be prevented. In addition, the resulting preservation of LV function would help prevent late infarct complications and heart failure.

References

1. De Lemos J, Braunwald E. ST segment resolution as a tool for assessing the efficacy of reperfusion therapy. J Am Coll Cardiol. 2001;38:1283–94.
2. Kumar S, Sivagangabalan G, Hsieh C, Ryding AD, Narayan A, Chan H, Burgess DC, Ong AT, Sadick N, Kovoor P. Predictive value of ST resolution analysis performed immediately versus at ninety minutes after primary percutaneous coronary intervention. Am J Cardiol. 2010;105(4):467–74.
3. Sejersten M, Valeur N, Grande P, Nielsen TT, Clemmensen P, DANAMI-2 Investigators. Long-term prognostic value of ST-segment resolution in patients treated with fibrinolysis or primary percutaneous coronary intervention results from the DANAMI-2 (Danish trial in acute myocardial infarction-2). J Am Coll Cardiol. 2009;54(19):1763–9.
4. Buller CE, Westerhout CM, Armstrong PW. ST-segment resolution and outcome in myocardial infarction. J Am Coll Cardiol. 2010;55(15):1646–7.
5. Buller CE, Fu Y, Mahaffey KW, Todaro TG, Adams P, et al. ST segment recovery and outcome after primary percutaneous coronary intervention for ST- elevation myocardial infarction: insights from the assessment of the pexelizumab in acute myocardial infarction (APEX-AMI trial). Circulation. 2008;118:1335–46.
6. Sorajja P, Gersh BJ, Costantini C, McLaughlin MG, et al. Combined prognostic utility of ST-segment recovery and myocardial blush after primary percutaneous coronary intervention in acute myocardial infarction. Eur Heart J. 2005;26(7):667–74. Epub 2005 Feb 25.
7. Nijveldt R, Beek AM, Hirsch A, Stoel MG, et al. Functional recovery after acute myocardial infarction. Comparison between angiography, electrocardiography, and cardiovascular magnetic resonance measures of microvascular injury. J Am Coll Cardiol. 2008;52:181–9.
8. Wu KC, Zerhouni EA, Judd RM, Lugo-Olivieri CH, et al. Prognostic significance of microvascular obstruction by magnetic resonance imaging in patients with acute myocardial infarction. Circulation. 1998;97:765–72.
9. Galiuto L, Garramore B, Scara A, Rebuzzi AG, for the AMICI investigators, et al. The extent of microvascular damage during myocardial contrast echocardiography is superior to other known indexes of post-infarct reperfusion in predicting left ventricular remodeling: results of the AMICI study. J Am Coll Cardiol. 2008;51:552–9.
10. Mehta RH, Starr AZ, Lopes RD, Hochman JS, for the APEX-AMI investigators, et al. Incidence of and outcomes associated with ventricular tachycardia or fibrillation in patients undergoing primary percutaneous coronary intervention. JAMA. 2009;301:1779–89.
11. Keeley EC, Boura JA, Grines CL. Primary angioplasty versus intravenous thrombolytic therapy for acute myocardial infarction: a quantitative review of 23 randomised trials. Lancet. 2003;361:13–20.
12. Gershlick AH, Stephens-Lloyd A, Hughes S, Abrams KR, (For the REACT trial investigators), et al. Rescue angioplasty after failed thrombolytic therapy for acute myocardial infarction. N Engl J Med. 2005;353:2758–68.
13. DiMario C, Dudek D, Piscione F, Mielecki W, et al. Immediate angioplasty versus standard therapy with rescue angioplasty after thrombolysis in the Combined Abciximab REteplase Stent Study in acute myocardial infarction. (CARESS in AMI). An open prospective randomized trial. Lancet. 2008;371:559–68.
14. Van't Hof AW, Ernst N, de Boer MJ, de Winter R, On-TIME study group, et al. Facilitation of primary coronary angioplasty by early start of a glycoprotein 2b/3a inhibitor. Results of the ongoing tirofiban in myocardial infarction evaluation (On-TIME) trial. Eur Heart J. 2004;25:837–46.
15. Gibson CM, Kirtane AJ, Murphy SA, Rohrbeck S, et al. Early initiation of eptifibatide in the emergency department before primary percutaneous coronary intervention for ST segment elevation myocardial infarction: results of the Time to Integrilin Therapy in Acute Myocardial Infarction (TITAN)-TIMI 34 trial. Am Heart J. 2006;152(4):668–75.

16. ASSENT-4 PCI Investigators. Assessment of the safety and efficacy of a new treatment strategy with percutaneous coronary intervention. Primary versus tenecteplase-facilitated percutaneous coronary intervention in patients with ST-segment elevation acute myocardial infarction (ASSENT-4 PCI): randomised trial. Lancet. 2006;367:569–78.
17. Ellis SG, Tendera M, de Belder MA, van Boven AJ, for the FINESSE investigators, et al. Facilitated PCI in patients with ST elevation myocardial infarction. N Engl J Med. 2008;358:2205–17.
18. De Luca G. Overview of contemporary reperfusion strategies in acute ST-elevation myocardial infarction. Cardiol Int. 2007;8:92–8.
19. Dzielicka E, Swanton H. Optimal reperfusion strategy for acute myocardial infarction. Br J Hosp Med (Lond). 2008;69(1):18–23.
20. Svilaas T, Vlaar PJ, van der Horst IC, Diercks GFH, et al. Thrombus aspiration during primary percutaneous coronary intervention. TAPAS trial. N Engl J Med. 2008;358:557–67.
21. Spaulding C, Teiger E, Commeau P, Varenne O, et al. Four year follow up of TYPHOON (trial to assess the use of cypher sirolimus-eluting coronary stent in acute myocardial infarction treated with balloon angioplasty). J Am Coll Cardiol. 2011;4:14–23.
22. Dangas G, for the HORIZONS-AMI trial investigators. Role of clopidogrel loading dose on patients with ST segment elevation myocardial infarction undergoing primary angioplasty: results from the HORIZONS-AMI (Harmonising Outcomes with Revascularisation and Stents in Acute Myocardial Infarction) trial. J Am Coll Cardiol. 2009;54:1438.
23. Freedman J, Hylek E. Clopidogrel, genetics, and drug responsiveness. N Eng J Med. 2009;360:411–3.
24. Wiviott SD, Braunwald E, McCabe CH, Montalescot G, for the TRITON-TIMI 38 investigators, et al. Prasugrel versus clopidogrel in patients with acute coronary syndromes. N Engl J Med. 2007;357:2001–15.
25. Ho PM, Maddox TM, Wang L, Fihn SD, Jesse RL, Peterson ED, Rumsfeld JS. Risk of adverse outcomes associated with concomitant use of clopidogrel and proton pump inhibitors following acute coronary syndrome. JAMA. 2009;301(9):937–44.
26. Bhatt DL, Cryer BL, Contant CF, Cohen M, for the COGENT investigators, et al. Clopidogrel with or without omeprazole in coronary artery disease. N Engl J Med. 2010; 363:1909–17.
27. Montalescot G, Wiviott S, Braunwald E, Murphy SA, et al. Prasugrel compared with clopidogrel in patients undergoing percutaneous coronary intervention for ST-elevation myocardial infarction (TRITON-TIMI 38): double blind randomised control trial. Lancet. 2009;373:723–32.
28. Bhatt DL, Lincoff AM, Gibson CM, Stone GW, for the CHAMPION PLATFORM investigators, et al. Intravenous platelet blockade with cangrelor during PCI. N Engl J Med. 2009;361:2330–41.
29. Wallentin L, Becker RC, Budaj A, Cannon CP, for the PLATO investigators, et al. Ticagrelor versus clopidogrel in patients with acute coronary syndromes. N Engl J Med. 2009;361:1045–57.
30. Niccoli G, Burzotta F, Galiuto L, Crea F. Myocardial no reflow in humans. J Am Coll Cardiol. 2009;54:281–92.
31. Niccoli G, Kharbanda RK, Crea F, Banning A. No reflow: again prevention is better than treatment. Eur Heart J. 2010;31(20):2449–55.
32. Kharbanda RK. Cardiac conditioning: a review of evolving strategies to reduce ischaemia-reperfusion injury. Heart. 2010;96(15):1179–86.
33. Burzotta F, Testa L, Giannico F, Biondi-Zoccai GG, et al. Adjunctive devices in primary or rescue PCI: a meta-analysis of randomised trials. Int J Cardiol. 2008;123:313–21.
34. Galiuto L, Garramore B, Burzotta F, Lombardo A, For the REMEDIA investigators, et al. Thrombus aspiration reduces microvascular obstruction after primary coronary intervention: a myocardial contrast echocardiographic substudy of the REMEDIA trial. J Am Coll Cardiol. 2006;48:1355–60.

35. Stone GW, Webb J, Cox DA, Brodie BR, For the: enhanced myocardial efficacy and recovery by aspiration of liberated debris (EMERALD) investigators, et al. Distal microcirculatory protection during percutaneous coronary intervention in acute ST-segment elevation myocardial infarction: a randomized controlled trial. JAMA. 2005;293:1063–72.
36. Kaltoft A, Kelbaek H, Klovgaard L, Terkelsen CJ, Clemmensen P, Helqvist S, Lassen JF, Theusen L. Increased rate of stent thrombosis and target lesion revascularisation after filter protection in primary percutaneous coronary intervention for ST segment elevation myocardial infarction: 15 month follow up of the DEDICATION (Drug Elution and Distal protection in ST Elevation Myocardial Infarction) trial. J Am Coll Cardiol. 2010;55:867–71.
37. Petronio AS, De Carlo M, Ciabtatti N, Amoroso G, et al. Left ventricular remodeling after primary coronary angioplasty in patients treated with abciximab or intracoronary adenosine. Am Heart J. 2005;150:1015.
38. Thiele H, Schinder K, Freudenberger J, Eitel I, et al. Intracoronary compared with intravenous bolus abciximab application in patients with ST- elevation myocardial infarction undergoing primary coronary intervention: the randomised Leipzig immediate percutaneous coronary intervention abciximab iv versus i.c in ST elevation myocardial infarct trial. Circulation. 2008;118:49–57.
39. Iwakura K, Ito H, Kawano S, Okamura A, Kurotobi T, Date M, Inoue K, Fujii K. Chronic pretreatment with statins is associated with a reduction of the no-reflow phenomenon in the patients with reperfused myocardial infarction. Eur Heart J. 2006;27(5):534–9.
40. Iwakura K, Ito H, Ikushima M, Kawano S, et al. Association between hyperglycaemia and the no-reflow phenomenon in patients with acute myocardial infarction. J Am Coll Cardiol. 2003;41:1–7.
41. Malmberg K, Ryden L, Efendic S, Herlitz J, et al. Randomised trial of insulin-glucose infusion followed by subcutaneous insulin treatment in diabetic patients with acute myocardial infarction (DIGAMI study). Effects on mortality at 1 year. J Am Coll Cardiol. 1995;26:56–65.
42. Ito H, Taniyama Y, Iwakura K, Nishikawa N, et al. Intravenous nicorandil can preserve microvascular integrity and myocardial viability in patients with reperfused anterior wall myocardial infarction. J Am Coll Cardiol. 1999;33:654–60.
43. Ishii H, Ichimiya S, Kanashiro M, Amano T, Imai K, Murohara T, Matsubara T. Impact of a single intravenous administration of nicorandil before reperfusion in patients with ST-segment-elevation myocardial infarction. Circulation. 2005;112:1284–8.
44. Amit G, Cafri C, Yaroslavstev S, Fuchs S, et al. Intracoronary nitroprusside for the prevention of the no reflow phenomenon after primary percutaneous coronary intervention in acute myocardial infarction. A randomised double blind placebo controlled clinical trial. Am Heart J. 2006;152:887 e9–14.
45. Marzilli M, Orsini E, Marraccini P, Testa R. Beneficial effects of intracoronary adenosine as an adjunct to primary angioplasty in acute myocardial infarction. Circulation. 2000;101:2154–9.
46. Mahaffey KW, Puma JA, Barbagelata NA, DiCarli MF, for the AMISTAD investigators, et al. Adenosine as an adjunct to thrombolytic therapy for acute myocardial infarction. J Am Coll Cardiol. 1999;34:1711–20.
47. Ross A, Gibbons RJ, Stone GW, Kloner RA, Alexander RW, for the AMISTAD II investigators. A randomised double blinded controlled multicenter trial of adenosine as an adjunct to reperfusion in the treatment of acute myocardial infarction (AMISTAD II). J Am Coll Cardiol. 2005;45:1775–80.
48. Werner GS, Lang K, Kuehnert H, Figulla HR. Intracoronary verapamil for reversal of no-reflow during coronary angioplasty for acute myocardial infarction. Catheter Cardiovasc Interv. 2002;57:444–51.
49. Piot C, Croisille P, Staat P, Thibault H, et al. Effect of cyclosporine on reperfusion injury in acute myocardial infarction. N Engl J Med. 2008;359:473–81.
50. Mewton N, Croisille P, Gahide G, Rioufol G, et al. Effect of cyclosporine on left ventricular remodeling after reperfused myocardial infarction. J Am Coll Cardiol. 2010;55:1200–5.

51. Kitakaze M, Asakura M, Kim J, Shintani Y, et al. Human atrial natriuretic peptide and nicorandil as adjuncts to reperfusion treatment for acute myocardial infarction (J-WIND). Two randomised trials. Lancet. 2007;370:1483–93.
52. Reimer KA, Jennings RB. The wavefront phenomenon of myocardial ischaemic cell death II. Transmural progression of necrosis within the framework of ischaemic bed size (myocardium at risk) and collateral flow. Lab Invest. 1979;40:633–44.
53. Hochman JS, Lamas GA, Buller CE, Dzavik V, for the Occluded Artery Trial investigators, et al. Coronary intervention for persistent occlusion after myocardial infarction. N Engl J Med. 2006;355:2395–407.
54. Alderman EL, Stadius M. The angiographic definitions of the by-pass angioplasty revascularisation investigation. Coron Artery Dis. 1992;3:1189–207.
55. Graham MM, Faris PD, Ghali WA, Galbraith PD, et al. Validation of three myocardial jeopardy scores in a population based cardiac catheterization cohort. Am Heart J. 2001;142: 254–61.
56. Ortiz-Perez JT, Meyers SN, Lee DC, Kansal P, et al. Angiographic estimates of myocardium at risk during acute myocardial infarction: validation study using cardiac magnetic resonance imaging. Eur Heart J. 2007;28:1750–8.
57. Gerber BL. Risk area, infarct size and the exposure of the wavefront phenomenon of myocardial necrosis in humans. Eur Heart J. 2007;28:1670–2.
58. Gibbons RJ, Holmes DR, Reeder GS, Bailey KR, Hopfenspirger MR, Gersh BJ. Immediate angioplasty compared with the administration of a thrombolytic agent followed by conservative treatment for myocardial infarction. N Engl J Med. 1993;328:685–91.
59. Appleby MA, Michaels AD, Chen NY, Gibson MC. Importance of the TIMI frame count: implications for future trials. Curr Control Trials Cardiovasc Med. 2000;1:31–4.
60. Gibson CM, Murphy SA, Morrow DA, Aroesty JM, Gibbons RJ, Gourlay SG, Barron HV, Giugliano RP, Antman EM, Braunwald E. Angiographic perfusion score: an angiographic variable that integrates both epicardial and tissue level perfusion before and after facilitated percutaneous coronary intervention in acute myocardial infarction. Am Heart J. 2004;148(2): 336–40.

Chapter 7
Echocardiography in Myocardial Reperfusion Injury

Mariana Mirabel and Denis Pellerin

Abstract Assessment of all parameters related to myocardial reperfusion injury can be obtained by echocardiography, an ultrasound-based, noninvasive, radiation-free, and widely available imaging technique. Echocardiography allows the measurement of left ventricular regional and global function, of the area at risk and the infarct size, and estimates microvascular flow. Two-dimensional echocardiography can be used either at the patient's bedside, either in isolation or combined to contrast agents and/or to dobutamine. The advent of three-dimensional echocardiography and Doppler strain, strain rate, and non-Doppler strain has more recently broadened the possibilities to assess myocardial reperfusion injury.

Keywords Ischemic heart disease • Myocardial reperfusion injury • Myocardial stunning • Microvascular obstruction • No-reflow phenomenon • Reperfusion arrhythmias • Lethal myocardial reperfusion injury • Cardiomyocyte death Echocardiography • Tissue Doppler velocity • Myocardial deformation imaging Doppler strain • Strain rate • Non-Doppler strain • Speckle tracking • Three-dimensional echocardiography • Contrast cavity opacification • Myocardial contrast echocardiography • Coronary flow reserve • Molecular ultrasound imaging

M. Mirabel, M.D.
Department of Cardiology, The Heart Hospital, University College London Hospitals, London, UK

Paris Cardiovascular Research Center, 4, rue du Pont Neuf, Paris 75001, France
e-mail: mariana.mirabel@inserm.fr

D. Pellerin, M.D., Ph.D. (✉)
Department of Cardiology, The Heart Hospital, University College London Hospitals, 16 Westmoreland Street, London W1G 8PH, UK
e-mail: denis.pellerin@uclh.nhs.uk

J.C. Kaski et al. (eds.), *Management of Myocardial Reperfusion Injury*,
DOI 10.1007/978-1-84996-019-9_7, © Springer-Verlag London 2012

Introduction

Ischemic heart disease is a major global health problem in developed and emerging countries [1]. Recognition of the prognostic relevance of malignant arrhythmias during the acute phase of myocardial infarction (MI) prompted the creation of intensive coronary care units in the 1950s and 1960s. After successful resolution of acute phase arrhythmias, it became clear that the extent of myocardial necrosis was a major determinant of long-term prognosis. Direct restoration of vessel patency in acute MI by thrombolysis and primary percutaneous coronary intervention (PCI) has undoubtedly had a major effect on outcomes. Nonetheless, clinical experience of coronary reperfusion has demonstrated that in approximately 50% of the patients, left ventricular dysfunction persists to a greater or lesser degree with a major impact upon both early and late outcomes. In many such patients, patency of the infarct-related artery is present, but there is a discrepancy between restoration of patency and myocardial perfusion. In this respect, evolving concepts including lethal reperfusion injury, microvascular dysfunction, "no-reflow" phenomenon, stunned myocardium, and hibernating myocardium have become the target of basic research and clinical investigation. Moreover, reperfusion itself is a cause of end-organ damage and accounts for a significant part of mortality and morbidity due to acute coronary syndromes.

Recent studies demonstrated that myocardial reperfusion injury results in four major categories (albeit interrelated) of cardiac dysfunction: myocardial stunning, which relates to a temporary dysfunction; no-reflow phenomenon due to a combination of endothelial dysfunction and microvascular obstruction in spite of epicardial coronary artery patency; reperfusion arrhythmias; and lethal myocardial reperfusion injury related to increased cardiomyocyte death secondary to the reperfusion itself. Therefore, the focus is on therapies that improve myocardial perfusion, promote functional recovery of viable muscle, and reduce infarct expansion.

Echocardiography is a noninvasive imaging technique that can be performed at the patient's bedside. Diagnostic capabilities have increased exponentially as a result of technical innovation. Several cardiac ultrasound imaging modalities are now available including two-dimensional imaging, tissue Doppler velocity, myocardial deformation imaging including myocardial Doppler strain and strain rate and myocardial non-Doppler strain, three-dimensional echocardiography, contrast cavity opacification, myocardial contrast echocardiography, coronary flow reserve, and molecular ultrasound imaging. Most modalities can be combined at rest and during stress. Echocardiography assesses myocardial stunning through regional wall motion abnormalities, microvascular obstruction is addressed by myocardial contrast perfusion echocardiography and coronary flow measurements, and lethal myocardial injury and cardiomyocyte death after reperfusion therapy are estimated by measuring the infarct size. This chapter reviews cardiac ultrasound imaging modalities and discusses currently available quantification tools and clinical applications that are relevant for the assessment of myocardial reperfusion injury, pre- and postconditioning.

Cardiac Ultrasound Imaging Modalities

Transthoracic echocardiography is the most widely available, radiation-free, and cost-effective cardiac imaging technique. It can be performed at the bedside during the acute phase of MI and can be repeated as many times as deemed necessary. Multiple technical advances during the past 20 years have significantly improved image quality. Echocardiography provides valuable information on LV cavity size and global and regional function and detects mechanical complications during the acute phase of MI. Echocardiography techniques have been developed to measure both the area at risk and the infarct size. Quantification of microcirculatory obstruction within the area at risk can also be obtained.

Left Ventricular Diameters, Volumes, and Global Ejection Fraction by Two-Dimensional Echocardiography

Assessment of global LV systolic function is paramount in risk stratification of patients with coronary artery disease, particularly after MI. Left ventricular global ejection fraction (LVEF) adds incremental value to clinical scores in predicting mortality [2]. The American and the European Societies of Echocardiography released documents to standardize LVEF assessment methods and, therefore, improve reproducibility among laboratories [3, 4].

Linear methods based on M-mode or bidimensional measurements from the parasternal long-axis view were first used. Although linear methods including the Teichholz method proved to be feasible and reproducible, they present major limitations in case of regional wall motion abnormalities [5].

Bidimensional LV volume methods proved to be more accurate than linear methods when compared to LV angiography. The most commonly used 2D measurement for LV volumes is the biplane method of disks or modified Simpson's rule (Fig. 7.1). For many years, Simpson's biplane method has been the most reliable noninvasive, non-irradiating method to quantify LVEF. Simpson's biplane method has been recommended by consensus in recent international echocardiography guidelines [3, 4]. Left ventricular remodeling is appreciated by measuring LV volumes.

Limitations of two-dimensional echocardiography in this situation are image quality partially due to the fact it is an operator-dependent technique. Observer variability in the assessment of LV volumes and global LVEF was due to the difficulty to visualize the endocardial border of the LV lateral and anterior walls, which are often located at the edge of the image sector.

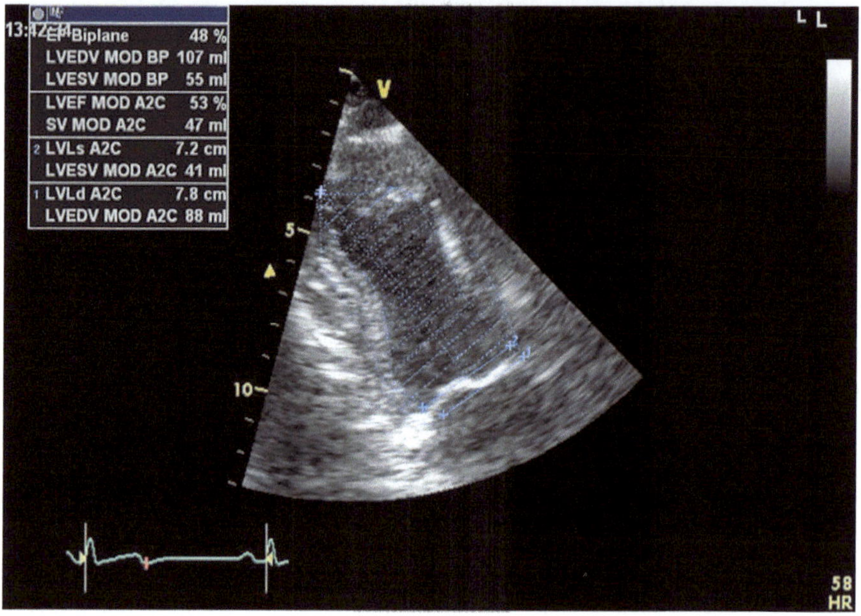

Fig. 7.1 Apical two-chamber view in end-systole in a patient with recent anterior MI and mild global LV systolic impairment according to LVEF by the Simpson's biplane method (48%)

Regional Wall Motion Assessment

Although the size of the infarct is a predominant factor in left ventricular dysfunction post-infarction, it is not the only aspect to be considered. Echocardiography has good temporal resolution allowing accurate and reproducible regional wall motion assessment. Thirty years ago, 2D echocardiography showed high sensitivity in detecting infarcted segments when compared to postmortem histology [6]. Wall motion score index (WMSI) has been widely used in an attempt to quantify regional abnormalities [7, 8]. Nomenclature standardization of myocardial segments makes possible intra- and inter-modality comparisons. Segments are scored as normal (score 1), hypokinetic (score 2), akinetic (score 3), or dyskinetic (score 4). Extent and severity of regional wall motion abnormalities at the acute phase of MI is well correlated with hemodynamic LV function. WMSI is a powerful 1-year mortality predictor after MI.

Regional wall motion abnormalities at rest after acute MI are due to a combination of infarcted and stunned myocardium. Differentiating viable from nonviable myocardium at an early stage is challenging. WMSI at rest at an early stage of MI is unable to accurately predict recovery and appreciate the transmural extent of necrosis [9, 10]. In contrast, 3 days after the acute phase or later, low-dose dobutamine infusion provides valuable information on myocardial viability as recommended by the American Heart Association [11]. Image quality and reader experience are key factors in interpreting wall motion abnormalities during dobutamine stress echocardiogram.

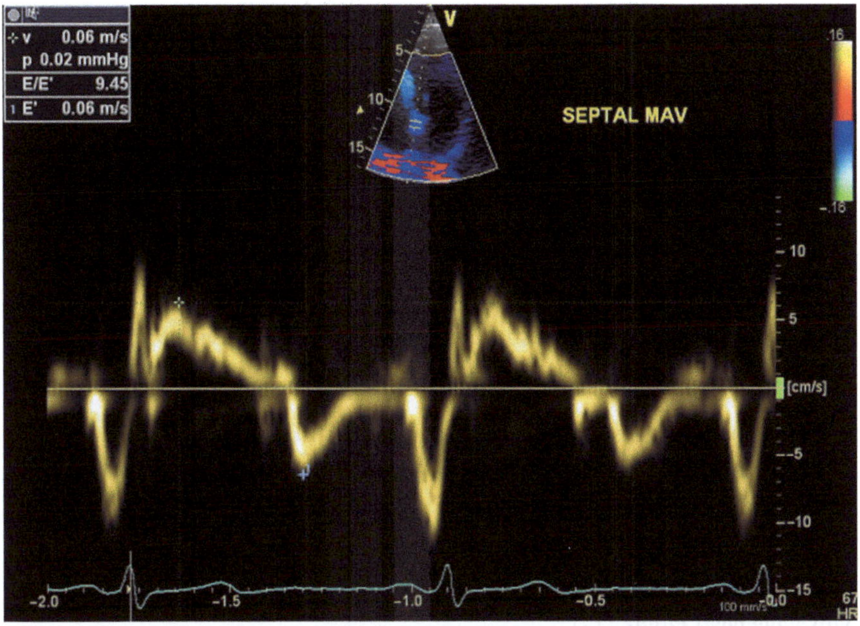

Fig. 7.2 Septal mitral annular velocity (*MAV*) recording. Calipers are located at peak systole measuring peak systolic mitral annular velocity 0.06 m/s and at early diastole (*E*′) also measuring 0.06 m/s. The ratio between peak early diastolic transmitral inflow velocity (*E*) and peak early septal mitral annular velocity (*E*′) is calculated at 9.45

Tissue Doppler Velocity

Tissue Doppler echocardiography is a real-time ultrasound technique that provides an objective mean to quantify global and regional left and right ventricular wall motions with high temporal and spatial resolution [12]. This modality is angle dependent and apical segments cannot be reliably analyzed. The main application of this imaging modality at present is the measurement of mitral annular velocity along the LV long axis to assess longitudinal LV systolic and diastolic functions [13, 14]. A quick and easy assessment of LVEF is obtained by mitral annular velocity measurement during a routine study, especially in patients with poor endocardial definition or abnormal septal motion (Fig. 7.2). Limitations are mitral annular calcification and severe mitral regurgitation.

Doppler Strain and Strain Rate and Non-Doppler Strain

Temporal resolution of the human eye is insufficient to detect events shorter than 90 ms such as postsystolic shortening [15]. Over the last decade, strain and strain rate imaging have emerged as valuable tools in quantifying LV function. Strain rate measures the rate of deformation of a myocardial segment and is measured in s^{-1}. Strain represents deformation of a myocardial segment over time. Strain is expressed as the percent change from the original dimension. Two modalities have been successively developed for the assessment of myocardial strain: color myocardial Doppler and speckle tracking. Color Doppler myocardial imaging is derived from myocardial velocities, while speckle tracking relies on natural ultrasound reflectors within the myocardium recorded during conventional imaging. Unlike Doppler strain, speckle tracking strain is not angle dependent, and therefore apical segments can be interrogated [12]. Speckle tracking provides information on radial, circumferential, and longitudinal deformation in real time. Cardiac motion is a complex mechanism that also includes torsion. Cyclic tissue compression and compound directions of myocardial fibers account for longitudinal and circumferential motion.

Global longitudinal strain correlates well with LVEF measured by magnetic resonance imaging (MRI) [16]. Several studies have shown the prognostic implication of speckle tracking strain in a wide range of cardiac conditions [17–20]. Longitudinal global systolic strain adds significant power into a model predicting mortality among a large unselected population [18]. When compared to 2D LVEF by the Simpson's method, global circumferential strain accurately predicted cardiac events in patients with acute heart failure [17].

In patients with coronary artery disease, strain rate and strain are particularly accurate in detecting subendocardial dysfunction [21]. The use of strain increases ischemia detection during stress echocardiography in experimental and clinical studies [22–24].

Studies have shown a good correlation between strain values and final infarct size. Weidemann and colleagues showed in an experimental model that radial peak systolic strain rate and systolic strain could differentiate non-transmural from transmural MI and estimate infarct size (Fig. 7.3). At rest, values were higher in the non-transmural MI group and increased slightly at low-dose dobutamine compared to unchanged values in the transmural MI regions [25]. In humans, global longitudinal systolic strain at rest early after MI correlates well with final infarct size measured by MRI [26–28]. Sjøli and coworkers found that global longitudinal strain with a cutoff value of −15% yields a higher sensitivity than LVEF in identifying large myocardial infarcts defined as late gadolinium enhancement of >20% of the myocardium by MRI [27]. Peak systolic strain and strain rate early after MI can precisely detect ischemic segments and accurately predict transmurality immediately after PCI [29]. Similarly Hoffmann and colleagues found that an increase in peak systolic strain rate (cutoff value −0.23/s) during low-dose dobutamine infusion discriminates viable from nonviable myocardium, as determined by 18F-fluorodeoxyglucose positron emission tomography with a sensitivity of 83% and a specificity of 84% [30]. The increment of strain rate during low-dose dobutamine in combination with WMSI predicts regional wall motion recovery after revascularization at 9 months follow-up [31]. In addition, longitudinal peak systolic strain at the acute phase of anterior MI predicts LV remodeling defined by LV enlargement [32].

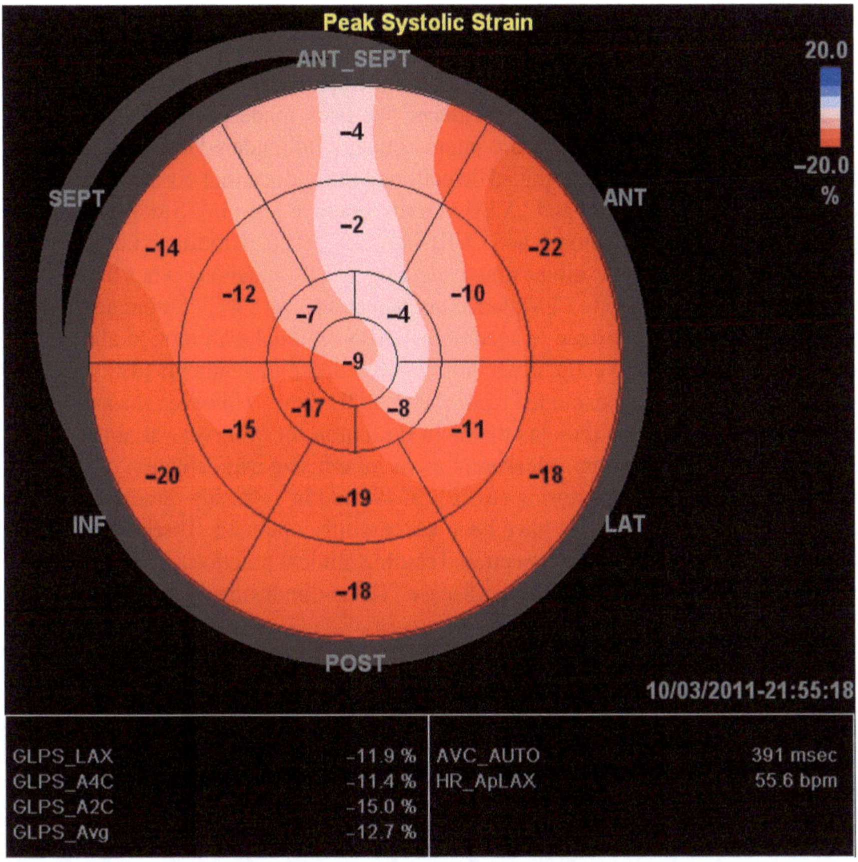

Fig. 7.3 Bull's eye representation of longitudinal peak systolic strain obtained from 2D apical views (4-, 2-, and 3-chamber views) by speckle tracking in a patient with a late presentation of anterior MI. In this case, peak systolic regional values were markedly reduced in the antero septum and resulted in global severe LV systolic impairment (global longitudinal strain –12.7%)

Speckle tracking strain imaging is a relatively recent, easy to perform, and already robust technique to quantify global and regional LV dysfunction. The ability of strain imaging to quantify regional myocardial function might overcome the limitations due to the reader's expertise. However, current post-processing analysis precludes from accurate analysis during exercise when heart rate is higher than 130/min [33].

Three-Dimensional Echocardiography

LV volumes and LVEF can be obtained by full volume acquisition of a three-dimensional left ventricular dataset. Three-dimensional echo measurements do not rely on artificially set 2D planes, avoiding geometric assumptions and errors caused by 2D foreshortened views. Early 3D technology required long and cumbersome off-line analysis. Engineering progress has dramatically improved its feasibility. The advent of a fully sampled matrix array transducer has been made possible by means of ultrasound, electronic, and software improvement with rendered online 3D images. Improvement of 3D semi-automated detection of the endocardial border has allowed us to measure LV volumes and LVEF in daily practice [34, 35]. Studies showed a good correlation in LV volumes and LVEF between 3D echo, radionuclide imaging, and MRI [36–39]. Three-dimensional imaging is advantageous when measuring volumes in case of distorted LV shape and aneurysms [40, 41]. Automated border detection process also proved to accurately detect regional wall motion abnormalities during real-time 3D echo, especially in basal and mid-segments [42], and may visualize parts of the LV excluded from classical 2D views. However, the automated border detection process remains the main limitation for observer variability when image quality is suboptimal. Measurement of infarct size and detection of regional wall motion abnormalities during stress [43, 44] and in assessing remote preconditioning during acute MI [45] have been successfully obtained. Three-dimensional echocardiography has already penetrated routine clinical practice and carries promising applications in ischemic heart disease. Three-dimensional echocardiography may gradually replace 2D echo in the future.

Contrast Cavity Opacification

Contrast cavity opacification is used to improve image quality during conventional 2D and during triplane imaging using a 3D probe (Fig. 7.4). A bolus injection of ultrasound contrast agent is administered in a peripheral vein. Ultrasound contrast agents are intravascular contrast agents, as the vessel wall is not permeable for microbubbles. Contrast microbubbles are smaller than red blood cells and cross lungs capillaries to opacity the LV cavity. Using modified settings including low frame rate, harmonic imaging, and low mechanical index, the myocardium appears black and the LV cavity is white. Contrast cavity opacification is based on the ability of microbubbles to remain stable within the vascular space. Second generation microbubbles contain high molecular weight gases that do not dissolve rapidly in the blood. Enhanced images last on average for 3 min in humans.

Myocardial Contrast Echocardiography

A team of investigators headed by Kevin Wei and Sanjiv Kaul at the University of Virginia, USA, made the landmark discovery that these ultrasound triggering techniques could be utilized to quantify myocardial blood flow, and examine the components responsible for myocardial blood flow [46]. This has led to clinical studies

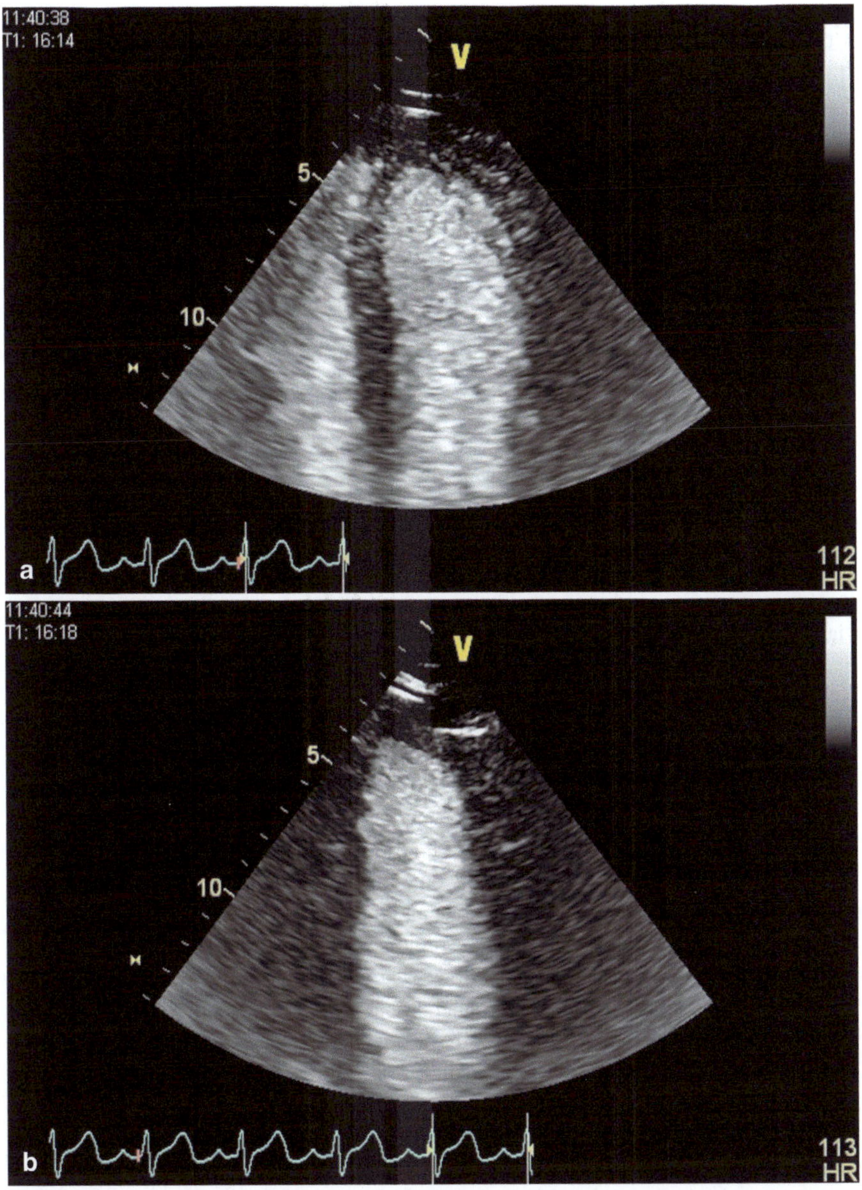

Fig. 7.4 Three apical 2D chamber views (**a**: 4 chamber view; **b**: 2 chamber view; **c**: 3 chamber view) using contrast cavity opacification to improve endocardial border detection, and thus, regional wall motion assessment in a patient with suboptimal image quality. Contrast cavity opacification can be used at rest and during stress

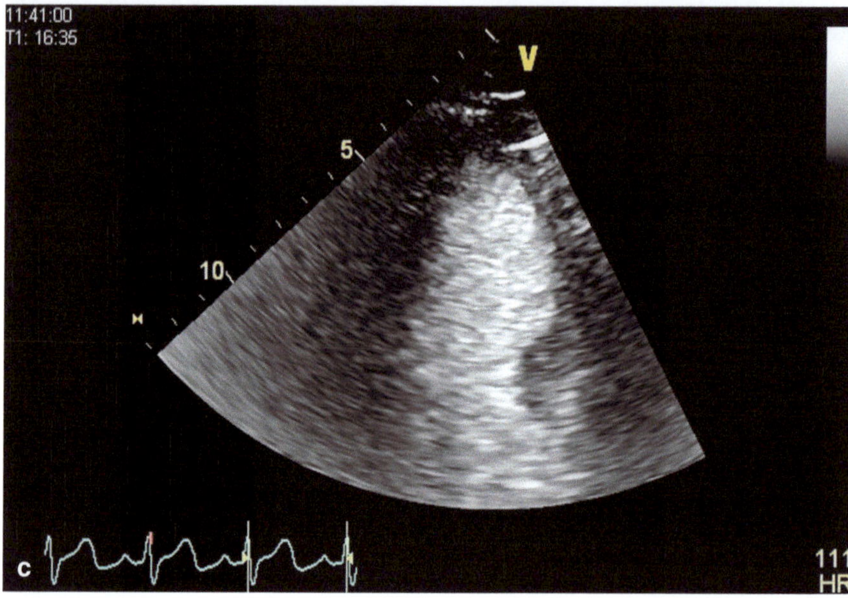

Fig 7.4 (continued)

demonstrating that myocardial contrast echocardiography (MCE) could visualize both the hypoperfused myocardium and regional wall motion abnormalities in acute coronary syndromes and chronic coronary artery disease. Direct visualization of myocardial microcirculation during MI experimental models was obtained by intracoronary injection of sonicated microbubbles and identified the area at risk and the final myocardial infarct size. Contrast defects on echocardiography obtained before coronary reflow denote the size of the risk area, and those obtained after successful epicardial coronary artery angioplasty denote regions of no-reflow [47, 48]. Engineering progress translated intracoronary injection to using venous administration by continuous infusion of contrast agents with transthoracic echocardiography [49–51].

High mechanical pulse (flash) destroys microbubbles in the myocardium, and one measures the delay before myocardial replenishment. The time-varying image intensity $\tilde{a}(t)$ in a specific region of interest, which corresponds to the ultrasound contrast agent concentration, can be modeled as γ(gamma)$(t) = A(1 - \exp - \beta$(beta)$t)$, where β(beta) represents the rate of the contrast agent replenishment and A is the steady intensity in the region of interest. A β(beta) is proportional to the myocardial blood flow through the specific region of interest, and A is proportional to the myocardial blood volume in the region of interest [46]. Myocardial blood flow reserve is the difference in flow velocity between rest and pharmacologically induced stress.

Myocardial perfusion has also been assessed without dedicated quantification software by counting the number of cardiac cycles required for myocardial replenishment after flash. Myocardial replenishment is visually estimated during real-time or triggered imaging taking into account that a normally perfused myocardium is homogeneously re-opacified after a maximum of six cardiac cycles. Visual estimation discriminates normal and homogenous opacification from heterogeneous or absent contrast opacification [52].

Janardhanan and colleagues compared MCE and MRI 7–10 days after MI. They found a good inverse correlation between MCE parameters and the infarct size defined by late gadolinium enhancement in MRI. MI transmurality was accurately estimated by several qualitative (myocardial contrast intensity) and quantitative MCE parameters (peak contrast intensity, microbubble velocity, and myocardial blood flow) [53]. The same authors showed the prognostic value of viability by MCE early after MI. A qualitative contrast intensity score after microbubble destruction was used to appreciate the extent of viable myocardium in a cohort of patients without systematic revascularization. This score was found to be independently associated with hard cardiac events (cardiac death or reinfarction) at follow-up [54].

Low-dose dobutamine can be combined with MCE when assessing contractile reserve and results in further improvement of specificity and positive predictive values in detecting viable myocardium [55–57] than those of each technique.

Although MCE has been thoroughly used to measure infarct size, seldom has it been used to assess the impact of interventions on myocardial reperfusion injury. The fact that only few investigators master this technique might have prevented its use in large multicenter randomized trials.

In spite of extensive research in MCE, this technique has not become part of clinical practice in ischemic heart disease. The U.S. Food and Drug Administration has not approved the use of ultrasound contrast for myocardial perfusion imaging. Several other factors account for this including: lack of standardization in investigation protocols, machine settings, and choice of contrast agent; lack of reproducibility and prolonged learning curve [58]; and tissue attenuation. Another major problem of MCE quantification is displacement of the successive images in the recorded sequence. This is mainly due to patient's motion, ultrasound probe, and breathing [59].

Coronary Flow Reserve

Coronary flow reserve (CRF) is the ratio between maximal artery flow induced by vasodilators (i.e., adenosine or dipyridamole) and baseline artery flow. CRF is a useful tool in assessing coronary function. It provides a functional estimate of microvascular integrity downstream of the patent infarct-related vessel. The direct measure of CRF can be obtained during coronary angiography and noninvasively from off-axis apical transthoracic views [60]. CRF is used for the quantification of epicardial coronary artery stenosis and microvascular obstruction.

Accurate measures of coronary blood flow velocity at rest and during vasodilator therapy are obtained by echocardiography from the distal left anterior descending coronary artery (LAD) by a combined approach of two-dimensional imaging and Doppler [61]. Results have initially been encouraging as to feasibility and reproducibility in an unselected population including patients with large body habitus [62].

Visualization of the LAD is improved by contrast agents [63]. Echocardiography CRF is accurate in detecting epicardial LAD stenosis proven by angiography and carries prognostic information [61, 62, 64–67]. However, there are limitations to the application of echocardiography CFR in clinical practice: measurement of the coronary flow by pulse-wave Doppler often requires angle correction; difficulties to complete Doppler spectral envelope throughout the cardiac cycle due to cardiac motion; and spatial resolution is insufficient to accurately measure the vessel diameter and therefore the absolute volumetric flow. Echocardiography CRF after myocardial reperfusion has not yet been addressed with serial measurements to quantify microvascular injury.

Molecular Ultrasound Imaging

The ability to bind microbubbles to a wide range of molecules has opened the area of molecular ultrasound research. Microbubbles are injected into the body through a venous cannula, and bubble destruction is obtained only in the area of drug delivery by high intensity ultrasound signals. A myriad of targeted microbubbles have been developed extending the investigational fields from tumor neoangiogenesis to transplant rejection and myocardial infarct size [68–70].

Targeted microbubbles may offer an ultrasound imaging technique for the detection of processes characterized by endothelial dysfunction. A hallmark of ischemia-reperfusion is the activation of the inflammatory cascade. Leukocyte-bound microbubbles have been injected in atherosclerosis and ischemic-reperfusion animal models [71–75]. An excellent relation was found between the ultrasound signal from retained microbubbles and the degree of renal inflammation, assessed by tissue myeloperoxidase activity. Microbubble persistence on contrast ultrasonography may be useful for the detection and monitoring of leukocyte adhesion in inflammatory diseases. Myocardial inflammation after ischemia-reperfusion can be characterized noninvasively by MCE imaging of leucocyte-targeted microbubbles [70]. After attaching to activated neutrophils and monocytes, intact microbubbles are phagocytosed. Despite viscoelastic damping, phagocytosed microbubbles remain responsive to ultrasound and can be detected by ultrasound in vivo after clearance of freely circulating microbubbles from the blood pool. Thus, contrast ultrasound has potential for imaging sites of inflammation. Retention of intravenously injected albumin microbubbles occurs in the setting of both global and regional endothelial dysfunction in large vessels and can be noninvasively imaged. Complement C3 binds to albumin-encapsulated microbubbles and mediates microbubble adherence to vascular endothelium both early and late in the atherosclerotic process. Selectin-bound microbubbles have been used to image recently ischemic myocardium by echocardiography opening the area of ischemic memory imaging. This may offer a new approach to the more timely and precise diagnosis of acute coronary syndrome in patients presenting with chest pain of uncertain cardiac origin [76]. To date, only experimental models have been used.

Transesophageal Examination and Combination of Imaging Modalities

Transesophageal echocardiography is complementary to transthoracic imaging in case of suboptimal image quality and need for high spatial resolution. Contrast cavity opacification is performed during 2D and 3D transthoracic and transesophageal studies. Coronary flow reserve is performed during 2D transthoracic and transesophageal studies. Recent studies have shown that contrast-enhanced 3D echocardiography is a promising technique to accurately detect and measure chronic MI scar [77]. However, contrast-enhanced 3D echocardiography remains in the research domain due to high bubble destruction rate and very low frame rate acquisition at present. One can hypothesize that it could become an invaluable noninvasive test in assessing ischemia, area at risk, and infarct size although further research is required to validate this promising technique. All these imaging modalities can be performed at rest and during stress.

Myocardial Reperfusion Injury

Myocardial reperfusion injury causes four types of cardiac dysfunction: myocardial stunning, microvascular obstruction and no-reflow phenomenon, reperfusion arrhythmias, and lethal myocardial reperfusion injury with increased cardiomyocyte death.

Myocardial Stunning

Myocardial stunning reflects a transient mechanical dysfunction related to ischemia that persists after reperfusion despite the absence of irreversible damage and despite restoration of normal or near-normal coronary flow. The stunning mechanism involves the generation of oxygen free radicals, calcium homeostasis, and changes in the structure of the contractile proteins. Myocardial stunning impacts systolic function at the acute phase of MI. A short ischemic episode might induce regional wall motion abnormalities due to myocardial stunning.

Microvascular Obstruction

Adverse outcome after acute MI may occur despite achieving epicardial coronary artery patency and has shifted investigators' attention toward the status of the microvasculature. Severe angiographic microvascular obstruction (MVO) is termed "no-reflow."

In reperfused myocardium, myocytes appear edematous and swollen from osmotic overload. Endothelial cells become voluminous, with large intraluminal endothelial protrusions into the vascular lumen, and together with swollen surrounding myocytes they occlude capillaries. The infiltration and activation of neutrophils and platelets and the deposition of fibrin also play an important role in reperfusion-induced microvascular damage and obstruction. In addition, coronary microembolization of atherosclerotic debris after percutaneous coronary intervention is responsible for a substantial part of clinically observed MVO. After reperfusion regions of hyperemia, impaired vasodilatory flow reserve and very low flow coexist, and these perfusion patterns vary over time as a result of reperfusion injury. MVO first appears centrally in the infarct core extending toward the epicardium over time. Microvascular dysfunction has been associated with larger infarct size, increased predisposition to ventricular arrhythmias, heart failure, cardiogenic shock, recurrent myocardial infarction, and death. It remains unclear whether this association is of direct mechanistic significance or whether the microcirculatory injury is an epiphenomenon and a manifestation of greater ischemic insult to the myocardium.

Several techniques for the detection of MVO are used clinically and experimentally (coronary angiography, MCE, cardiovascular MRI, electrocardiography) and measure slightly different biological and functional parameters. Currently, there is no consensus as to how and when MVO should be evaluated after acute MI. Direct visualization of MVO has been achieved in both experimental models and clinical studies through intracoronary injections of ultrasound contrast agents. In experimental models, the area at risk relates to the perfusion defect, while the coronary artery remains occluded. The measurements are then repeated once the artery is reopened detecting the area of MVO [47, 78]. This finding was followed by clinical investigations where the area of MVO correlated well with the infarcted area at follow-up in patients with acute MI and successful PCI of the infarct-related artery [79, 80]. Ito and colleagues demonstrated the no-reflow phenomenon on echocardiogram after thrombolysis for acute MI. Lack of myocardial perfusion after intracoronary injection of microbubbles in the patent infarct-related coronary artery predicts poor global and regional LV wall motion recovery [79, 81, 82]. Lepper and colleagues demonstrated that intravenous MCE at the acute phase of MI accurately defined the no-reflow area within the area at risk. Their findings were consistent with CFR measurements at baseline and segmental motion recovery at follow-up [83]. The contrast score index by MCE at the acute phase is a good predictor of regional wall motion recovery at long-term follow-up [52, 84, 85]. In addition, persistent perfusion defect after revascularization of MI is correlated to adverse LV remodeling [86, 87]. MVO following reperfusion of acute MI is an independent predictor of adverse outcome. Other reports have highlighted the value of CFR measured by transthoracic echocardiography after reperfused acute anterior MI [88, 89]. Ueno et al. showed that CFR correlated well with regional wall motion at discharge [88]. Lower CFR values are obtained in patients with acute anterior MI who subsequently develop LV dilatation. Patients with acute MI and pre-infarct angina had better outcomes than patients without prior angina suggesting the benefit of preconditioning. In the subgroup of patients with anterior MI treated by PCI, those with pre-infarct angina had higher transthoracic CFR at the acute phase and improved regional function at follow-up [89]. Although echocardiography may provide information on microcirculation patency, angiographic methods still prevail in clinical practice during PCI due to the accuracy and availability of intracoronary Doppler wire velocity measurements.

Different strategies have been explored to reduce MVO including vasodilators, antiplatelet therapy, thrombolysis, thrombus aspiration and embolic protection devices, intracoronary hyperoxic reperfusion therapies, and cytoprotection.

Imaging technology developments made it possible to demonstrate that microvascular obstruction occurs in 40% of patients who underwent primary angioplasty. Kunichika and colleagues showed that glycoprotein IIb/IIIa inhibitors reduced the infarct-related perfusion defect in an experimental porcine model of acute MI [90]. In clinical studies, MCE has been used to assess the impact of vasodilators at the acute phase of MI. Intracoronary verapamil injection during PCI and followed by oral treatment improved myocardial perfusion and regional left ventricular wall motion [91]. Micari and colleagues have shown that adenosine may reduce the infarct size as a ratio to the risk area measured 3–5 days post-MI [92]. Available devices for clinical use aiming at reducing distal embolization during coronary angioplasty and stent placement include thrombus aspiration and thrombectomy catheters. Initial studies did not have the expected impact, but the number of patients was limited. A recent series involving more than 1,000 AMI patients undergoing coronary angioplasty and thrombus aspiration has shown an improvement of myocardial perfusion indices and a reduction of mortality at 30 days [93]. Distal embolization protection systems aim to prevent the embolic material entering the circulation and causing macro- or microembolization.

Lethal Reperfusion Injury

Lethal reperfusion injury involves different pathways leading to cardiomyocyte death. The complexity of its mechanism involves among others oxygen paradox, calcium paradox, inflammation, and metabolic modulation.

Differences encountered between animal and clinical models as to the benefit of interventions aiming to prevent lethal reperfusion injury are potentially due to the methods used for infarct size measurement. The measurement of infarct size is accurate in experimental models. In humans, infarct size determination is more challenging despite major improvements in imaging techniques. For example, unlike experimental models, there is wide variability of epicardial coronary artery occlusion location, timing, collateral arteries, and global atheroma burden among humans admitted for acute MI. Thus, it is of the outmost importance to normalize infarct size to the size of the area at risk. The rationale for this adjustment is that for two infarcts with the same apparent size, the infarct that represents a larger proportion of the area at risk corresponds to a greater amount of ischemic injury. This principle should be applied when assessing interventions aiming to reduce infarct size and when choosing an imaging modality.

Pre- and Postconditioning

The concept of preconditioning, defined experimentally in 1986, establishes that multiple brief episodes of ischemia may protect the heart from a subsequent and prolonged infarction [94]. Several observations have proved that preconditioning occurs in cardiac patients, for example, during coronary angioplasty and coronary bypass graft surgery. Regional wall motion scores have been used to measure the impact of interventions aiming to reduce ischemia. Leesar and colleagues showed no differences on regional wall motion abnormalities during preconditioning by repeated short lasting coronary occlusions in patients referred for elective PCI of a single vessel [95, 96].

The concept of preconditioning was enlarged by the experimental demonstration that producing ischemia in a vascular bed could induce preconditioning in another vascular bed. Ischemia resulting from repeated successive insufflations of a blood pressure cuff on a limb reduces myocardial necrosis after coronary angioplasty or coronary bypass graft surgery. This remote preconditioning seemed to be a safe and effective noninvasive way of reducing the reperfusion injury. MacAllister and colleagues have demonstrated the concept of remote ischemic preconditioning in the clinical setting using the application of forearm ischemia to confer protection in endothelial function of the contralateral arm [97]. Several research teams have recently used strain imaging to assess the effects of interventions aiming at the reduction of reperfusion injury [45, 98, 99]. However, Hoole and coworkers showed that remote ischaemic preconditioning by forearm ischemia does not attenuate ischaemic left ventricular dysfunction induced by dobutamine stress echocardiography [98]. Munk and colleagues found no overall benefit of remote preconditioning in LVEF and global longitudinal strain during acute MI treated by PCI. However, there was a slight benefit in patients with LAD culprit lesions that are prone to develop large MI [45].

More recently, the concept of ischemic postconditioning has been described where the cardioprotective stimulus is applied after the index ischemia and at the time of reperfusion [100]. This has also been borne out by several studies in different animal and cellular models. Ischemic postconditioning can be readily applied to the acute setting of myocardial infarction and has therefore attracted great interest for cardioprotective strategies directed to the myocardial reperfusion phase. Postconditioning at the acute phase of MI has been beneficial in terms of LV systolic function assessed by Simpson's biplane LVEF, WMSI, and longitudinal strain within the area at risk in a recent 1-year follow-up study [101].

In the last 15 years, a large number of clinical studies have been carried with different pharmacologic groups to assess the effects of pre- and postconditioning. Four agents were studied in particular: adenosine, nicorandil, atrial natriuretic peptide, and statins. The cardioprotective effects of desflurane have also been tested in patients undergoing elective coronary artery bypass surgery. The use of desflurane provided a pharmacological preconditioning so as to reduce myocardial necrosis and improve the cardiac performance in the postoperative period [102]. Cyclosporine, recently tested, opens a new field of investigation since it inhibits mitochondrial permeability and may directly attenuate the reperfusion injury [103].

In the clinical setting, the study of cardioprotective strategies in acute myocardial infarction is beset with technical and logistical difficulties predominantly due to the

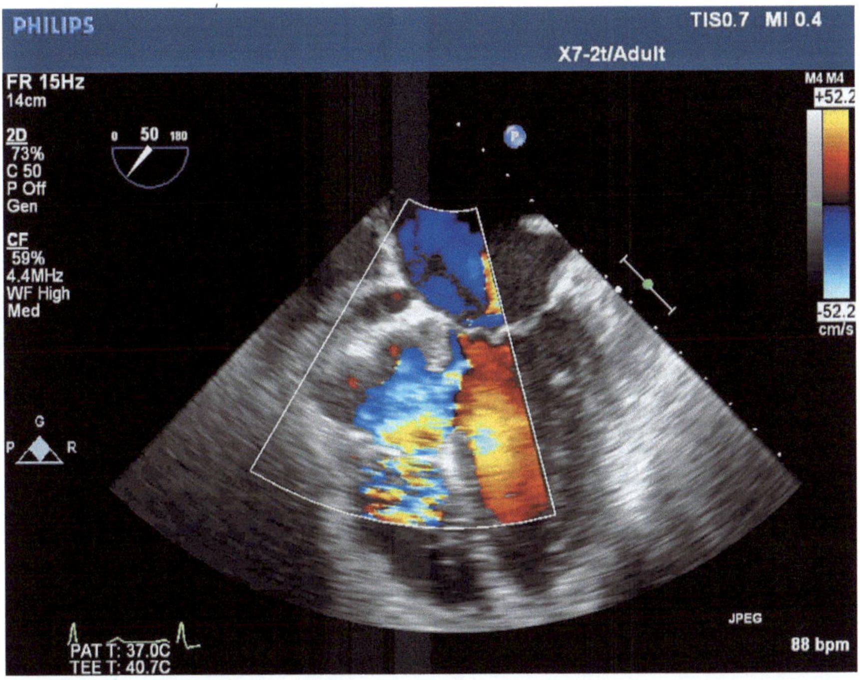

Fig. 7.5 Transesophageal echocardiogram performed 3 days after acute and large inferoposterior MI showing ischemic ventricular septal defect with left to right shunt

precipitous nature of its occurrence and the overbearing need to ensure that reperfusion of the infarcting myocardium is given utmost priority. Some of the surrogate models that have been studied include warm-up angina in which a patient is able to exercise for longer without symptoms following an episode of angina [104] preinfarction angina in which antecedent angina improves clinical outcome following a myocardial infarction [105], percutaneous transluminal coronary angioplasty in which intracoronary inflation lasting longer than 60–90 s improves indicators of myocardial ischemia for subsequent inflations [106], and cardiac surgery in which intermittent aortic cross-clamping prior to a sustained period of global ischemia required for the insertion of bypass grafts was cardioprotective [107].

Echocardiography in Clinically Unstable Patients

The group of unstable patients at the acute phase of MI requires special attention. Cardiogenic shock is a complication in 7% of acute MI and heavily impacts on outcomes [108–111]. Early mortality rate of 48–70% is reduced by early revascularization [112–114]. In the setting of hemodynamically unstable patients, bedside echocardiography detects mechanical complications including acute mitral regurgitation, pericardial effusion, ventricular septal defects (Fig. 7.5), and myocardial rupture [115]. However, severity of ischemic mitral regurgitation may be underestimated by transthoracic color Doppler flow mapping in the situation of low cardiac index. During mechanical ventilatory support, transthoracic windows may be difficult to obtain and transesophageal echocardiogram is carried out in the intensive care unit. Echocardiography, either transthoracic or transesophageal, is the only noninvasive imaging modality that can be performed in emergency situations and provide the serial assessments needed for the management of critically ill patients.

Conclusion and Perspectives

Reduction of infarct size has been the main objective of research on ischemic myocardial disease during the last 40 years. Myocardial revascularization at the acute phase of MI has markedly improved outcomes. However, restoring epicardial coronary flow does not always imply optimal myocardial perfusion and has therefore been the field of active research. Up to now, no specific marker of myocardial reperfusion injury has been found. Thus, effects of interventions aiming at limiting myocardial reperfusion injury are evaluated by surrogate markers of myocardial damage as infarct size normalized to the size of the area at risk. The final infarct size is the cornerstone of risk stratification.

Cardiac imaging assesses LV regional and global function, LV remodeling, measures the area at risk and the infarct size, and estimates microvascular flow. Echocardiography is a noninvasive, radiation-free, widely available, and bedside technique with high spatial and temporal resolutions, and it is highly cost-effective. Significant improvement in image quality has been responsible for the widespread of imaging modalities. The advent of 3D echo has ensured accurate LV volumes and LVEF measurements. Strain imaging provides valuable prognostic information to quantify regional myocardial function and differentiate viable from nonviable myocardium. Direct measurement of coronary flow reserve in the LAD territory is useful in assessing microvascular function after anterior MI. Although MCE is a valuable tool in assessing infarct size and the area at risk, it has not fulfilled practitioners' expectations and has remained a research tool used in highly specialized centers. Recently developed new contrast agents may achieve reliable detection of myocardial perfusion in the near future. Contrast agent-led molecular imaging is another promising area in the field of myocardial reperfusion injury. Molecular imaging may become a therapeutic approach through drug, gene delivery, or sonothrombolysis.

Cost-effectiveness of new technologies must be evaluated. It is no longer sufficient to provide test performance only as compared with established techniques but rather to determine whether they significantly affect patient treatment and ultimately patient outcomes. The use of any investigation tool requires awareness of its limitations.

Assessment of all parameters related to myocardial reperfusion injury can be obtained by echocardiography. Its widespread availability and reproducibility should prompt its use in large multicenter studies that are needed in the area of myocardial reperfusion injury.

References

1. Murray CJ, Lopez AD. Alternative projections of mortality and disability by cause 1990-2020: Global Burden of Disease study. Lancet. 1997;349(9064):1498–504.
2. Singh M, Reeder GS, Jacobsen SJ, Weston S, Killian J, Roger VL. Scores for post-myocardial infarction risk stratification in the community. Circulation. 2002;106(18):2309–14.
3. Lang RM, Bierig M, Devereux RB, et al. Recommendations for chamber quantification: a report from the American Society of Echocardiography's Guidelines and Standards Committee and the Chamber Quantification Writing Group, developed in conjunction with the European Association of Echocardiography, a branch of the European Society of Cardiology. J Am Soc Echocardiogr. 2005;18(12):1440–63.
4. Lang RM, Bierig M, Devereux RB, et al. Recommendations for chamber quantification. Eur J Echocardiogr. 2006;7(2):79–108.
5. Teichholz LE, Kreulen T, Herman MV, Gorlin R. Problems in echocardiographic volume determinations: echocardiographic-angiographic correlations in the presence of absence of asynergy. Am J Cardiol. 1976;37(1):7–11.
6. Weiss JL, Bulkley BH, Hutchins GM, Mason SJ. Two-dimensional echocardiographic recognition of myocardial injury in man: comparison with postmortem studies. Circulation. 1981;63(2):401–8.
7. Schiller NB, Shah PM, Crawford M, et al. Recommendations for quantitation of the left ventricle by two-dimensional echocardiography. American Society of Echocardiography Committee on Standards, Subcommittee on Quantitation of Two-Dimensional Echocardiograms. J Am Soc Echocardiogr. 1989;2(5):358–67.
8. Cerqueira MD, Weissman NJ, Dilsizian V, et al. Standardized myocardial segmentation and nomenclature for tomographic imaging of the heart: a statement for healthcare professionals from the Cardiac Imaging Committee of the Council on Clinical Cardiology of the American Heart Association. Circulation. 2002;105(4):539–42.
9. Nixon JV, Narahara KA, Smitherman TC. Estimation of myocardial involvement in patients with acute myocardial infarction by two-dimensional echocardiography. Circulation. 1980;62(6):1248–55.
10. Visser CA, Lie KI, Kan G, Meltzer R, Durrer D. Detection and quantification of acute, isolated myocardial infarction by two dimensional echocardiography. Am J Cardiol. 1981;47(5):1020–5.
11. Cheitlin MD, Armstrong WF, Aurigemma GP, et al. ACC/AHA/ASE 2003 guideline update for the clinical application of echocardiography: summary article: a report of the American College of Cardiology/American Heart Association Task Force on Practice Guidelines (ACC/AHA/ASE Committee to Update the 1997 Guidelines for the Clinical Application of Echocardiography). Circulation. 2003;108(9):1146–62.
12. Pellerin D, Sharma R, Elliott P, Veyrat C. Tissue Doppler, strain, and strain rate echocardiography for the assessment of left and right systolic ventricular function. Heart. 2003;89 Suppl 3:iii9–17.
13. Price DJ, Wallbridge DR, Stewart MJ. Tissue Doppler imaging: current and potential clinical applications. Heart. 2000;84 Suppl 2:ii11–8.
14. Quinones MA, Otto CM, Stoddard M, Waggoner A, Zoghbi WA. Recommendations for quantification of Doppler echocardiography: a report from the Doppler Quantification Task Force of the Nomenclature and Standards Committee of the American Society of Echocardiography. J Am Soc Echocardiogr. 2002;15(2):167–84.
15. Kvitting JP, Wigstrom L, Strotmann JM, Sutherland GR. How accurate is visual assessment of synchronicity in myocardial motion? An in vitro study with computer-simulated regional delay in myocardial motion: clinical implications for rest and stress echocardiography studies. J Am Soc Echocardiogr. 1999;12(9):698–705.
16. Brown J, Jenkins C, Marwick TH. Use of myocardial strain to assess global left ventricular function: a comparison with cardiac magnetic resonance and 3-dimensional echocardiography. Am Heart J. 2009;157(1):102; e1–5.

17. Cho GY, Marwick TH, Kim HS, Kim MK, Hong KS, Oh DJ. Global 2-dimensional strain as a new prognosticator in patients with heart failure. J Am Coll Cardiol. 2009;54(7):618–24.
18. Stanton T, Leano R, Marwick TH. Prediction of all-cause mortality from global longitudinal speckle strain: comparison with ejection fraction and wall motion scoring. Circ Cardiovasc Imaging. 2009;2(5):356–64.
19. Popovic ZB, Kwon DH, Mishra M, et al. Association between regional ventricular function and myocardial fibrosis in hypertrophic cardiomyopathy assessed by speckle tracking echocardiography and delayed hyperenhancement magnetic resonance imaging. J Am Soc Echocardiogr. 2008;21(12):1299–305.
20. Iwahashi N, Nakatani S, Kanzaki H, Hasegawa T, Abe H, Kitakaze M. Acute improvement in myocardial function assessed by myocardial strain and strain rate after aortic valve replacement for aortic stenosis. J Am Soc Echocardiogr. 2006;19(10):1238–44.
21. Hashimoto I, Li X, Hejmadi Bhat A, Jones M, Zetts AD, Sahn DJ. Myocardial strain rate is a superior method for evaluation of left ventricular subendocardial function compared with tissue Doppler imaging. J Am Coll Cardiol. 2003;42(9):1574–83.
22. Pasquet A, Armstrong G, Beachler L, Lauer MS, Marwick TH. Use of segmental tissue Doppler velocity to quantitate exercise echocardiography. J Am Soc Echocardiogr. 1999; 12(11):901–12.
23. Fathi R, Cain P, Nakatani S, Yu HC, Marwick TH. Effect of tissue Doppler on the accuracy of novice and expert interpreters of dobutamine echocardiography. Am J Cardiol. 2001;88(4): 400–5.
24. Voigt JU, Exner B, Schmiedehausen K, et al. Strain-rate imaging during dobutamine stress echocardiography provides objective evidence of inducible ischemia. Circulation. 2003;107(16): 2120–6.
25. Weidemann F, Dommke C, Bijnens B, et al. Defining the transmurality of a chronic myocardial infarction by ultrasonic strain-rate imaging: implications for identifying intramural viability: an experimental study. Circulation. 2003;107(6):883–8.
26. Vartdal T, Brunvand H, Pettersen E, et al. Early prediction of infarct size by strain Doppler echocardiography after coronary reperfusion. J Am Coll Cardiol. 2007;49(16):1715–21.
27. Sjoli B, Orn S, Grenne B, et al. Comparison of left ventricular ejection fraction and left ventricular global strain as determinants of infarct size in patients with acute myocardial infarction. J Am Soc Echocardiogr. 2009;22(11):1232–8.
28. Gjesdal O, Helle-Valle T, Hopp E, et al. Noninvasive separation of large, medium, and small myocardial infarcts in survivors of reperfused ST-elevation myocardial infarction: a comprehensive tissue Doppler and speckle-tracking echocardiography study. Circ Cardiovasc Imaging. 2008;1(3):189–96.
29. Weidemann F, Wacker C, Rauch A, et al. Sequential changes of myocardial function during acute myocardial infarction, in the early and chronic phase after coronary intervention described by ultrasonic strain rate imaging. J Am Soc Echocardiogr. 2006;19(7):839–47.
30. Hoffmann R, Altiok E, Nowak B, et al. Strain rate measurement by Doppler echocardiography allows improved assessment of myocardial viability in patients with depressed left ventricular function. J Am Coll Cardiol. 2002;39(3):443–9.
31. Hanekom L, Jenkins C, Jeffries L, et al. Incremental value of strain rate analysis as an adjunct to wall-motion scoring for assessment of myocardial viability by dobutamine echocardiography: a follow-up study after revascularization. Circulation. 2005;112(25):3892–900.
32. Park YH, Kang SJ, Song JK, et al. Prognostic value of longitudinal strain after primary reperfusion therapy in patients with anterior-wall acute myocardial infarction. J Am Soc Echocardiogr. 2008;21(3):262–7.
33. Davidavicius G, Kowalski M, Williams RI, et al. Can regional strain and strain rate measurement be performed during both dobutamine and exercise echocardiography, and do regional deformation responses differ with different forms of stress testing? J Am Soc Echocardiogr. 2003;16(4):299–308.

34. Kuhl HP, Schreckenberg M, Rulands D, et al. High-resolution transthoracic real-time three-dimensional echocardiography: quantitation of cardiac volumes and function using semi-automatic border detection and comparison with cardiac magnetic resonance imaging. J Am Coll Cardiol. 2004;43(11):2083–90.
35. Jacobs LD, Salgo IS, Goonewardena S, et al. Rapid online quantification of left ventricular volume from real-time three-dimensional echocardiographic data. Eur Heart J. 2006;27(4): 460–8.
36. Nosir YF, Fioretti PM, Vletter WB, et al. Accurate measurement of left ventricular ejection fraction by three-dimensional echocardiography. A comparison with radionuclide angiography. Circulation. 1996;94(3):460–6.
37. Siu SC, Rivera JM, Guerrero JL, et al. Three-dimensional echocardiography. In vivo validation for left ventricular volume and function. Circulation. 1993;88(4Pt1):1715–23.
38. Altmann K, Shen Z, Boxt LM, et al. Comparison of three-dimensional echocardiographic assessment of volume, mass, and function in children with functionally single left ventricles with two-dimensional echocardiography and magnetic resonance imaging. Am J Cardiol. 1997;80(8):1060–5.
39. Arai K, Hozumi T, Matsumura Y, et al. Accuracy of measurement of left ventricular volume and ejection fraction by new real-time three-dimensional echocardiography in patients with wall motion abnormalities secondary to myocardial infarction. Am J Cardiol. 2004;94(5): 552–8.
40. Jiang L, Vazquez de Prada JA, Handschumacher MD, et al. Quantitative three-dimensional reconstruction of aneurysmal left ventricles. In vitro and in vivo validation. Circulation. 1995;91(1):222–30.
41. Buck T, Hunold P, Wentz KU, Tkalec W, Nesser HJ, Erbel R. Tomographic three-dimensional echocardiographic determination of chamber size and systolic function in patients with left ventricular aneurysm: comparison to magnetic resonance imaging, cineventriculography, and two-dimensional echocardiography. Circulation. 1997;96(12):4286–97.
42. Corsi C, Lang RM, Veronesi F, et al. Volumetric quantification of global and regional left ventricular function from real-time three-dimensional echocardiographic images. Circulation. 2005;112(8):1161–70.
43. Takeuchi M, Otani S, Weinert L, Spencer KT, Lang RM. Comparison of contrast-enhanced real-time live 3-dimensional dobutamine stress echocardiography with contrast 2-dimensional echocardiography for detecting stress-induced wall-motion abnormalities. J Am Soc Echocardiogr. 2006;19(3):294–9.
44. Ahmad M, Xie T, McCulloch M, Abreo G, Runge M. Real-time three-dimensional dobutamine stress echocardiography in assessment stress echocardiography in assessment of ischemia: comparison with two-dimensional dobutamine stress echocardiography. J Am Coll Cardiol. 2001;37(5):1303–9.
45. Munk K, Andersen NH, Schmidt MR, et al. Remote ischemic conditioning in patients with myocardial infarction treated with primary angioplasty: impact on left ventricular function assessed by comprehensive echocardiography and gated single-photon emission CT. Circ Cardiovasc Imaging. 2010;3(6):656–62.
46. Wei K, Jayaweera AR, Firoozan S, Linka A, Skyba DM, Kaul S. Quantification of myocardial blood flow with ultrasound-induced destruction of microbubbles administered as a constant venous infusion. Circulation. 1998;97(5):473–83.
47. Kaul S, Gillam LD, Weyman AE. Contrast echocardiography in acute myocardial ischemia. II. The effect of site of injection of contrast agent on the estimation of area at risk for necrosis after coronary occlusion. J Am Coll Cardiol. 1985;6(4):825–30.
48. Kaul S, Glasheen W, Ruddy TD, Pandian NG, Weyman AE, Okada RD. The importance of defining left ventricular area at risk in vivo during acute myocardial infarction: an experimental evaluation with myocardial contrast two-dimensional echocardiography. Circulation. 1987;75(6):1249–60.

49. Grayburn PA, Erickson JM, Escobar J, Womack L, Velasco CE. Peripheral intravenous myocardial contrast echocardiography using a 2% dodecafluoropentane emulsion: identification of myocardial risk area and infarct size in the canine model of ischemia. J Am Coll Cardiol. 1995;26(5):1340–7.
50. Scherrer-Crosbie M, Liel-Cohen N, Otsuji Y, et al. Myocardial perfusion and wall motion in infarction border zone: assessment by myocardial contrast echocardiography. J Am Soc Echocardiogr. 2000;13(5):353–7.
51. Coggins MP, Sklenar J, Le DE, Wei K, Lindner JR, Kaul S. Noninvasive prediction of ultimate infarct size at the time of acute coronary occlusion based on the extent and magnitude of collateral-derived myocardial blood flow. Circulation. 2001;104(20):2471–7.
52. Janardhanan R, Swinburn JM, Greaves K, Senior R. Usefulness of myocardial contrast echocardiography using low-power continuous imaging early after acute myocardial infarction to predict late functional left ventricular recovery. Am J Cardiol. 2003;92(5):493–7.
53. Janardhanan R, Moon JC, Pennell DJ, Senior R. Myocardial contrast echocardiography accurately reflects transmurality of myocardial necrosis and predicts contractile reserve after acute myocardial infarction. Am Heart J. 2005;149(2):355–62.
54. Dwivedi G, Janardhanan R, Hayat SA, Swinburn JM, Senior R. Prognostic value of myocardial viability detected by myocardial contrast echocardiography early after acute myocardial infarction. J Am Coll Cardiol. 2007;50(4):327–34.
55. Agati L, Voci P, Autore C, et al. Combined use of dobutamine echocardiography and myocardial contrast echocardiography in predicting regional dysfunction recovery after coronary revascularization in patients with recent myocardial infarction. Eur Heart J. 1997;18(5):771–9.
56. Iliceto S, Galiuto L, Marchese A, Colonna P, Oliva S, Rizzon P. Functional role of microvascular integrity in patients with infarct-related artery patency after acute myocardial infarction. Eur Heart J. 1997;18(4):618–24.
57. Iliceto S, Galiuto L, Marchese A, Cavallari D, Colonna P, Biasco G, et al. Analysis of microvascular integrity, contractile reserve, and myocardial viability after acute myocardial infarction by dobutamine echocardiography and myocardial contrast echocardiography. Am J Cardiol. 1996;77(7):441–5.
58. Villanueva FS. Myocardial perfusion imaging using ultrasound contrast agents: now or never? JACC Cardiovasc Imaging. 2010;3(9):944–6.
59. http://www.fda.gov/Drugs/DrugSafety/PostmarketDrugSafetyInformationforPatientsandProviders/ucm125574.htm. Accessed on July 17, 2008.
60. Dimitrow PP. Transthoracic Doppler echocardiography—noninvasive diagnostic window for coronary flow reserve assessment. Cardiovasc Ultrasound. 2003;1:4.
61. Hozumi T, Yoshida K, Ogata Y, et al. Noninvasive assessment of significant left anterior descending coronary artery stenosis by coronary flow velocity reserve with transthoracic color Doppler echocardiography. Circulation. 1998;97(16):1557–62.
62. Caiati C, Montaldo C, Zedda N, et al. Validation of a new noninvasive method (contrast-enhanced transthoracic second harmonic echo Doppler) for the evaluation of coronary flow reserve: comparison with intracoronary Doppler flow wire. J Am Coll Cardiol. 1999;34(4):1193–200.
63. Caiati C, Montaldo C, Zedda N, Bina A, Iliceto S. New noninvasive method for coronary flow reserve assessment: contrast-enhanced transthoracic second harmonic echo Doppler. Circulation. 1999;99(6):771–8.
64. Pizzuto F, Voci P, Mariano E, Puddu PE, Sardella G, Nigri A. Assessment of flow velocity reserve by transthoracic Doppler echocardiography and venous adenosine infusion before and after left anterior descending coronary artery stenting. J Am Coll Cardiol. 2001;38(1):155–62.
65. Nohtomi Y, Takeuchi M, Nagasawa K, et al. Simultaneous assessment of wall motion and coronary flow velocity in the left anterior descending coronary artery during dipyridamole stress echocardiography. J Am Soc Echocardiogr. 2003;16(5):457–63.

66. Lowenstein J, Tiano C, Marquez G, Presti C, Quiroz C. Simultaneous analysis of wall motion and coronary flow reserve of the left anterior descending coronary artery by transthoracic Doppler echocardiography during dipyridamole stress echocardiography. J Am Soc Echocardiogr. 2003;16(6):607–13.
67. Rigo F, Sicari R, Gherardi S, Djordjevic-Dikic A, Cortigiani L, Picano E. Prognostic value of coronary flow reserve in medically treated patients with left anterior descending coronary disease with stenosis 51% to 75% in diameter. Am J Cardiol. 2007;100(10):1527–31.
68. Ellegala DB, Leong-Poi H, Carpenter JE, et al. Imaging tumor angiogenesis with contrast ultrasound and microbubbles targeted to alpha(v)beta3. Circulation. 2003;108(3):336–41.
69. Weller GE, Lu E, Csikari MM, et al. Ultrasound imaging of acute cardiac transplant rejection with microbubbles targeted to intercellular adhesion molecule-1. Circulation. 2003;108(2): 218–24.
70. Christiansen JP, Leong-Poi H, Klibanov AL, Kaul S, Lindner JR. Noninvasive imaging of myocardial reperfusion injury using leukocyte-targeted contrast echocardiography. Circulation. 2002;105(15):1764–7.
71. Lindner JR, Song J, Xu F, et al. Noninvasive ultrasound imaging of inflammation using microbubbles targeted to activated leukocytes. Circulation. 2000;102(22):2745–50.
72. Lindner JR, Dayton PA, Coggins MP, et al. Noninvasive imaging of inflammation by ultrasound detection of phagocytosed microbubbles. Circulation. 2000;102(5):531–8.
73. Lindner JR, Coggins MP, Kaul S, Klibanov AL, Brandenburger GH, Ley K. Microbubble persistence in the microcirculation during ischemia/reperfusion and inflammation is caused by integrin- and complement-mediated adherence to activated leukocytes. Circulation. 2000; 101(6):668–75.
74. Tsutsui JM, Xie F, Cano M, et al. Detection of retained microbubbles in carotid arteries with real-time low mechanical index imaging in the setting of endothelial dysfunction. J Am Coll Cardiol. 2004;44(5):1036–46.
75. Anderson DR, Tsutsui JM, Xie F, Radio SJ, Porter TR. The role of complement in the adherence of microbubbles to dysfunctional arterial endothelium and atherosclerotic plaque. Cardiovasc Res. 2007;73(3):597–606.
76. Villanueva FS, Lu E, Bowry S, et al. Myocardial ischemic memory imaging with molecular echocardiography. Circulation. 2007;115(3):345–52.
77. Montant P, Chenot F, Goffinet C, et al. Detection and quantification of myocardial scars by contrast-enhanced 3D echocardiography. Circ Cardiovasc Imaging. 2010;3(4):415–23.
78. Kemper AJ, O'Boyle JE, Cohen CA, Taylor A, Parisi AF. Hydrogen peroxide contrast echocardiography: quantification in vivo of myocardial risk area during coronary occlusion and of the necrotic area remaining after myocardial reperfusion. Circulation. 1984;70(2): 309–17.
79. Ito H, Tomooka T, Sakai N, et al. Lack of myocardial perfusion immediately after successful thrombolysis. A predictor of poor recovery of left ventricular function in anterior myocardial infarction. Circulation. 1992;85(5):1699–705.
80. Sakuma T, Hayashi Y, Sumii K, Imazu M, Yamakido M. Prediction of short- and intermediate-term prognoses of patients with acute myocardial infarction using myocardial contrast echocardiography one day after recanalization. J Am Coll Cardiol. 1998;32(4):890–7.
81. Sakuma T, Hayashi Y, Shimohara A, Shindo T, Maeda K. Usefulness of myocardial contrast echocardiography for the assessment of serial changes in risk area in patients with acute myocardial infarction. Am J Cardiol. 1996;78(11):1273–7.
82. Nanto S, Lim YJ, Masuyama T, Hori M, Nagata S. Diagnostic performance of myocardial contrast echocardiography for detection of stunned myocardium. J Am Soc Echocardiogr. 1996;9(3):314–9.
83. Lepper W, Hoffmann R, Kamp O, et al. Assessment of myocardial reperfusion by intravenous myocardial contrast echocardiography and coronary flow reserve after primary percutaneous transluminal coronary angioplasty [correction of angiography] in patients with acute myocardial infarction. Circulation. 2000;101(20):2368–74.

84. Ragosta M, Camarano G, Kaul S, Powers ER, Sarembock IJ, Gimple LW. Microvascular integrity indicates myocellular viability in patients with recent myocardial infarction. New insights using myocardial contrast echocardiography. Circulation. 1994;89(6):2562–9.
85. Greaves K, Dixon SR, Fejka M, et al. Myocardial contrast echocardiography is superior to other known modalities for assessing myocardial reperfusion after acute myocardial infarction. Heart. 2003;89(2):139–44.
86. Ujino K, Hillis GS, Mulvagh SL, Hagen ME, Oh JK. Usefulness of real-time intravenous myocardial contrast echocardiography in predicting left ventricular dilation after successfully reperfused acute myocardial infarction. Am J Cardiol. 2005;96(1):17–21.
87. Kamp O, Lepper W, Vanoverschelde JL, et al. Serial evaluation of perfusion defects in patients with a first acute myocardial infarction referred for primary PTCA using intravenous myocardial contrast echocardiography. Eur Heart J. 2001;22(16):1485–95.
88. Ueno Y, Nakamura Y, Kinoshita M, Fujita T, Sakamoto T, Okamura H. Can coronary flow velocity reserve determined by transthoracic Doppler echocardiography predict the recovery of regional left ventricular function in patients with acute myocardial infarction? Heart. 2002;88(2):137–41.
89. Colonna P, Cadeddu C, Montisci R, et al. Reduced microvascular and myocardial damage in patients with acute myocardial infarction and preinfarction angina. Am Heart J. 2002;144(5): 796–803.
90. Kunichika H, Ben-Yehuda O, Lafitte S, Kunichika N, Peters B, DeMaria AN. Effects of glycoprotein IIb/IIIa inhibition on microvascular flow after coronary reperfusion. A quantitative myocardial contrast echocardiography study. J Am Coll Cardiol. 2004;43(2):276–83.
91. Taniyama Y, Ito H, Iwakura K, et al. Beneficial effect of intracoronary verapamil on microvascular and myocardial salvage in patients with acute myocardial infarction. J Am Coll Cardiol. 1997;30(5):1193–9.
92. Micari A, Belcik TA, Balcells EA, et al. Improvement in microvascular reflow and reduction of infarct size with adenosine in patients undergoing primary coronary stenting. Am J Cardiol. 2005;96(10):1410–5.
93. Svilaas T, Vlaar PJ, van der Horst IC, et al. Thrombus aspiration during primary percutaneous coronary intervention. N Engl J Med. 2008;358(6):557–67.
94. Murry CE, Jennings RB, Reimer KA. Preconditioning with ischemia: a delay of lethal cell injury in ischemic myocardium. Circulation. 1986;74(5):1124–36.
95. Leesar MA, Stoddard MF, Xuan YT, Tang XL, Bolli R. Nonelectrocardiographic evidence that both ischemic preconditioning and adenosine preconditioning exist in humans. J Am Coll Cardiol. 2003;42(3):437–45.
96. Leesar MA, Stoddard M, Ahmed M, Broadbent J, Bolli R. Preconditioning of human myocardium with adenosine during coronary angioplasty. Circulation. 1997;95(11):2500–7.
97. Kharbanda RK, Mortensen UM, White PA, et al. Transient limb ischemia induces remote ischemic preconditioning in vivo. Circulation. 2002;106(23):2881–3.
98. Hoole SP, Khan SN, White PA, et al. Remote ischaemic pre-conditioning does not attenuate ischaemic left ventricular dysfunction in humans. Eur J Heart Fail. 2009;11(5):497–505.
99. Sadigh B, Quintana M, Sylven C, Berglund M, Brodin LA. The ischemic preconditioning effect of adenosine in patients with ischemic heart disease. Cardiovasc Ultrasound. 2009;7:52.
100. Zhao ZQ, Corvera JS, Halkos ME, et al. Inhibition of myocardial injury by ischemic postconditioning during reperfusion: comparison with ischemic preconditioning. Am J Physiol Heart Circ Physiol. 2003;285(2):H579–88.
101. Thibault H, Piot C, Staat P, et al. Long-term benefit of postconditioning. Circulation. 2008;117(8):1037–44.
102. Meco M, Cirri S, Gallazzi C, Magnani G, Cosseta D. Desflurane preconditioning in coronary artery bypass graft surgery: a double-blinded, randomised and placebo-controlled study. Eur J Cardiothorac Surg. 2007;32(2):319–25.
103. Piot C, Croisille P, Staat P, et al. Effect of cyclosporine on reperfusion injury in acute myocardial infarction. N Engl J Med. 2008;359(5):473–81.

104. Williams DO, Bass TA, Gewirtz H, Most AS. Adaptation to the stress of tachycardia in patients with coronary artery disease: insight into the mechanism of the warm-up phenomenon. Circulation. 1985;71(4):687–92.
105. Rezkalla SH, Kloner RA. Ischemic preconditioning and preinfarction angina in the clinical arena. Nat Clin Pract Cardiovasc Med. 2004;1(2):96–102.
106. Deutsch E, Berger M, Kussmaul WG, Hirshfeld Jr JW, Herrmann HC, Laskey WK. Adaptation to ischemia during percutaneous transluminal coronary angioplasty. Clinical, hemodynamic, and metabolic features. Circulation. 1990;82(6):2044–51.
107. Jenkins DP, Steare SE, Yellon DM. Preconditioning the human myocardium: recent advances and aspirations for the development of a new means of cardioprotection in clinical practice. Cardiovasc Drugs Ther. 1995;9(6):739–47.
108. Holmes Jr DR, Berger PB, Hochman JS, et al. Cardiogenic shock in patients with acute ischemic syndromes with and without ST-segment elevation. Circulation. 1999;100(20):2067–73.
109. Goldberg RJ, Samad NA, Yarzebski J, Gurwitz J, Bigelow C, Gore JM. Temporal trends in cardiogenic shock complicating acute myocardial infarction. N Engl J Med. 1999;340(15):1162–8.
110. Holmes Jr DR, Bates ER, Kleiman NS, et al. Contemporary reperfusion therapy for cardiogenic shock: the GUSTO-I trial experience. The GUSTO-I Investigators. Global Utilization of Streptokinase and Tissue Plasminogen Activator for Occluded Coronary Arteries. J Am Coll Cardiol. 1995;26(3):668–74.
111. Babaev A, Frederick PD, Pasta DJ, Every N, Sichrovsky T, Hochman JS. Trends in management and outcomes of patients with acute myocardial infarction complicated by cardiogenic shock. JAMA. 2005;294(4):448–54.
112. Hochman JS, Boland J, Sleeper LA, et al. Current spectrum of cardiogenic shock and effect of early revascularization on mortality. Results of an International Registry. SHOCK Registry Investigators. Circulation. 1995;91(3):873–81.
113. Hochman JS, Sleeper LA, Webb JG, et al. Early revascularization in acute myocardial infarction complicated by cardiogenic shock. SHOCK Investigators. Should we emergently revascularize occluded coronaries for cardiogenic shock. N Engl J Med. 1999;341(9):625–34.
114. Carnendran L, Abboud R, Sleeper LA, et al. Trends in cardiogenic shock: report from the SHOCK study. SHould we emergently revascularize Occluded Coronaries for cardiogenic shocK? Eur Heart J. 2001;22(6):472–8.
115. Lamia B, Ochagavia A, Monnet X, Chemla D, Richard C, Teboul JL. Echocardiographic prediction of volume responsiveness in critically ill patients with spontaneously breathing activity. Intensive Care Med. 2007;33(7):1125–32.

Chapter 8
Nuclear Imaging to Assess Infarction, Reperfusion, No-Reflow, and Viability

Victoria Delgado, Arend F.L. Schinkel, Kai-Hang Yiu, and Jeroen J. Bax

Abstract Thrombolytic therapy and primary percutaneous coronary have improved the survival of patients with acute myocardial infarction. However, this superior survival leads to an increased prevalence of left ventricular systolic dysfunction and development of heart failure at follow-up. Nuclear imaging permits comprehensive evaluation of patients with coronary artery disease. In the setting of acute myocardial infarction, ^{99m}Tc-sestamibi SPECT provides information on myocardium at risk, infarct size and myocardial salvage, well-known measures of the efficacy of reperfusion therapy, and important prognostic markers. In addition, nuclear imaging permits the assessment of no-reflow phenomenon that may take place during thrombolysis or percutaneous revascularization techniques. Timely detection of this phenomenon may help to select the most appropriate therapies to improve the microcirculation of the infarcted areas and, consequently, to improve the contractile function of the myocardium at follow-up. Furthermore, nuclear imaging plays a central role in the evaluation of ischemic heart failure patients with a substantial amount of dysfunctional but viable myocardium who may benefit from coronary revascularization with significant improvements in left ventricular function, heart failure symptoms, and prognosis.

V. Delgado, M.D., Ph.D. (✉) • K.-H. Yiu, MBBS • J.J. Bax, M.D., Ph.D.
Cardiology Department, Leiden University Medical Center,
Albinusdreef 2, Leiden 2300 RC, The Netherlands
e-mail: v.delgado@lumc.nl; k.h.yiu@lumc.nl; j.j.bax@lumc.nl

A.F.L. Schinkel, M.D., Ph.D.
Department of Cardiology, Thoraxcenter, Erasmus MC,
Rotterdam, The Netherlands

Division of Pharmacology, Vascular and Metabolic Diseases,
Department of Internal Medicine, Erasmus MC,
Rotterdam, The Netherlands
e-mail: a.schinkel@erasmusmc.nl

J.C. Kaski et al. (eds.), *Management of Myocardial Reperfusion Injury*,
DOI 10.1007/978-1-84996-019-9_8,

This chapter will review the role of nuclear imaging in acute myocardial infarction, with special focus on the relevance of this technique to assess the efficacy of reperfusion therapy. In addition, a detailed appraisal of multimodality imaging for noninvasive assessment of hibernating myocardium will be provided.

Keywords Nuclear imaging • Myocardial infarction • No-reflow • Myocardial viability.

Introduction

Coronary artery disease is currently the leading cause of left ventricular systolic dysfunction and heart failure in the Western countries [1]. The widespread use of thrombolytic therapy, the increasing number of primary percutaneous coronary interventions, and advances in antithrombotic therapies have improved the clinical outcome of patients with acute coronary syndromes [2].

The efficacy of these therapies is commonly evaluated with the measurement of left ventricular ejection fraction, left ventricular end-systolic volume, and infarct size, well-known determinants of short- and long-term survival after myocardial infarction [3–5]. Radionuclide imaging, especially single-photon emission computed tomography (SPECT) myocardial perfusion imaging with ^{99m}Tc-sestamibi, is considered the gold standard to measure the efficacy of reperfusion therapy in myocardial infarction by means of infarct size and myocardial salvage [4]. In addition, early coronary arterial patency has been used in randomized controlled trials as a measure of the efficacy of reperfusion therapies [6]. However, the restoration of epicardial blood flow does not always imply restoration of myocardial perfusion. The "no-reflow" or microvascular obstruction phenomenon indicates myocardial tissue hypoperfusion in the presence of a patent epicardial coronary artery and it has been related to progressive left ventricular remodeling and impaired prognosis after myocardial infarction [7–9]. Late-gadolinium contrast-enhanced magnetic resonance imaging (MRI) provides high-spatial-resolution images to identify this phenomenon, but SPECT myocardial perfusion and positron emission tomography (PET) can also provide useful information.

Finally, the superior survival after myocardial infarction is also associated with increased prevalence of left ventricular systolic dysfunction and development of heart failure. Evaluation of myocardial viability is fundamental in the assessment and management of patients with coronary artery disease and left ventricular dysfunction. Myocardial revascularization improves regional and global left ventricular function in as much as 40% of patients with ischemic left ventricular dysfunction [10–12]. This potentially reversible condition, known as myocardial hibernation, is characterized by reduced myocardial contractility due to sustained reduction in myocardial arterial supply [13]. Timely identification and revascularization of patients who show dysfunctional but viable myocardium will improve left ventricular systolic function and clinical outcome. Multimodality imaging plays a central role in the clinical diagnosis and management of patients with coronary artery disease and left ventricular dysfunction. A number of imaging modalities including nuclear imaging (SPECT and PET), echocardiography (rest and stress; contrast-enhanced), and MRI have shown to be sensitive and specific for identification of patients with chronic ischemic heart failure and viable myocardium.

This chapter will review the role of nuclear imaging in acute myocardial infarction, with special focus on the relevance of this technique to assess the efficacy of reperfusion therapy. In addition, a detailed appraisal of multimodality imaging for noninvasive assessment of hibernating myocardium will be provided.

Myocardial Infarction: Role of ^{99m}Tc-Sestamibi SPECT

Early reperfusion therapy with intravenous thrombolytic agents or percutaneous coronary intervention in patients with acute myocardial infarction has been demonstrated to provide superior short- and long-term outcomes [14]. The superior prognosis is related to myocardial salvage and patency of the infarct-related artery achieved with reperfusion therapies [15]. The efficacy of these therapies is commonly assessed by means of infarct size, left ventricular ejection fraction, and end-systolic volume, well-established prognostic markers after acute myocardial infarction [5, 16–18]. SPECT imaging with ^{99m}Tc-sestamibi is a comprehensive imaging tool to assess the efficacy of reperfusion therapies in acute myocardial infarction since it provides information on the extent of myocardium at risk, infarct size, and myocardial salvage [19]. The acute perfusion defect measured by injection of ^{99m}Tc-sestamibi during coronary occlusion estimates the extent of myocardium at risk whereas the measurement of the perfusion defect by injection of ^{99m}Tc-sestamibi at least 120 h after epicardial coronary blood flow restoration provides an estimate of infarct size [20, 21]. The difference between these two measurements reflects the amount of myocardial salvage, and the ratio between the amount of myocardial salvage and the amount of myocardium at risk provides the myocardial salvage index.

Myocardium at Risk

Myocardium at risk is a measurement of the amount of jeopardized myocardium for infarction if a coronary artery occludes. Several experimental and clinical studies have confirmed the role of ^{99m}Tc-sestamibi for the measurement of myocardium at risk [20–24]. Myocardial uptake of this radiopharmaceutical is proportional to myocardial blood flow, and therefore the infarct area will appear as a perfusion defect.

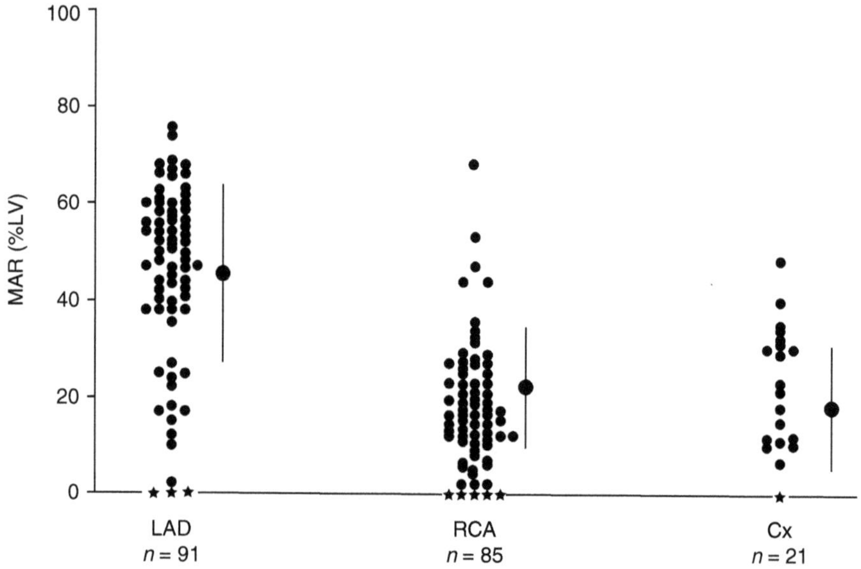

Fig. 8.1 Myocardium at risk by infarct-related coronary artery. The amount of myocardium at risk (*MAR*) is highly variable. Patients with inferior myocardial infarction (with right coronary artery [*RCA*] or left circumflex coronary artery [*Cx*] as infarct-related arteries) show smaller amount of myocardium at risk as compared with patients with anterior myocardial infarction (infarct-related artery, left anterior descending artery [*LAD*]). However, significant overlap between these patients can be observed (Reprinted from Klarich et al. [26]. With kind permission of Elsevier Limited)

Once the ^{99m}Tc-sestamibi has been taken up by the myocardium, the washout rate is very slow, and the redistribution of the radiopharmaceutical is minimal, permitting the measurement of myocardium at risk. To assess the amount of myocardium at risk, ^{99m}Tc-sestamibi is injected during coronary occlusion before reperfusion therapy. The tomographic images can be acquired 1–8 h after reperfusion therapy, providing accurate estimation of the myocardial perfusion defect or myocardium at risk at the time of the initial injection. Therefore, this imaging modality permits evaluation of the myocardium at risk without delaying the reperfusion therapy.

The extent of myocardium at risk is a major determinant of infarct size and long-term prognosis [22, 25]. However, it has been demonstrated that the amount of myocardium at risk is highly variable even when the coronary occlusion occurs in a similar location [22, 23]. In several clinical series evaluating the role of ^{99m}Tc-sestamibi SPECT to assess myocardium at risk in acute myocardial infarction, the extent of hypoperfusion varied from 9% to 68% of the left ventricle (Fig. 8.1) [23, 26]. In addition, the amount of myocardium at risk is usually larger in patients with anterior acute myocardial infarction as compared to inferior myocardial infarction [27]. In a series of 43 patients with acute myocardial infarction (20 with anterior infarction and 23 with inferior infarction), the area of myocardium at risk was evaluated with ^{99m}Tc-sestamibi SPECT. Patients with anterior myocardial infarction showed larger areas of myocardium at risk as compared to patients with inferior myocardial infarction

(52 ± 9% vs. 18 ± 10%, $p < 0.001$). The variability in the myocardial territory supplied by the coronary arteries and the effect of collateral flow in patients with chronic coronary artery disease may account for the reported wide spectrum of myocardium at risk [22, 23].

Infarct Size and Myocardial Salvage

The assessment of infarct size with ^{99m}Tc-sestamibi SPECT imaging after reperfusion therapy is an important surrogate to evaluate the efficacy of reperfusion therapy and has been related to long-term survival [16, 17]. To quantify infarct size, patients are imaged with ^{99m}Tc-sestamibi SPECT at least 120 h after reperfusion therapy. The presence of a perfusion defect as assessed with ^{99m}Tc-sestamibi SPECT imaging several days after the index infarction provides an accurate measurement of the final infarct size. Extensive evidence supports ^{99m}Tc-sestamibi SPECT imaging as a valid technique to assess infarct size.

First, a close correlation between infarct size, as measured with ^{99m}Tc-sestamibi SPECT imaging, and histological infarct size has been demonstrated in several animal models (of permanent coronary occlusion or reperfused myocardial infarction) [20, 21, 28]. In addition, various clinical studies have shown the close association between extent of tomographic defects and pathologic infarction by histology [29, 30]. For example, in a series of 30 patients with stenosis of the left anterior descending coronary artery and anterior wall motion abnormalities, Maes et al. demonstrated a close relationship between ^{99m}Tc-sestamibi uptake and myocardial fibrosis (assessed in perioperative transmural biopsies) [30]. More recently, gadolinium contrast-enhanced MRI has showed a close agreement to ^{99m}Tc-sestamibi SPECT imaging for infarct size quantification early after reperfused acute myocardial infarction [31]. Gadolinium contrast agents diffuse across the extracellular space; in irreversible injured myocardial tissue (myocardial scar), the extracellular space increases, and the contrast agent is trapped in these regions and visualized on contrast-enhanced MRI as bright hyperenhanced areas. A recent series of 30 patients with reperfused acute myocardial infarction showed a good correlation between gadolinium contrast-enhanced MRI and ^{99m}Tc-sestamibi SPECT for measurement of infarct size ($r = 0.86$, $p < 0.0001$) (Fig. 8.2) [31].

Furthermore, infarct size as assessed with ^{99m}Tc-sestamibi SPECT is related to other surrogates of infarct size commonly used in clinical practice such as left ventricular ejection fraction and end-systolic volume, wall motion score index, and levels of creatinine kinase [19]. Data from the Collaborative Organization for RheothRx Evaluation (CORE) trial showed that infarct size significantly correlated with left ventricular ejection fraction ($r = -0.67$, $p < 0.0001$) and end-systolic volume ($r = 0.57$, $p < 0.0001$) [16]. Importantly, infarct size measured with ^{99m}Tc-sestamibi SPECT imaging at hospital discharge is not affected by the presence of stunning or compensatory hyperkinesia, factors that may reduce the accuracy of left ventricular ejection fraction as a surrogate of infarct size [21, 32]. Indeed, several studies

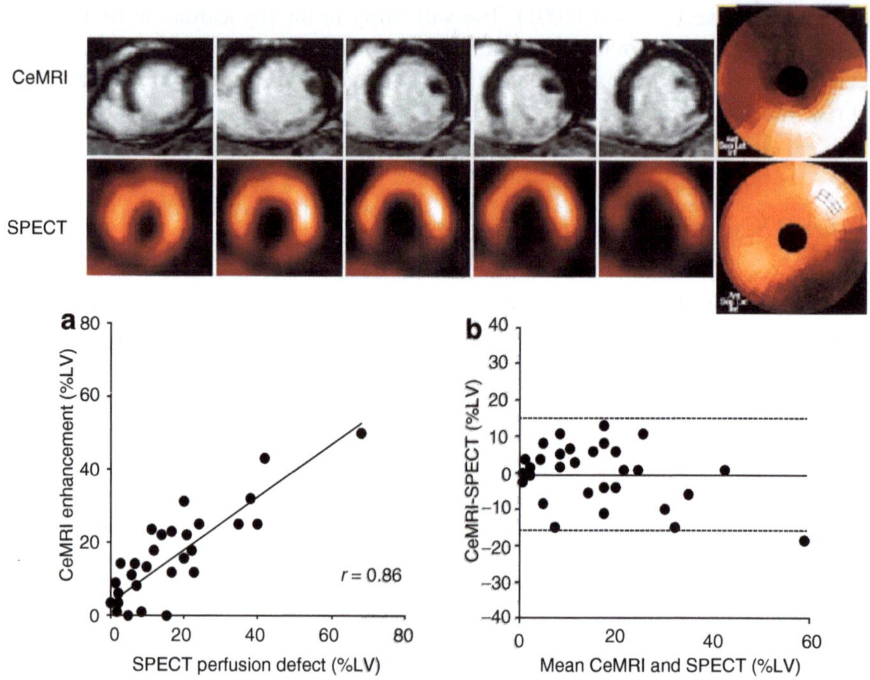

Fig. 8.2 Comparison between gadolinium contrast-enhanced MRI and ^{99m}Tc-tetrofosmin SPECT imaging to quantify infarct size. An inferoposterior transmural myocardial infarction visualized with contrast-enhanced MRI (CeMRI) and ^{99m}Tc-tetrofosmin SPECT imaging is shown in the *upper panel*. Short-axis slices (from apical [*left*] to basal [*right*]) of the left ventricle show a transmural area of hyperenhancement with MRI in the inferoposterior segments. On ^{99m}Tc-tetrofosmin SPECT short-axis views and polar maps, these areas are visualized as perfusion defect. The close correlation between contrast-enhanced MRI and ^{99m}Tc-tetrofosmin SPECT imaging to quantify infarct size is shown in *panel* (**a**). In addition, the agreement between the two techniques is shown in the Bland–Altman plot (*panel* **b**) (Reprinted from Ibrahim et al. [31]. With kind permission from Elsevier Ltd)

have shown that left ventricular ejection fraction may significantly increase at 6 weeks follow-up after index infarction [32]. The presence of stunning at discharge may explain the lower left ventricular ejection fraction than expected based on the perfusion defect size. In contrast, other series have shown a decrease in left ventricular ejection fraction at follow-up, indicating that, at discharge, the presence of compensatory hyperkinesia may result in a higher left ventricular ejection fraction than expected based on the perfusion defect size.

In addition, infarct size measured with ^{99m}Tc-sestamibi SPECT at discharge is a strong predictor of all-cause and cardiac mortality [16, 17, 33]. The largest series reporting the association between infarct size as assessed with ^{99m}Tc-sestamibi SPECT and 6-month outcome included 1,164 patients with acute myocardial infarction treated with thrombolysis (chi-square value = 9.05, p = 0.003) [16]. The mortality rate was 4.5% in patients with infarct size exceeding 35% of the left ventricle [16].

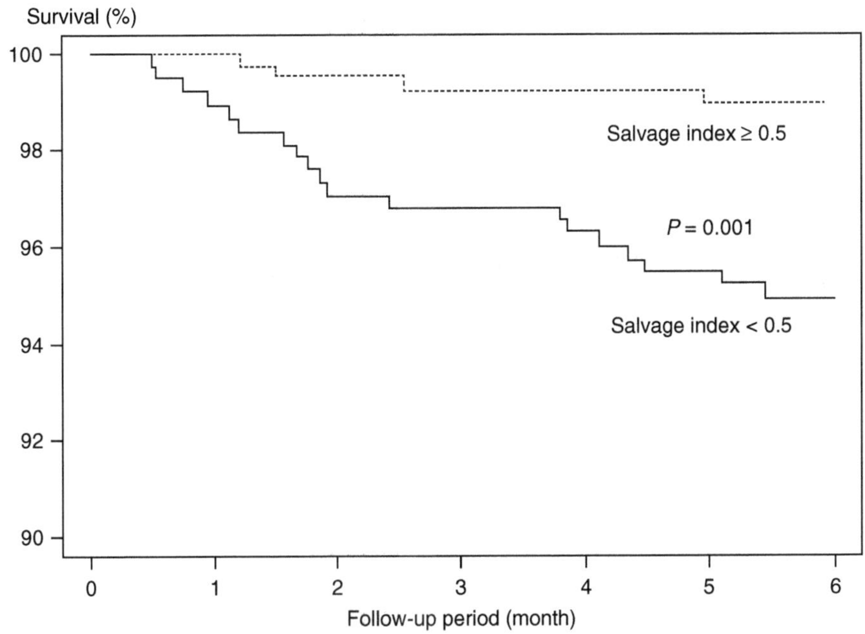

Fig. 8.3 Six months survival and myocardial salvage. The Kaplan–Meier curves show that patients with greater myocardial salvage indices (≥0.5) had superior 6-month survival with patients with lower myocardial salvage indices (<0.5) (Reprinted by permission of the Society of Nuclear Medicine from Ndrepepa et al. [35], Figure 1)

Finally, ^{99m}Tc-sestamibi SPECT permits the assessment of myocardial salvage, an index that may be more interesting rather than the measurement of infarct size alone. The difference between myocardial perfusion defect measured before reperfusion therapy (myocardium at risk) and the final infarct size (measured at discharge) results in myocardial salvage. Most studies have demonstrated that anterior myocardial infarction showed larger areas of myocardium at risk and larger infarct size as compared to inferior myocardial infarction, indicating that the benefit of reperfusion therapy is greater in patient with anterior myocardial infarction. However, after reperfusion therapy, the myocardial salvage was not significantly different (anterior myocardial infarction: 0.49 ± 0.34 vs. inferior myocardial infarction: 0.59 ± 0.35; p=NS) [27]. Importantly, myocardial salvage has been related to clinical outcome in several randomized trials [34]. Reperfusion strategies that result in smaller infarct size and greater myocardial salvage portend improved clinical outcomes [35]. Pooled data from three randomized trials evaluating different reperfusion strategies in 765 patients with acute myocardial infarction demonstrated that myocardial salvage index was independently associated with 6-month mortality (chi-square = 11.4, $p < 0.0007$) (Fig. 8.3). Patients with a salvage index ≥0.5 showed superior survival at 6 months follow-up as compared to patients with lower salvage indices [35].

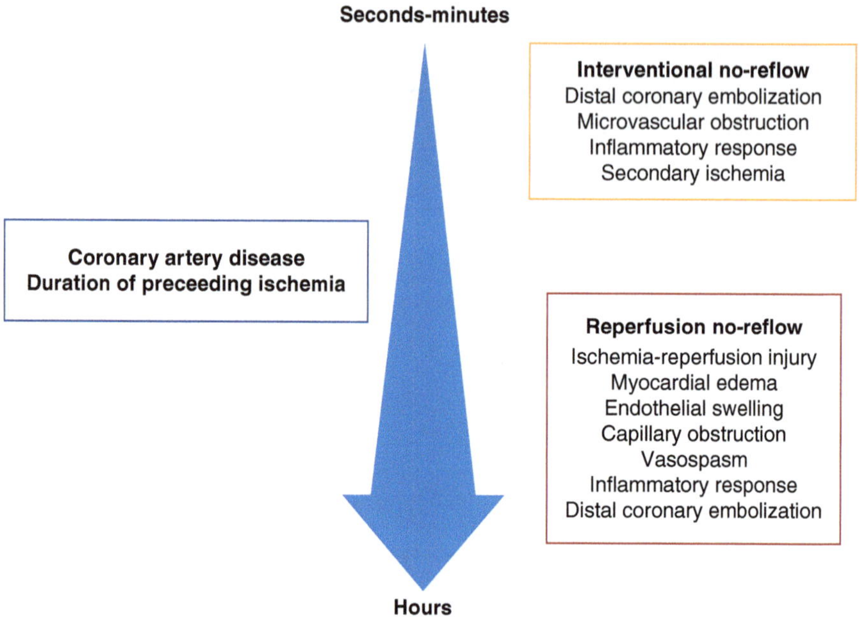

Fig. 8.4 Effect of duration of preceding myocardial ischemia on no-reflow phenomenon and underlying pathophysiological mechanisms. During interventional no-reflow, distal coronary embolization is the main mechanism of secondary ischemia. In contrast, during reperfusion no-reflow, the microvasculature within the necrotic zone is subjected to additional injury after reperfusion. Both mechanisms lead to myocardial ischemia and cell death (Adapted with permission from Jaffe et al. [7])

However, both infarct size and myocardial salvage are influenced by other markers of successful revascularization. The presence of adequate perfusion at the tissue level within the jeopardized myocardium has been associated with smaller infarct size and greater myocardial salvage [36]. In contrast, the presence of impaired myocardial perfusion despite a patent infarct-related artery is associated with larger infarct size and reduced salvage indexes. This phenomenon, also known as no-reflow phenomenon, will be discussed in the following paragraphs.

Microvascular Obstruction: Role of Nuclear Imaging

The concept of microvascular obstruction or "no-reflow" phenomenon is defined by myocardial tissue hypoperfusion in the presence of a patent epicardial coronary artery [7, 37]. Various pathophysiological mechanisms are involved in the no-reflow phenomenon (Fig. 8.4). Duration and severity of ischemia are the main determinants of microvascular damage. It has been demonstrated that endothelial cells are more resistant to ischemia than myocardial cells [9]. During the first 20 min of ischemic injury, the microcirculation remains structurally preserved whereas the myocardium may show reversible damage [38]. However, after 40 min of ischemia, the endothelium shows the first sign of damage (swollen cells), and the myocardium is irreversibly damaged. After 90 min of ischemia, both the endothelium and the myocardium show severe structural damage with obliteration of the vascular lumen and consequently myocardial tissue hypoperfusion. Early revascularization will reduce the area at risk, salvage myocardium, and improve long-term outcome [7]. However, myocardial hypoperfusion and infarct size may also increase after revascularization.

Reperfusion of the areas with damaged endothelium may lead to an acute inflammatory response with rapid release of oxygen free radicals, intracellular calcium overload, increased mitochondrial permeability, and intravascular plugging of red cells, platelets, and leukocytes. The adhesion of these cells to the vessel wall aggravates further the microvascular obstruction.

The no-reflow phenomenon can be observed during reperfusion of acute myocardial infarction in up to 35% of patients ("reperfusion no-reflow") or, less frequently, during elective percutaneous coronary intervention (<2% of patients) ("interventional no-reflow") [7, 39]. In patients with preexisting microvascular dysfunction, such as diabetic patients or patients with dyslipidemia, this phenomenon may be exacerbated.

Timely recognition of the no-reflow phenomenon has important prognostic implications [8]. Semiquantitative scoring with invasive coronary angiography is a common method to evaluate the epicardial coronary flow. The Thrombolysis in Myocardial Infarction (TIMI) score 3 indicates normal epicardial coronary flow whereas scores 0–2 indicate absence or reduced flow. It has been shown that patients with a Thrombolysis in Myocardial Infarction (TIMI) flow grade 3 have superior long-term outcome as compared to patients with TIMI flow grades 0–2 [8]. However, angiographic epicardial flow is a poor surrogate of tissue perfusion. Several noninvasive imaging modalities have shown that despite TIMI flow 3 after percutaneous coronary intervention, microvascular obstruction occurs frequently [37, 40, 41]. Myocardial contrast echocardiography, MRI techniques, and nuclear imaging have shown better diagnostic accuracy in characterizing myocardial tissue hypoperfusion in patients with TIMI flow 3 [37, 40, 41]. Particularly, nuclear imaging techniques can investigate myocardial perfusion, cell membrane integrity, and metabolic activity of the areas with no-reflow phenomenon (Table 8.1). The images obtained before percutaneous coronary intervention characterize the area at risk whereas the images obtained after revascularization indicate the degree of reflow and the extent of myocardial salvage (in the setting of an acute myocardial infarction).

Single-Photon Emission Computed Tomography

Several studies have shown the role of ^{201}Tl and ^{99m}Tc-sestamibi or ^{99m}Tc-tetrofosmin SPECT to evaluate the infarct size and the presence of microvascular obstruction or no-reflow phenomenon [42–44]. In patients with myocardial infarction treated with

Table 8.1 Radionuclide imaging techniques to evaluate microvascular obstruction

Imaging technique	Markers of microvascular obstruction
SPECT	
^{201}Tl/^{99m}Tc-microalbumin aggregates	Myocardial blood flow
^{99m}Tc-tetrofosmin	Myocardial blood flow
^{201}Tl/^{123}I-BMIPP	Perfusion–metabolism mismatch
PET	
Myocardial perfusion imaging/^{18}F-FDG	Perfusion–metabolism mismatch
^{13}N-ammonia	Myocardial blood flow
^{15}O-labeled water	Myocardial blood flow
^{82}Rb	Myocardial blood flow

^{18}FDG fluorodeoxyglucose, *^{123}I-BMIPP* beta-methyl-iodophenyl pentadecanoic acid, *^{13}N* nitrogen, *^{15}O* oxygen, *^{82}Rb* rubidium, *^{99}Tc* technetium, *^{201}Tl* thallium

revascularization (thrombolysis or percutaneous coronary intervention), patency of the epicardial coronary blood flow but impaired microvascular perfusion will be detected as a scintigraphic defect.

With intracoronary injection of ^{201}Tl- or ^{99m}Tc-microalbumin aggregates, Schofer et al. described the presence of scintigraphic no-reflow phenomenon in patients with first acute myocardial infarction [44]. The microalbumin aggregates permit evaluation of the blood flow at the precapillary or capillary level, and, therefore, microvascular dysfunction can be identified. In 12 patients with first acute myocardial infarction, ^{201}Tl or ^{99m}Tc-SPECT imaging was performed before and immediately after intracoronary thrombolysis [44]. In six patients, there were no changes in the perfusion defects after successful thrombolysis, suggesting that the absence of new uptake of the radionuclide tracers reflects the presence of impaired microvascular flow or no-reflow phenomenon [44]. Hamada et al. confirmed and extended these results by evaluating the area at risk, myocardial salvage, and infarct size with ^{99m}Tc-tetrofosmin SPECT imaging in 35 patients with first myocardial infarction treated with primary percutaneous coronary angioplasty [42]. The use of ^{99m}Tc-tetrofosmin permitted image acquisition before primary percutaneous coronary intervention (15 min after tracer injection). The SPECT scan was repeated immediately after successful revascularization of the culprit vessel and at 1 month follow-up. The defect score obtained before primary coronary intervention defined the area at risk whereas the defect score obtained at 1 month follow-up defined the final infarct size. The no-reflow phenomenon was defined by no significant change in the defect score between the first and the second radionuclide scan (before and after primary percutaneous coronary intervention). Figure 8.5 shows representative images of a patient with normal flow after revascularization and a patient with no-reflow phenomenon. A total of 15 (43%) patients showed no significant change in the defect score (the no-reflow group) [42]. Importantly, despite similar elapsed times between admission and coronary revascularization, collateral grade or TIMI flow grade and area at risk, the group of patients with microvascular obstruction showed significantly larger final infarct size at 1 month follow-up as compared to the group of patients with restoration of the microvascular flow (8.1 ± 4.3 vs. 4.9 ± 3.0, $p < 0.001$) [42].

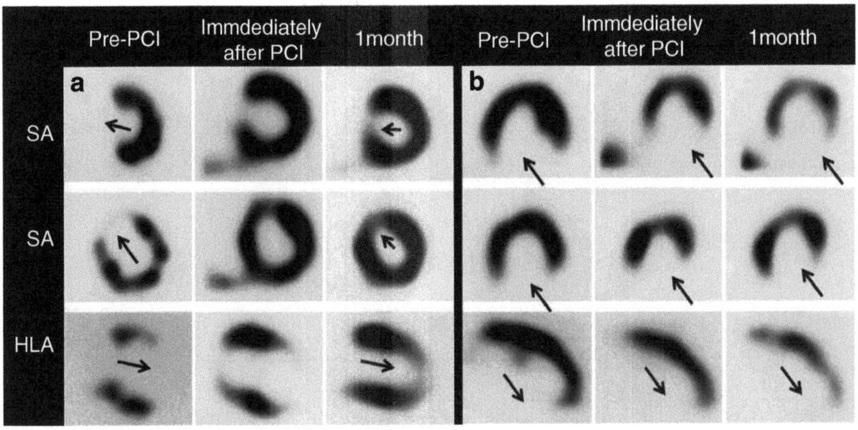

Fig. 8.5 Evaluation of no-reflow phenomenon with ^{99m}Tc-tetrofosmin single-photon emission computed tomography. *Panel* (**a**) Representative example of a patient with an anterior acute myocardial infarction and successful primary percutaneous coronary intervention to the left anterior descending coronary artery. Perfusion defects observed in the anteroseptal and apical regions improved immediately after revascularization and at 1 month follow-up. Therefore, TIMI flow grade 3 was achieved together with microvascular perfusion. *Panel* (**b**) Representative example of a patient with an inferior acute myocardial infarction. Despite TIMI flow grade 3 after primary percutaneous coronary intervention to the right coronary artery, the perfusion defects observed in the inferior and posterior walls (*arrows*) did not improve immediately after intervention and at 1-month follow-up, suggesting the presence of no-reflow phenomenon. *HLA* horizontal long-axis slice, *PCI* percutaneous coronary intervention, *SA* short-axis slice (Adapted from Hamada et al. [42]. With kind permission from Springer)

More recently, combination of metabolic and perfusion imaging has provided further characterization of the no-reflow phenomenon [45]. Dual-isotope myocardial SPECT using ^{99m}Tc or ^{201}Tl-label tracers and ^{123}I-beta-methyl-iodophenyl pentadecanoic acid (BMIPP) has demonstrated to be a valuable imaging technique to assess the efficacy of reperfusion therapies for acute myocardial infarction [45, 46]. In the clinical setting of successfully revascularized acute myocardial infarction, the myocardial areas with less uptake of ^{123}I-BMIPP relative to the uptake of ^{99m}Tc or ^{201}Tl-label tracers (perfusion–metabolism mismatch) indicate restored microvascular perfusion and have been related to inotropic reserve and further improvement in regional myocardial function at follow-up [45]. In contrast, the presence of microvascular obstruction or no-reflow phenomenon will result in similar areas of reduced ^{123}I-BMIPP and ^{99m}Tc or ^{201}Tl-label tracers uptake (smaller perfusion–metabolism mismatch). Shimizu et al. provided further relevant information by characterizing the presence of no-reflow phenomenon with ^{201}Tl-chloride/^{123}I-BMIPP dual-isotope myocardial SPECT in 73 patients with first myocardial infarction who underwent percutaneous revascularization [46]. All patients underwent ^{201}Tl-chloride/^{123}I-BMIPP dual-isotope myocardial SPECT within 1 week after percutaneous coronary intervention. The perfusion–metabolism mismatch ratios were significantly lower in the no-reflow subgroup as compared to the reflow subgroup (0.2 ± 0.1 vs. 0.4 ± 0.2,

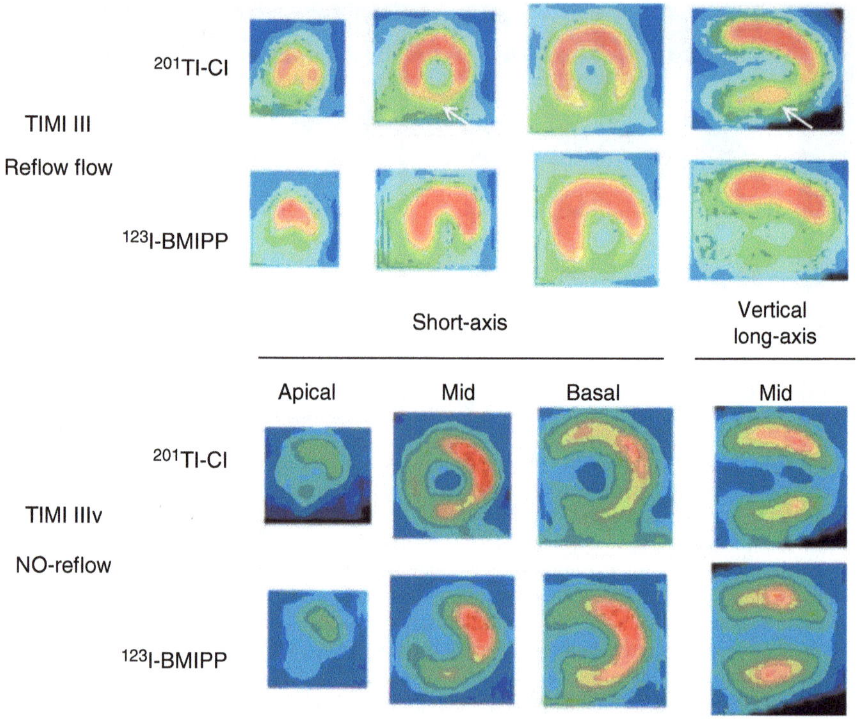

Fig. 8.6 Perfusion–metabolism mismatch with ^{201}Tl-chloride and ^{123}I-beta-methyl-iodophenyl pentadecanoic acid SPECT to evaluate no-reflow phenomenon. Vertical long-axis and short-axis slices of ^{201}Tl-chloride/^{123}I-BMIPP SPECT in two patients with acute myocardial infarction. The *upper panel* shows the example of a patient with an inferior acute myocardial infarction successfully treated with primary percutaneous coronary intervention. The metabolism defects as assessed with ^{123}I-BMIPP SPECT are larger as compared to the perfusion defects as evaluated with ^{201}Tl-chloride SPECT (*arrows*). This indicates restoration of blood flow at microvascular level. The *lower panels* show the example of a patient with an anterior myocardial infarction treated with primary percutaneous coronary intervention. Similar defects were identified in both the ^{201}Tl-chloride and the ^{123}I-BMIPP SPECT images. The absence of perfusion–metabolism mismatch indicates the presence of microvascular obstruction despite patency of the epicardial coronary flow. *^{123}I-BMIPP* ^{123}I-beta-methyl-iodophenyl pentadecanoic acid, *^{201}Tl-Cl* ^{201}thallium-chloride, *TIMI* Thrombolysis in Myocardial Infarction (Adapted from Shimizu et al. [46]. With kind permission from The Medical Association of Nippon Medical School)

$p < 0.001$) [46]. Figure 8.6 shows two representative examples of two patients with acute myocardial infarction treated with percutaneous coronary intervention and different perfusion–metabolism mismatch pattern.

Positron Emission Tomography

Positron emission tomography permits comprehensive evaluation of microvascular function and myocardial viability. Water labeled with oxygen-15 (^{15}O) and ammonia labeled with nitrogen-13 (^{13}N) and rubidium-82 (^{82}Rb) have been used to evaluate myocardial perfusion and quantify myocardial blood flow and coronary flow reserve [47]. Particularly, the measurement of myocardial blood flow and coronary flow reserve provides information on the macrocirculation (epicardial coronary arteries) and microcirculation. In patients with patent epicardial coronary arteries, the presence of a reduced coronary flow reserve indicates the presence of abnormal microvascular function.

In the setting of acute myocardial infarction, PET imaging has been used to evaluate the efficacy of coronary reperfusion. The no-reflow phenomenon has been demonstrated by PET in experimental and clinical studies [40, 48]. In 30 patients with an acute myocardial infarction and TIMI flow grade 3 after thrombolytic therapy, myocardial perfusion and metabolism were evaluated with ^{13}N-ammonia and ^{18}F-fluorodeoxyglucose (^{18}F-FDG) PET imaging, respectively [29]. In 73% of patients, a PET perfusion–metabolism match (proportional decrease of myocardial perfusion and metabolism) was observed within 24 h after coronary revascularization whereas the remaining 27% of patients showed a significant PET perfusion–metabolism mismatch (decreased myocardial perfusion with preserved ^{18}F-FDG uptake). Patients with severely impaired myocardial blood flow showed no functional improvement at 3 months follow-up whereas patients with mildly reduced or preserved myocardial blood flow showed significant functional improvement. Interestingly, patients with moderately reduced myocardial blood flow and perfusion–metabolism mismatch showed a significant functional improvement [29]. Therefore, the assessment of myocardial perfusion with PET early after successful thrombolysis has important prognostic implications since it predicts left ventricular functional recovery. In addition, the assessment of myocardial metabolism permits identification of dysfunctional but viable myocardium that may benefit from additional therapies that aim to improve the microcirculation of the reperfused myocardium.

Assessment of Myocardial Viability

Chronic heart failure is most often caused by ischemic left ventricular dysfunction as a consequence of chronic coronary artery disease [1]. Patients with chronic ischemic left ventricular dysfunction generally have a poor prognosis. The prognosis is related to the severity and cause of left ventricular function and the presence of comorbidity. Although the prognosis of these patients is poor, significant progress has been made in medical therapy, coronary revascularization and additional surgical procedures, device therapy, and cardiac transplant. It has become clear that coronary revascularization may substantially improve left ventricular function and prognosis in a subset of these patients [49, 50]. However, patients with chronic ischemic left ventricular dysfunction are at an increased risk of periprocedural complications, and not all patients benefit from coronary revascularization. Therefore, a careful selection of patients for coronary revascularization is required. Noninvasive assessment of myocardial viability may improve selection of patients with chronic ischemic left ventricular dysfunction for coronary revascularization.

Concept of Hibernating Myocardium

In 1978, Diamond et al. demonstrated in an animal model that ischemic noninfarcted myocardium could exist in a state of hibernation [51]. Rahimtoola was the first who described hibernating myocardium in patients with chronic ischemic left ventricular dysfunction [13, 52]. Myocardial hibernation is defined as a condition of chronic left ventricular dysfunction due to chronic hypoperfusion in patients with coronary artery disease in whom coronary revascularization causes recovery of left ventricular contractile function [13, 52]. The pathophysiological mechanisms involved in hibernating myocardium are not fully clear; the phenomenon may be caused by cardiomyocytes reducing their activity level to match a reduced perfusion supply. In biopsy samples of hibernating myocardium, signs of a reduced activity level have been demonstrated including loss of contractile filaments, small mitochondria, nuclei with uniformly distributed chromatin, and a severely reduced sarcoplasmic reticulum [53, 54]. Patients with ischemic left ventricular dysfunction often have coexisting areas of viable myocardium with myocardial hibernation and myocardial stunning and irreversibly scarred areas because of myocardial infarction. Myocardial stunning is defined as viable myocardium exhibiting prolonged contractile dysfunction in the presence of (near) normal resting blood flow. Myocardial infarction is characterized by dysfunctional, irreversibly scarred myocardium as a consequence of myocardial ischemia.

Which Noninvasive Imaging Techniques?

Various noninvasive imaging have been developed to evaluate myocardial viability in patients with ischemic left ventricular dysfunction [49, 50]. These noninvasive imaging techniques probe different features of dysfunctional but viable myocardium, and therefore, the diagnostic accuracy of the noninvasive imaging techniques varies [50, 55]. Dobutamine stress echocardiography and dobutamine stress MRI can be used to evaluate contractile reserve. Contractile reserve is an improvement of myocardial contractility and can be elicited by exercise or pharmacological stimulation. Cardiac metabolism can be evaluated by nuclear imaging techniques such as SPECT and PET. Intact cell membranes and intact mitochondria also can be evaluated by SPECT and PET. More recently, contrast-enhanced MRI has been developed for assessment of scar tissue and the transmurality of scar tissue. The noninvasive imaging techniques that are currently used for evaluation of myocardial viability are summarized in Table 8.2 and will be sequentially discussed in more detail.

Dobutamine Stress Echocardiography

Dobutamine stress echocardiography is a widely available and extensively used noninvasive imaging technique for the evaluation of myocardial viability and myocardial

Table 8.2 Viability characteristics, imaging modalities, and viability criteria

Characteristic	Imaging modality	Viability criteria
Contractile reserve	Dobutamine echo/MRI	Improved contraction during infusion of low-dose dobutamine
Scar tissue	Contrast-enhanced MRI	Non-transmural hyperenhancement
Glucose metabolism	^{18}F-FDG PET/SPECT	Normal perfusion/FDG uptake
		Perfusion–FDG mismatch
Intact cell membrane	^{201}Tl-SPECT	Redistribution
		Activity >50%
Intact mitochondria	^{99m}Tc-sestamibi/tetrofosmin SPECT	Activity >50%
		Improved tracer uptake post-nitrates

Table based on Schinkel et al. [56]
^{18}*FDG* fluorodeoxyglucose, *MRI* magnetic resonance imaging, ^{99}*Tc* technetium, ^{201}*Tl* thallium

ischemia [49, 50]. The technique evaluates the changes in contractile function during pharmacological stimulation with dobutamine. Dobutamine is a sympathicomimetic amine that was developed for its positive inotropic and chronotropic effects in patients with heart failure. During low-dose (5–10 μg/kg/min) dobutamine infusion, cardiac output typically increases because of an increase in stroke volume and a decrease of systemic vascular resistance, and additionally, a slight increase in heart frequency usually occurs. At higher doses of dobutamine (up to 40 μg/kg/min), the chronotropic effects predominate, and myocardial ischemia may be elicited. Dobutamine stress echocardiography is a safe test, but complications may occur and are more frequently observed in patients with previous myocardial infarction or impaired left ventricular function [57].

Image acquisition is performed at rest, during low-dose dobutamine infusion, at high-dose dobutamine infusion, and in the recovery phase (Fig. 8.7). Subsequently, the wall motion and wall thickening are scored visually using a semiquantitative grading scale. This method is dependent on the experience of the reader; therefore, quantitative analysis of myocardial contractility has been developed [58]. However until now, quantitative scoring has not been used on a routine basis in most echocardiography laboratories.

Viability analysis: Low-dose dobutamine infusion may improve contractile function in dysfunctional but viable myocardium, which has been referred to as contractile reserve. Irreversibly scarred nonviable myocardium does not show contractile reserve during low-dose dobutamine infusion. Incremental doses of dobutamine can be administered to evaluate stress-induced myocardial ischemia, which is characterized by worsening of wall motion during high-dose dobutamine stress. A biphasic response during low- and high-dose dobutamine stress echocardiography is characterized by improvement of wall motion and contractility during low-dose dobutamine infusion and subsequent worsening of wall motion at high-dose dobutamine infusion. This biphasic response is indicative of a hemodynamically significant coronary stenosis, and revascularization of segments with a biphasic response pattern is associated with a relatively high chance of improvement of segmental wall motion following coronary revascularization [59].

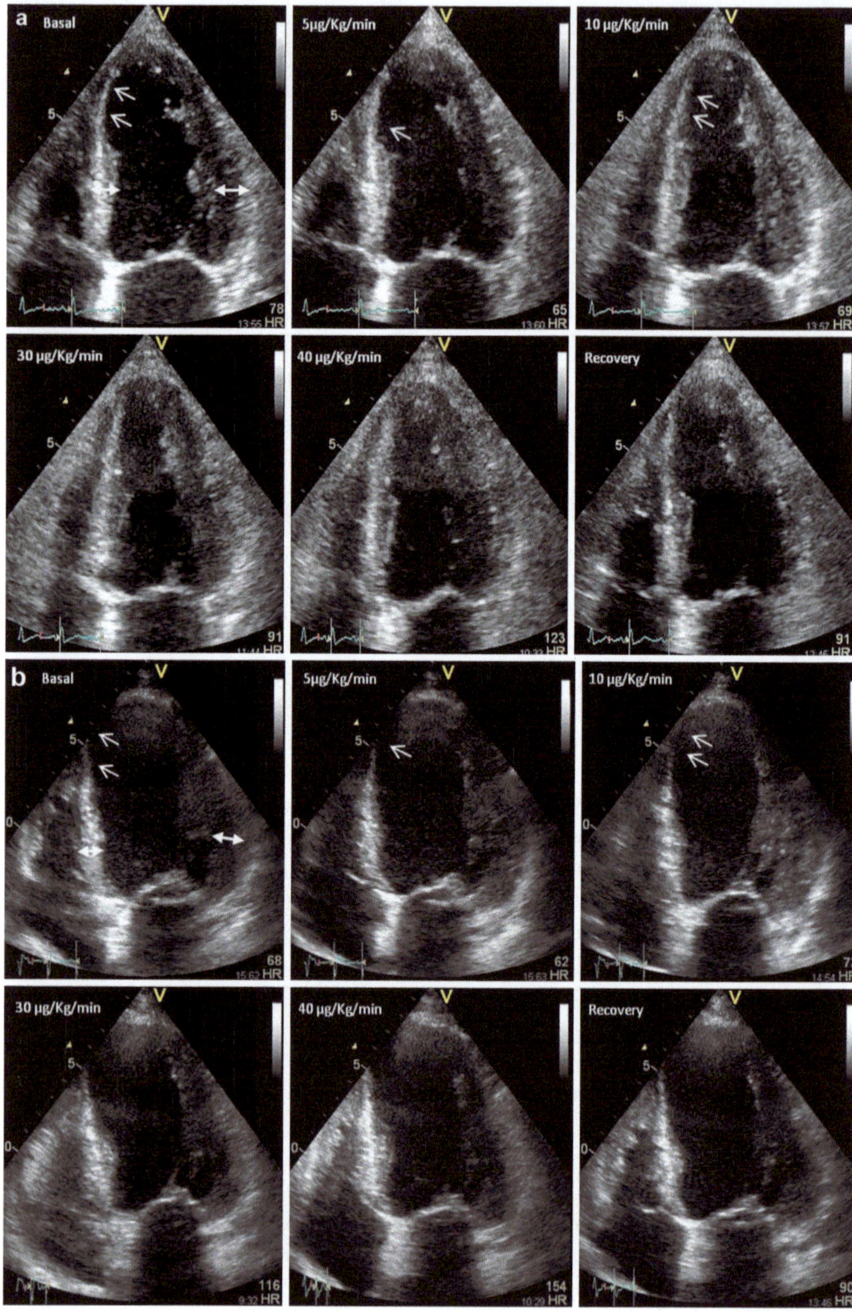
a
Basal
5μg/Kg/min
10 μg/Kg/min
30 μg/Kg/min
40 μg/Kg/min
Recovery
b
Basal
5μg/Kg/min
10 μg/Kg/min
30 μg/Kg/min
40 μg/Kg/min
Recovery

Magnetic Resonance Imaging

Three MRI techniques are currently used in clinical practice for the noninvasive evaluation of myocardial viability [60, 61]. Resting MRI can be used to measure end-diastolic wall thickness, dobutamine MRI is used in a similar way to dobutamine stress echocardiography to evaluate contractile reserve, and contrast-enhanced MRI allows precise detection of scar tissue. Cardiac MRI has several advantages, including a high-spatial resolution which allows evaluation of the transmurality of myocardial scar tissue. Cardiac MRI can be used in the majority of patients with chronic ischemic left ventricular dysfunction, except those with cardiac pacemakers or defibrillators. The three-dimensional data acquisition allows reconstruction in any required plane.

Viability analysis: A first impression on the absence of myocardial viability can be obtained by measuring end-diastolic wall thickness in the dysfunctional segments. An end-diastolic wall thickness <6 mm indicates nonviable myocardium (Fig. 8.8) [50]. In dysfunctional segments with a preserved end-diastolic wall thickness, additional information is needed to estimate the chances of recovery following coronary revascularization.

Dobutamine stress MRI can be performed in a similar way to dobutamine stress echocardiography. Changes in wall motion and wall thickening during low- and high-dose dobutamine infusions can be quantified using MRI tagging techniques.

Contrast-enhanced MRI is mostly performed using a gadolinium-based contrast agent. Gadolinium contrast agents are retained in the intercellular compartment of infarcted myocardium, which allows precise evaluation of scar tissue (see Fig. 8.8). The transmural extent of gadolinium enhancement on cardiac MRI is an important predictor of the chances of recovery of left ventricular function following coronary revascularization [50, 55].

Fig. 8.7 Assessment of myocardial viability with resting and dobutamine stress echocardiography. Resting and dobutamine stress echocardiographies permit evaluation of myocardial thinning, contractile reserve, and myocardial ischemia. *Panel* (**a**) Example of a patient with ischemic cardiomyopathy (left ventricular ejection fraction 35%). At baseline, the resting echocardiography shows areas of thinning (<1 cm markers) in the mid and apical segments of the septal wall (*arrows*) whereas the lateral wall and the basal segment of the septum show preserved thickness (*double arrows*). During low-dose and peak-dose dobutamine stress echocardiography, the mid and apical segments of the septal wall show improved thickening (*arrows*) consistent with myocardial viability. *Panel* (**b**) Example of patient with ischemic cardiomyopathy (left ventricular ejection fraction 32%). Resting echocardiography shows extensive areas of thinning in the left ventricular apex (*arrows*). The lateral wall and the mid and basal segments of the septum show normal thickening. In contrast to the example of *panel* (**a**), low-dose dobutamine stress echocardiography does not show improvement in regional thickening of these areas consistent with absence of myocardial viability

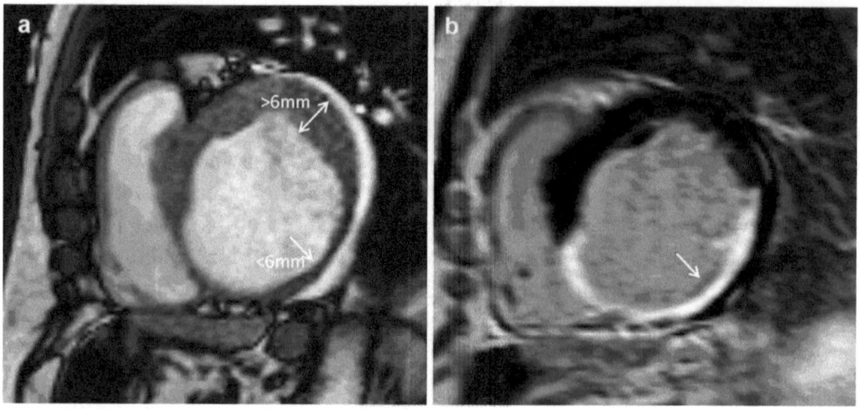

Fig. 8.8 Cardiac magnetic resonance imaging to evaluate myocardial viability. Magnetic resonance imaging techniques provide comprehensive information on myocardial viability. Left ventricular segments with end-diastolic wall thickness <6 mm indicate the presence of transmural scar and low likelihood of functional improvement after revascularization (*panel* **a**). Late-gadolinium enhancement provides exact information on the location and transmurality of myocardial scar tissue (*arrow*) (*panel* **b**)

Single-Photon Emission Computed Tomography

Nuclear imaging with SPECT has been extensively studied for the evaluation of myocardial viability. Traditionally, ^{201}Tl has been used to assess myocardial perfusion; several imaging protocols have been developed for evaluation of myocardial viability. Early after intravenous administration, myocardial uptake of ^{201}Tl is relatively high. In the hours after initial uptake, myocardial redistribution of ^{201}Tl may occur because of a different clearance of the tracer between normal and ischemic myocardium. The ^{201}Tl uptake over longer time is dependent on integrity of the cell membrane and thus indicates myocardial viability. Usually, image acquisition is performed early after ^{201}Tl injection to optimize the detection of flow heterogeneity. Subsequently, image acquisition is repeated after 3–4 h to allow tracer redistribution that becomes more apparent over time.

Viability analysis ^{201}Tl: In clinical practice, ^{201}Tl rest-redistribution and stress-redistribution-reinjection protocols are both used (Fig. 8.9). The rest-redistribution protocol (early and 3–4 h acquisition) provides information on myocardial perfusion at rest and myocardial redistribution which indicates myocardial viability. The stress-redistribution-reinjection protocol consists of initial image acquisition early after tracer injection during exercise or pharmacological stress and delayed (3–4 h) image acquisition to evaluate redistribution. Finally, a third image set is acquired 1 h after tracer reinjection. The stress-redistribution-reinjection protocol provides information on both myocardial ischemia and myocardial viability.

Myocardial viability is indicated by:

1. Normal ^{201}Tl uptake at stress
2. Stress defects with redistribution (reversible defects) at the 3–4 h delayed image sets

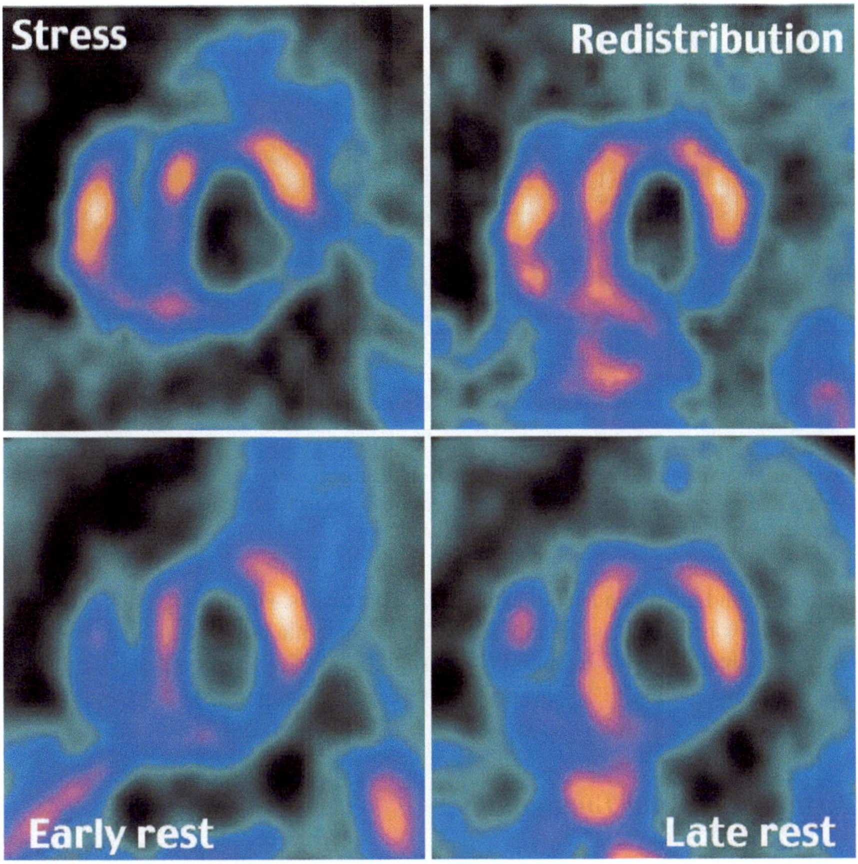

Fig. 8.9 Myocardial viability assessment with thallium-201. The stress-redistribution-reinjection protocol was employed in this example. The short-axis ^{201}Tl tomograms show stress-induced perfusion abnormalities in the septum and the anterior wall and a fixed defect in the infero-lateral wall in the conventional stress and redistribution images (*top row*). On a separate occasion, ^{201}Tl was injected at rest with immediate and delayed imaging (*bottom row*), demonstrating reduced perfusion in the septum and a fixed infero-lateral defect. Therefore, the anteroseptal region is viable and will recover function after revascularization. The infero-lateral wall is infarcted, and it will not recover (Adapted from Anagnostopoulos et al. [62]. With kind permission from Oxford University Press)

3. Redistribution in fixed defects at redistribution following reinjection or delayed rest images (frequently a threshold of 10% increase in tracer uptake is used)
4. Tracer uptake >50% at the redistribution/reinjection images or the delayed rest images

Viability analysis ^{99m}Tc: To overcome some of the basic limitations of ^{201}Tl, the ^{99m}Tc-based tracers (^{99m}Tc-sestamibi and ^{99m}Tc-tetrofosmin) were introduced to improve imaging physics and minimize radiation. Myocardial accumulation of these tracers is mainly determined by passive diffusion and depends on the cell

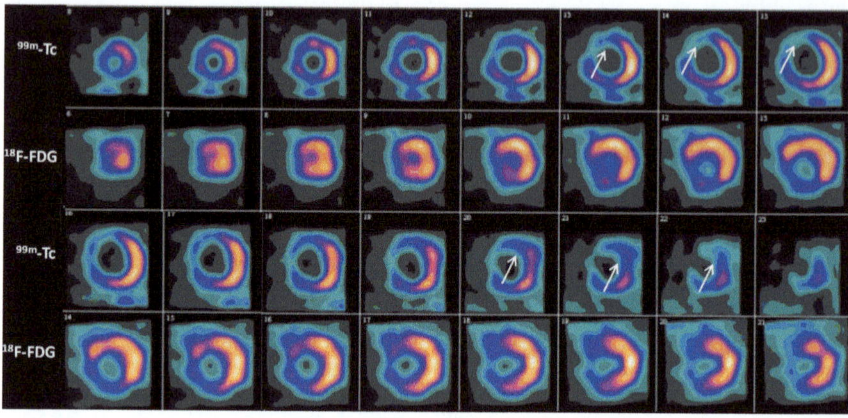

Fig. 8.10 Dual-isotope simultaneous acquisition ^{99m}Tc-tetrofosmin/^{18}F-FDG SPECT to evaluate myocardial perfusion and myocardial metabolism. The left ventricular short-axis slices show extensive areas of perfusion–metabolism mismatch (*arrows*), indicating viable myocardium in the anteroseptal, anterior, lateral, and posterior regions

membrane and mitochondrial transmembrane potentials. For assessment of myocardial viability, both ^{99m}Tc-sestamibi and ^{99m}Tc-tetrofosmin are used; most experience has been obtained with resting ^{99m}Tc-sestamibi SPECT. Myocardial viability is defined as myocardial ^{99m}Tc-sestamibi or ^{99m}Tc-tetrofosmin uptake >50–60%.

Positron Emission Tomography

^{18}F-fluorodeoxyglucose PET imaging is a reliable quantitative method for assessment of myocardial viability. Myocardial uptake of ^{18}F-FDG is comparable to glucose uptake; subsequently, the tracer is trapped in the myocytes, providing a strong signal for imaging. Myocardial ^{18}F-FDG uptake highly depends on metabolic circumstances: insulin stimulates cardiac glucose (and ^{18}F-FDG) uptake, whereas free fatty acids inhibit glucose (and ^{18}F-FDG) accumulation. Usually, oral glucose loading is used to optimize ^{18}F-FDG PET image quality. However, this approach may result in suboptimal image quality in patients with impaired glucose tolerance or diabetes mellitus. In these patients, hyperinsulinemic euglycemic clamping or oral administration of nicotinic acid derivatives can be used to improve image quality [63].

Viability analysis: Hibernating myocardium is characterized by a reduced perfusion and relatively preserved ^{18}F-FDG uptake (perfusion–metabolism mismatch pattern). Nonviable myocardium exhibits a perfusion–metabolism match pattern. Subendocardial and transmural scar tissue can be distinguished by the percentage of tracer uptake. The availability of PET imaging for assessment of myocardial viability is limited. Dual-isotope simultaneous acquisition SPECT enables evaluation of myocardial perfusion using ^{99m}Tc-sestamibi or ^{99m}Tc-tetrofosmin and myocardial metabolism using ^{18}F-FDG (Fig. 8.10). Despite the differences between PET and

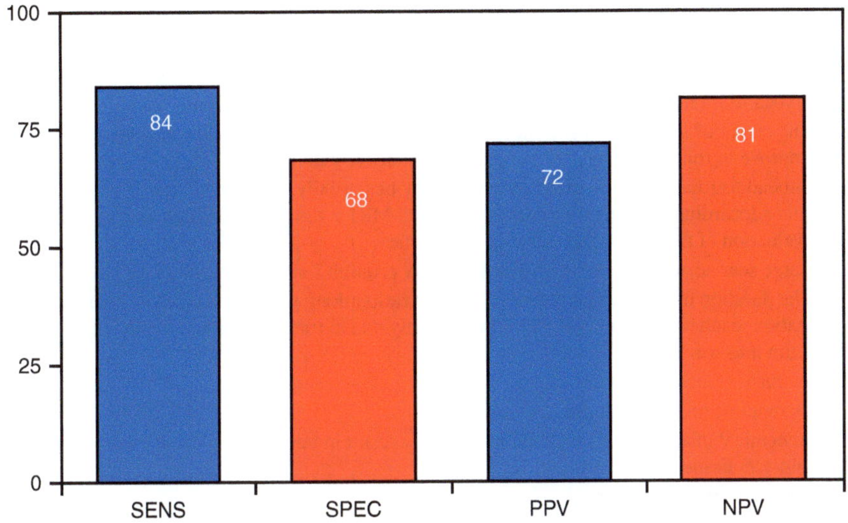

Fig. 8.11 Results of a pooled analysis of 143 studies including 4,437 patients on the diagnostic accuracy of noninvasive imaging techniques for the prediction of improvement of regional contractile function following coronary revascularization. *SENS* sensitivity, *SPEC* specificity, *PPV* positive predictive value, *NPV* negative predictive value (Data based on Schinkel et al. [50])

SPECT in terms of image resolution, dual-isotope simultaneous acquisition SPECT provides similar information.

Prediction of Improvement of Regional Function

Most studies that have evaluated the diagnostic accuracy of noninvasive imaging techniques have focused on the prediction of recovery of regional contractile dysfunction following coronary revascularization. Pooled analysis of the available literature (143 studies involving 4,437 patients) for the prediction of improvement of regional function following coronary revascularization demonstrated a sensitivity of 84% (9,635/11,500 segments) and a specificity of 68% (8,011/11,770 segments) (Fig. 8.11) [50]. Clearly, this pooled analysis has inherent limitations, as different noninvasive imaging techniques were pooled using arbitrary cutoffs for the classification of myocardial viability. In general, specificities were lower than sensitivities, indicating that a substantial percentage of segments that are classified as viable by the imaging techniques do not improve in function after revascularization. This does not necessarily mean that noninvasive imaging techniques overestimate recovery of function. Multiple factors may explain why viable segments do not improve in function after revascularization [50]. These can be divided into issues before, during, and after revascularization (Table 8.3).

Table 8.3 Factors influencing recovery of function following coronary revascularization

Factors before revascularization
1. The severity of cellular damage in the hibernating myocardium: too severely damaged myocardium may no longer improve in function after revascularization
2. The extent of left ventricular remodeling: severely dilated left ventricles may no longer improve in function despite the presence of extensive viability
3. Subendocardial scar formation: a segment may be partially viable (with scar limited to the subendocardium). Currently, contrast-enhanced MRI is the only technique that permits evaluation of the transmural extent of scar tissue
4. Large scar adjacent to viable myocardium may prohibit functional recovery
5. The duration of hibernation before revascularization; long waiting time before revascularization resulted in absence of recovery, probably due to transition of hibernating myocardium into scar tissue.
Factors during revascularization
1. Incomplete revascularization
2. Ischemic damage during revascularization may result in transition of viable myocardium into scar tissue
Factors after revascularization
1. Graft occlusion or restenosis may result in lack of recovery
2. Timing of assessment of function after revascularization; severely damaged myocardium may take up to 1 year to improve in function after coronary revascularization

Table based on Schinkel et al. [50]
MRI magnetic resonance imaging

Prediction of Improvement of Global Function, Heart Failure Symptoms, and Prognosis

Besides improvement of regional contractile function following coronary revascularization, other endpoints have been studied. A total of 13 studies have evaluated various noninvasive imaging techniques for the prediction of recovery of global contractile function (left ventricular ejection fraction) following coronary revascularization [50]. Pooled analysis of the 13 available studies demonstrated a sensitivity of 76% (246/322 patients) and a specificity of 66% (212/319 patients) for the prediction of improvement of global contractile function following coronary revascularization (Fig. 8.12). It should be noted, however, that treatment decisions were not standardized in these studies, and most studies had a retrospective design.

Improvement of heart failure symptoms has been studied as an alternative endpoint in a few studies [50]. These studies indicated that improvement of heart failure symptoms and exercise capacity may occur in patients with a substantial amount of dysfunctional but viable myocardium who undergo coronary revascularization. Currently, it is not clear how much dysfunctional but viable myocardium is needed for improvement of symptoms and exercise capacity. Moreover, it is not clear if an improvement in global left ventricular function will result in an improvement of symptoms [50].

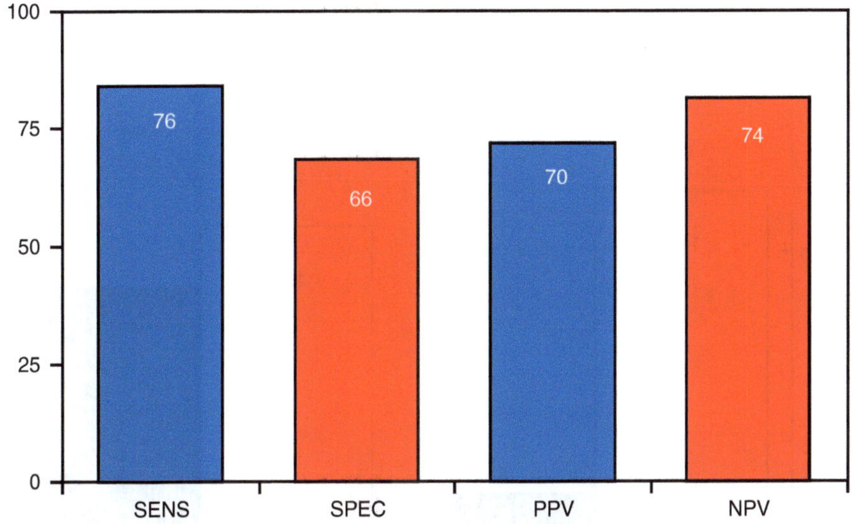

Fig. 8.12 Results of a pooled analysis of 13 studies including 641 patients on the diagnostic accuracy of noninvasive imaging techniques for the prediction of improvement of global contractile function (left ventricular ejection fraction) following coronary revascularization. *SENS* sensitivity, *SPEC* specificity, *PPV* positive predictive value, *NPV* negative predictive value (Data based on Schinkel et al. [50])

Improvement of long-term prognosis may be the ultimate goal of revascularization of dysfunctional but viable myocardium. A total of 29 studies have evaluated the results of noninvasive viability techniques in relation to therapy (medical therapy or coronary revascularization). Pooled analysis of these results revealed that patients with viability who underwent revascularization had the best long-term prognosis (Fig. 8.13). Conversely, the pooled results revealed that patients with viable myocardium who were treated medically had a high mortality rate. The patients without viable myocardium had a poor prognosis irrespective of the chosen therapy.

These observations have been recently confronted by the results of the randomized STICH (Surgical Treatment for Ischemic Heart Failure) trial [64]. A total of 1,212 patients with left ventricular ejection fraction ≤35% and coronary artery disease amenable to surgical revascularization were randomized to optimized medical treatment alone or medical treatment plus coronary artery bypass surgery. There were no differences in the primary endpoint of all-cause mortality between the two study groups. However, cardiovascular mortality and heart failure hospitalization rates were significantly reduced in the group of patients who were revascularized. These findings indicate that in patients with ischemic heart failure, angiographic assessment of coronary artery disease should be considered in order to evaluate the potential benefit of surgical revascularization. However, the presence of myocardial viability may be another important predictor of survival benefit from revascularization.

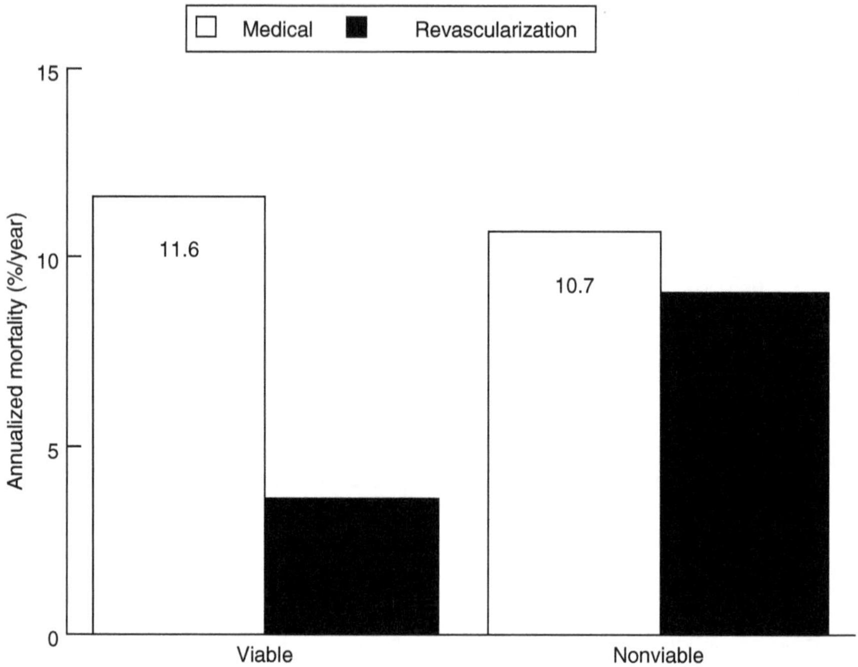

Fig. 8.13 Pooled analysis of data from 29 prognostic studies using different viable techniques that showed the annualized mortality rate in patient with and without substantial viable myocardium according to treatment strategy (medical therapy vs. revascularization). Patients with viable myocardium who underwent coronary revascularization had the lowest annualized mortality rate (Data based on Schinkel et al. [50])

Indeed, the results of the subanalysis of the STICH trial evaluating the interaction between presence of viable myocardium and treatment effect in 601 patients demonstrated that patients with myocardial viability had lower all-cause mortality rates than patients without viability (hazard ratio: 0.64; 95% confidence interval 0.48–0.86; $p=0.003$) [65]. However, at multivariate analysis, after correcting for other prognostic variables, presence of myocardial viability was not an independent predictor of all-cause mortality ($p=0.21$). There was no significant interaction between myocardial viability and treatment for any of the study endpoints. These findings suggest that, besides the selection bias, other variables included in the multivariate analysis, that may be also influenced by the presence of viable myocardium such as left ventricular volumes or ejection fraction, may have had a stronger influence on long-term survival. Therefore, evaluation of myocardial viability may be reserved for patients with high operative risk and more reduced left ventricular ejection fraction in order to identify the patients who will benefit from surgical revascularization.

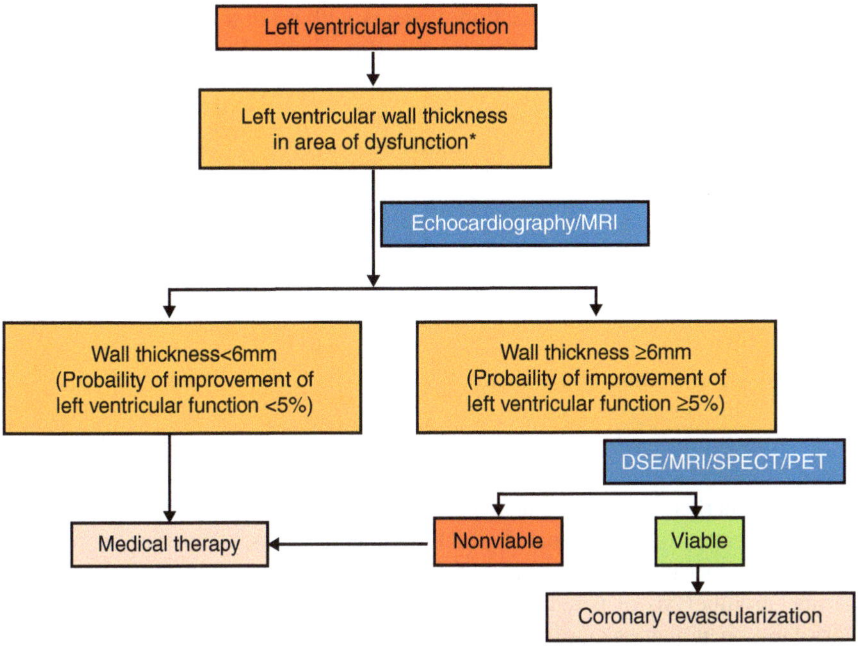

Fig. 8.14 Algorithm for the evaluation of myocardial viability and the need for coronary revascularization in patients with ischemic left ventricular dysfunction. *All patients need intensive medical therapy by standards of current era. *DSE* dobutamine stress echocardiography, *MRI* magnetic resonance imaging, *PET* positron emission tomography, *SPECT* single-photon emission computed tomography (Algorithm adapted from Rahimtoola et al. [55]. With kind permission from Elsevier Ltd.)

Integration of Noninvasive Imaging Results in Patient Management

The clinical data, results from noninvasive imaging, coronary angiography, and treatment options are preferably evaluated in a heart team conference by cardiologists, cardiac surgeons, and anesthesiologists to optimize therapy. Several models have been proposed to integrate the information on myocardial viability obtained with noninvasive imaging in clinical patient management [55, 66]. A suggested algorithm for the evaluation of myocardial viability and the need for coronary revascularization is shown in Fig. 8.14.

In patients with suspected ischemic left ventricular dysfunction, echocardiography is usually the first noninvasive imaging modality to assess left ventricular function and volumes and evaluate concomitant valvular disease. Echocardiography or MRI can be used to assess wall thickness in the dysfunctional areas for initial evaluation of myocardial viability. If end-diastolic wall thickness is <6 mm, recovery of function is unlikely. In dysfunctional regions with a preserved end-diastolic wall thickness, additional diagnostic testing is needed to estimate the benefits of coronary revascularization. Patients with no or a very limited amount of viable tissue and severe left ventricular dysfunction will not benefit from coronary revascularization and should proceed with optimal medical therapy. Patients with a substantial amount of dysfunctional viable tissue, and a coronary anatomy that is amendable to coronary revascularization, may be candidates for coronary revascularization.

Conclusion

Nuclear imaging permits comprehensive evaluation of patients with coronary artery disease. In the setting of acute myocardial infarction, ^{99m}Tc-sestamibi SPECT provides information on myocardium at risk, infarct size, and myocardial salvage. These parameters are valid measures of reperfusion efficacy therapy and important prognostic markers. However, patency of the epicardial coronary flow after revascularization therapy does not equate to restoration of microvascular perfusion. Nuclear imaging also permits the assessment of no-reflow phenomenon that may take place during thrombolysis or percutaneous revascularization techniques. Timely detection of this phenomenon may help to select the most appropriate therapies to improve the microcirculation of the infarcted areas and, consequently, to improve the contractile function of the myocardium at follow-up. Finally, patients with a substantial amount of dysfunctional but viable myocardium may improve in regional and global left ventricular function and experience a reduction in heart failure symptoms and improvement of prognosis after coronary revascularization. Accurate assessment of viable myocardium with multimodality imaging may help the clinical management and long-term outcomes of these patients.

Disclosures The Department of Cardiology received grants from Biotronik, Medtronic, Boston Scientific Corporation, Lantheus Medical Imaging, St. Jude Medical, GE Healthcare, and Edwards Lifesciences. Dr. Victoria Delgado received consulting fees from Medtronic and St. Jude Medical. Dr. Kai-Hang Yiu is financially supported by the Hong Kong Heart Foundation.

References

1. Gheorghiade M, Sopko G, De LL, et al. Navigating the crossroads of coronary artery disease and heart failure. Circulation. 2006;114:1202–13.
2. Camici PG, Prasad SK, Rimoldi OE. Stunning, hibernation, and assessment of myocardial viability. Circulation. 2008;117:103–14.
3. Bonow RO. Prognostic assessment in coronary artery disease: role of radionuclide angiography. J Nucl Cardiol. 1994;1:280–91.
4. Gibbons RJ, Christian TF, Hopfenspirger M, Hodge DO, Bailey KR. Myocardium at risk and infarct size after thrombolytic therapy for acute myocardial infarction: implications for the design of randomized trials of acute intervention. J Am Coll Cardiol. 1994;24:616–23.

5. Risk stratification and survival after myocardial infarction. Multicenter Postinfarction Research Group. N Engl J Med. 1983;309:331–6.
6. Smalling RW, Bode C, Kalbfleisch J, et al. More rapid, complete, and stable coronary thrombolysis with bolus administration of reteplase compared with alteplase infusion in acute myocardial infarction. RAPID Investigators. Circulation. 1995;91:2725–32.
7. Jaffe R, Charron T, Puley G, Dick A, Strauss BH. Microvascular obstruction and the no-reflow phenomenon after percutaneous coronary intervention. Circulation. 2008;117:3152–6.
8. Morishima I, Sone T, Okumura K, et al. Angiographic no-reflow phenomenon as a predictor of adverse long-term outcome in patients treated with percutaneous transluminal coronary angioplasty for first acute myocardial infarction. J Am Coll Cardiol. 2000;36:1202–9.
9. Rezkalla SH, Kloner RA. No-reflow phenomenon. Circulation. 2002;105:656–62.
10. Bonow RO. The hibernating myocardium: implications for management of congestive heart failure. Am J Cardiol. 1995;75(3):17A–25.
11. Dilsizian V, Bonow RO, Cannon III RO, et al. The effect of coronary artery bypass grafting on left ventricular systolic function at rest: evidence for preoperative subclinical myocardial ischemia. Am J Cardiol. 1988;61:1248–54.
12. Elefteriades JA, Tolis Jr G, Levi E, Mills LK, Zaret BL. Coronary artery bypass grafting in severe left ventricular dysfunction: excellent survival with improved ejection fraction and functional state. J Am Coll Cardiol. 1993;22:1411–7.
13. Rahimtoola SH. The hibernating myocardium. Am Heart J. 1989;117:211–21.
14. Antman EM, Van de WF. Pharmacoinvasive therapy: the future of treatment for ST-elevation myocardial infarction. Circulation. 2004;109:2480–6.
15. Braunwald E. Myocardial reperfusion, limitation of infarct size, reduction of left ventricular dysfunction, and improved survival. Should the paradigm be expanded? Circulation. 1989;79:441–4.
16. Burns RJ, Gibbons RJ, Yi Q, et al. The relationships of left ventricular ejection fraction, end-systolic volume index and infarct size to six-month mortality after hospital discharge following myocardial infarction treated by thrombolysis. J Am Coll Cardiol. 2002;39:30–6.
17. Miller TD, Christian TF, Hopfenspirger MR, Hodge DO, Gersh BJ, Gibbons RJ. Infarct size after acute myocardial infarction measured by quantitative tomographic 99mTc sestamibi imaging predicts subsequent mortality. Circulation. 1995;92:334–41.
18. White HD, Norris RM, Brown MA, Brandt PW, Whitlock RM, Wild CJ. Left ventricular end-systolic volume as the major determinant of survival after recovery from myocardial infarction. Circulation. 1987;76:44–51.
19. Gibbons RJ, Miller TD, Christian TF. Infarct size measured by single photon emission computed tomographic imaging with (99m)Tc-sestamibi: a measure of the efficacy of therapy in acute myocardial infarction. Circulation. 2000;101:101–8.
20. De Coster PM, Wijns W, Cauwe F, Robert A, Beckers C, Melin JA. Area-at-risk determination by technetium-99m-hexakis-2-methoxyisobutyl isonitrile in experimental reperfused myocardial infarction. Circulation. 1990;82:2152–62.
21. Sinusas AJ, Trautman KA, Bergin JD, et al. Quantification of area at risk during coronary occlusion and degree of myocardial salvage after reperfusion with technetium-99m methoxyisobutyl isonitrile. Circulation. 1990;82:1424–37.
22. Feiring AJ, Johnson MR, Kioschos JM, Kirchner PT, Marcus ML, White CW. The importance of the determination of the myocardial area at risk in the evaluation of the outcome of acute myocardial infarction in patients. Circulation. 1987;75:980–7.
23. Gibbons RJ, Verani MS, Behrenbeck T, et al. Feasibility of tomographic 99mTc-hexakis-2-methoxy-2-methylpropyl-isonitrile imaging for the assessment of myocardial area at risk and the effect of treatment in acute myocardial infarction. Circulation. 1989;80:1277–86.
24. O'Connor MK, Hammell T, Gibbons RJ. In vitro validation of a simple tomographic technique for estimation of percentage myocardium at risk using methoxyisobutyl isonitrile technetium 99m (sestamibi). Eur J Nucl Med. 1990;17:69–76.
25. Christian TF, Schwartz RS, Gibbons RJ. Determinants of infarct size in reperfusion therapy for acute myocardial infarction. Circulation. 1992;86:81–90.

26. Klarich KW, Christian TF, Higano ST, Gibbons RJ. Variability of myocardium at risk for acute myocardial infarction. Am J Cardiol. 1999;83:1191–5.
27. Christian TF, Gibbons RJ, Gersh BJ. Effect of infarct location on myocardial salvage assessed by technetium-99m isonitrile. J Am Coll Cardiol. 1991;17:1303–8.
28. Verani MS, Jeroudi MO, Mahmarian JJ, et al. Quantification of myocardial infarction during coronary occlusion and myocardial salvage after reperfusion using cardiac imaging with technetium-99m hexakis 2-methoxyisobutyl isonitrile. J Am Coll Cardiol. 1988;12:1573–81.
29. Maes AF, Borgers M, Flameng W, et al. Assessment of myocardial viability in chronic coronary artery disease using technetium-99m sestamibi SPECT. Correlation with histologic and positron emission tomographic studies and functional follow-up. J Am Coll Cardiol. 1997;29:62–8.
30. Medrano R, Lowry RW, Young JB, et al. Assessment of myocardial viability with 99mTc sestamibi in patients undergoing cardiac transplantation. A scintigraphic/pathological study. Circulation. 1996;94:1010–7.
31. Ibrahim T, Nekolla SG, Hornke M, et al. Quantitative measurement of infarct size by contrast-enhanced magnetic resonance imaging early after acute myocardial infarction: comparison with single-photon emission tomography using Tc99m-sestamibi. J Am Coll Cardiol. 2005;45:544–52.
32. Christian TF, Gitter MJ, Miller TD, Gibbons RJ. Prospective identification of myocardial stunning using technetium-99m sestamibi-based measurements of infarct size. J Am Coll Cardiol. 1997;30:1633–40.
33. Miller TD, Hodge DO, Sutton JM, et al. Usefulness of technetium-99m sestamibi infarct size in predicting posthospital mortality following acute myocardial infarction. Am J Cardiol. 1998;81:1491–3.
34. Schomig A, Kastrati A, Dirschinger J, et al. Coronary stenting plus platelet glycoprotein IIb/IIIa blockade compared with tissue plasminogen activator in acute myocardial infarction. Stent versus Thrombolysis for Occluded Coronary Arteries in Patients with Acute Myocardial Infarction Study Investigators. N Engl J Med. 2000;343:385–91.
35. Ndrepepa G, Mehilli J, Schwaiger M, et al. Prognostic value of myocardial salvage achieved by reperfusion therapy in patients with acute myocardial infarction. J Nucl Med. 2004;45:725–9.
36. Dibra A, Mehilli J, Dirschinger J, et al. Thrombolysis in myocardial infarction myocardial perfusion grade in angiography correlates with myocardial salvage in patients with acute myocardial infarction treated with stenting or thrombolysis. J Am Coll Cardiol. 2003;41:925–9.
37. Bekkers SC, Yazdani SK, Virmani R, Waltenberger J. Microvascular obstruction: underlying pathophysiology and clinical diagnosis. J Am Coll Cardiol. 2010;55:1649–60.
38. Kloner RA, Ganote CE, Jennings RB. The "no-reflow" phenomenon after temporary coronary occlusion in the dog. J Clin Invest. 1974;54:1496–508.
39. Niccoli G, Burzotta F, Galiuto L, Crea F. Myocardial no-reflow in humans. J Am Coll Cardiol. 2009;54:281–92.
40. Galiuto L, Natale L, Leccisotti L, et al. Non-invasive imaging of microvascular damage. J Nucl Cardiol. 2009;16:811–31.
41. Tan KT. Pathology, imaging and treatment of cardiac microvascular obstruction. Thromb Res. 2010;125:107–9.
42. Hamada S, Nakamura S, Sugiura T, et al. Early detection of the no-reflow phenomenon in reperfused acute myocardial infarction using technetium-99m tetrofosmin imaging. Eur J Nucl Med. 1999;26:208–14.
43. Kondo M, Nakano A, Saito D, Shimono Y. Assessment of "microvascular no-reflow phenomenon" using technetium-99m macroaggregated albumin scintigraphy in patients with acute myocardial infarction. J Am Coll Cardiol. 1998;32:898–903.
44. Schofer J, Montz R, Mathey DG. Scintigraphic evidence of the "no reflow" phenomenon in human beings after coronary thrombolysis. J Am Coll Cardiol. 1985;5:593–8.
45. Taki J, Matsunari I. Metabolic imaging using SPECT. Eur J Nucl Med Mol Imaging. 2007;34:S34–48.

46. Shimizu Y, Kumita S, Cho K, et al. Evaluation of no-reflow phenomenon using 201TlCl/123I-BMIPP dual-isotope myocardial SPECT. J Nippon Med Sch. 2006;73:258–64.
47. Bax JJ, Beanlands RS, Klocke FJ, et al. Diagnostic and clinical perspectives of fusion imaging in cardiology: is the total greater than the sum of its parts? Heart. 2007;93:16–22.
48. Jeremy RW, Links JM, Becker LC. Progressive failure of coronary flow during reperfusion of myocardial infarction: documentation of the no reflow phenomenon with positron emission tomography. J Am Coll Cardiol. 1990;16:695–704.
49. Bax JJ, Poldermans D, Elhendy A, Boersma E, Rahimtoola SH. Sensitivity, specificity, and predictive accuracies of various noninvasive techniques for detecting hibernating myocardium. Curr Probl Cardiol. 2001;26:147–86.
50. Schinkel AF, Bax JJ, Poldermans D, Elhendy A, Ferrari R, Rahimtoola SH. Hibernating myocardium: diagnosis and patient outcomes. Curr Probl Cardiol. 2007;32:375–410.
51. Diamond GA, Forrester JS, deLuz PL, Wyatt HL, Swan HJ. Post-extrasystolic potentiation of ischemic myocardium by atrial stimulation. Am Heart J. 1978;95:204–9.
52. Rahimtoola SH. A perspective on the three large multicenter randomized clinical trials of coronary bypass surgery for chronic stable angina. Circulation. 1985;72:V123–35.
53. Depre C, Vanoverschelde JL, Gerber B, Borgers M, Melin JA, Dion R. Correlation of functional recovery with myocardial blood flow, glucose uptake, and morphologic features in patients with chronic left ventricular ischemic dysfunction undergoing coronary artery bypass grafting. J Thorac Cardiovasc Surg. 1997;113:371–8.
54. Elsasser A, Muller KD, Skwara W, Bode C, Kubler W, Vogt AM. Severe energy deprivation of human hibernating myocardium as possible common pathomechanism of contractile dysfunction, structural degeneration and cell death. J Am Coll Cardiol. 2002;39:1189–98.
55. Rahimtoola SH, Dilsizian V, Kramer CM, Marwick TH, Vanoverschelde JL. Chronic ischemic left ventricular dysfunction: from pathophysiology to imaging and its integration into clinical practice. JACC Cardiovasc Imaging. 2008;1:536–55.
56. Schinkel AF, Bax JJ, Poldermans D. Clinical assessment of myocardial hibernation. Heart. 2005;91:111–7.
57. Geleijnse ML, Krenning BJ, Nemes A, et al. Incidence, pathophysiology, and treatment of complications during dobutamine-atropine stress echocardiography. Circulation. 2010;121:1756–67.
58. Bountioukos M, Schinkel AF, Bax JJ, et al. Pulsed-wave tissue Doppler quantification of systolic and diastolic function of viable and nonviable myocardium in patients with ischemic cardiomyopathy. Am Heart J. 2004;148:1079–84.
59. Rizzello V, Schinkel AF, Bax JJ, et al. Individual prediction of functional recovery after coronary revascularization in patients with ischemic cardiomyopathy: the scar-to-biphasic model. Am J Cardiol. 2003;91:1406–9.
60. Kim RJ, Fieno DS, Parrish TB, et al. Relationship of MRI delayed contrast enhancement to irreversible injury, infarct age, and contractile function. Circulation. 1999;100:1992–2002.
61. Kim RJ, Wu E, Rafael A, et al. The use of contrast-enhanced magnetic resonance imaging to identify reversible myocardial dysfunction. N Engl J Med. 2000;343:1445–53.
62. Anagnostopoulos C, Henein MY, Underwood SR. Non-invasive investigations. Br Med Bull. 2001;59:29–44.
63. Schinkel AF, Bax JJ, Valkema R, et al. Effect of diabetes mellitus on myocardial 18F-FDG SPECT using acipimox for the assessment of myocardial viability. J Nucl Med. 2003;44:877–83.
64. Velazquez EJ, Lee KL, Deja MA, et al. Coronary-artery bypass surgery in patients with left ventricular dysfunction. N Engl J Med. 2011;364:1607–16.
65. Bonow RO, Maurer G, Lee KL, et al. Myocardial viability and survival in ischemic left ventricular dysfunction. N Engl J Med. 2011;364:1617–25.
66. Nelson C, Marwick TH. Clinical decision-making and myocardial viability: current perspectives. Intern Med J. 2005;35:118–25.

Chapter 9
Role of Cardiovascular Magnetic Resonance in the Assessment of Patients with Acute Myocardial Infarction

Andreas Kumar and Matthias G. Friedrich

Abstract This chapter describes the utility of cardiovascular magnetic resonance (CMR) imaging in patients with acute myocardial infarction.

Next to issues related to patient safety during CMR scans, special attention is given to the added value of CMR to characterize tissue abnormalities as markers for reversible and irreversible myocardial injury in reperfused myocardial infarction. In the context of clinical application, the role for imaging myocardial edema, the area at risk, myocardial salvage, microvascular obstruction, and – as a novel marker – myocardial hemorrhage, are discussed and compared with other imaging modalities. The chapter also addresses current limitations of CMR.

Keywords Cardiovascular magnetic resonance • Acute myocardial infarction • Myocardial edema • Myocardial area at risk • Myocardial salvage • Myocardial hemorrhage

A. Kumar, M.D., M.Sc.
Department of Cardiology, The Quebec Heart and Lung Institute, Laval University, Hopital Laval, Pavillon de Recherche, Room U-4794, 2725 Chemin Ste-Foy, Quebec G1V 4G5, Canada
e-mail: andreas.kumar@mac.com

M.G. Friedrich, M.D. (✉)
Department of Cardiac Sciences and Radiology, Foothills Medical Centre, SSB 700, 1403-29 St. NW, Calgary, AB T2V 5E7, Canada
e-mail: matthias.friedrich@ucalgary.ca

J.C. Kaski et al. (eds.), *Management of Myocardial Reperfusion Injury*,
DOI 10.1007/978-1-84996-019-9_9,

Cardiovascular MR: Clinical Potential and Safety Aspects

Cardiovascular magnetic resonance (CMR) can contribute a wide range of diagnostic information for the work-up of the patient with acute myocardial infarction and ischemia/reperfusion injury. As described in detail below, this includes qualitative, quantitative, or semiquantitative measurements of left ventricular size and function, structure and anatomy, and tissue characterization including edema, necrosis, fibrosis, microvascular obstruction, hemorrhage, and valvular function. For most its clinical applications, it is considered the noninvasive gold standard.

A large European multicenter registry has demonstrated that CMR is very safe, with severe complications occurring in 0.05% of patients only [1]. Taking into consideration the abovementioned factors, CMR can be safely performed in patients with an acutely reperfused myocardial infarction, as long as the patient is clinically stable and a number of precautions for patient safety and monitoring are respected.

CMR suites allow for continuous monitoring of the patients' vital signs including blood pressure, heart rate, ECG, respiratory rate, and oxygen saturation. Intercom systems ensure communication with the patient during the study, and video cameras and direct view of the patient add to the safety. Vital sign monitors come equipped with the usual alarms for values measured beyond normal range, and patients are given an alarm system to alert medical staff if needed.

For imaging patients with acute coronary syndromes, it is recommended to use a detachable patient tray that can be disconnected from the scanner manually in the event of a cardiac arrest and wheeled outside the magnet in seconds for resuscitation with non-MRI compatible equipment. Also, a resuscitation trolley with a defibrillator and an on-site cardiac arrest team should be provided to ensure patient safety.

Numerous studies have confirmed the safety of CMR data in patients with acute coronary syndrome and myocardial infarction [2–8], and CMR has also been used to detect acute coronary syndromes in patients without frank ST-elevation myocardial infarction without complications [9–11].

In summary, CMR can be safely performed in patients with an acute myocardial infarction, as long as the patient is clinically stable enough to undergo such a study. Appropriate measures for patient safety, including monitoring and backup for cardiac emergencies, must be provided.

Role of CMR in Patients with Reperfused ST-Elevation MI

Assessment of Cardiac Wall Motion Abnormalities and Stunning

Steady-state-free-precession cine sequences allow for visualization and quantification of left ventricular function with a robustness and accuracy which cannot be achieved by other imaging methods such as echocardiography or nuclear imaging. Typical in-plane resolution reaches up to 1.3 × 1.0 mm with a slice thickness of 5–10 mm.

Short-axis slice summation and multiple long-axis methods are used for quantification of global function, and regional wall thickening is easily visualized and quantified on short- and long-axis views, showing both infarcted and non-infarcted tissue. Furthermore, CMR has a consistently low inter- and intra-observer variability [12–14]. The European Society of Cardiology considers CMR the gold standard method for the assessment ventricular volumes and systolic function [15]. It is important to realize that, in patients with ischemia-reperfusion injury, left ventricular structure, anatomy, and regional and global function can be acquired within 3–10 min of acquisition time.

CMR of Left Ventricular Function as a Predictor of Long-Term Functional Recovery

Several studies have demonstrated that left ventricular systolic function in the acute phase after myocardial infarction predicts long-term left ventricular function.

Because, however, global function does not account for reversibility of dysfunction, the amount of viable and nonviable tissue as assessed by late gadolinium enhancement is a stronger prognostic marker for functional recovery after acute myocardial infarction [16].

Functional recovery can also be predicted by low-dose dobutamine protocols. Importantly, the wall motion index is not superior in the prediction of functional recovery than late gadolinium enhancement (see below).

Outcome

Several studies have demonstrated that left ventricular systolic dysfunction predicts major adverse clinical events (MACE). In a recent prospective trial in 250 patients after reperfused STEMI, abnormalities of resting wall motion and transmural necrosis were both identified as independent predictors of adverse outcome, while microvascular obstruction (by visual assessment on late enhancement) was not [4, 17].

Imaging of Myocardial Infarction

"Late gadolinium enhancement imaging" (LGE-CMR) (also "late enhancement," "delayed enhancement imaging," or "late hyperenhancement") [18, 19] has become the noninvasive gold standard for visualization and quantification of myocardial infarction and as such is recognized by leading North American and European Societies for Cardiology [20].

The contrast is generated by the fact that remote, non-infarcted myocardium has a very small volume of distribution, while infarcted myocardium (acute as well as chronic) is characterized by permeable cell membranes or fibrosis with a subsequently increased volume of distribution for Gadolinium-DTPA. Around 10 min after injection of Gadolinium-based contrast, the contrast agent is largely washed out from remote but not from the infarcted myocardium. For maximizing the contrast between viable and nonviable tissue, a so-called inversion-recovery gradient-echo sequence is applied: A specific inversion pulse inverts the direction of the spin vector to null signal from remote, non-infarcted myocardium, when applied at a specific time (inversion time). Infarcted tissue remains bright and allows for precise quantitative assessment of even small (<1 g) areas of irreversible injury [21]. The method is well validated in experimental [22] and animal models [18–25]. It was shown to be more sensitive to detect small and subendocardial infarction than nuclear imaging methods using single-proton emission computed tomography with Thallium or sestamibi [26].

Clinical studies have demonstrated a close correlation between infarct size measured by late gadolinium enhancement CMR and Troponin levels [27–29] as well with infarct size on SPECT [26] and FDG-PET [30].

Several important differences between Troponin measurements, nuclear imaging methods, and LE-CMR need to be mentioned.

Troponin elevation is not specific to myocardial infarction as it can be also observed in several other clinical scenarios, i.e., pulmonary embolism, acute exacerbation of chronic obstructive pulmonary disease, pneumonia, status after cardioversion/defibrillation, myocarditis, stress-induced cardiomyopathy (also termed Takotsubo cardiomyopathy), and other diseases and states causing myocardial strain [20].

In stable patients CMR can therefore be useful for:

- Verification or exclusion as well as quantitative assessment of recent or remote myocardial infarction
- Differentiation and localization of acute versus chronic infarction by combining T2-weighted sequences (see below) with LGE [31, 32]
- Differentiation of ischemic versus nonischemic cardiomyopathies based on specific patterns of regional distribution of fibrosis (in contrast to infarction, nonischemic injuries characteristically do not involve the subendocardium, are mostly mid-myocardial or epicardial, and not necessarily restricted to a perfusion bed) [33–36]

Recent guidelines on the diagnosis of myocardial infarction endorse the use of LGE-CMR in situations of diagnostic uncertainty [20], and studies applying CMR in the emergency room in patients with chest pain and elevated troponin have underlined the diagnostic utility of this method in the setting of acute chest pain [9, 11, 35].

Multiple studies have shown that infarct size as measured by LGE-CMR predicts functional recovery in acute myocardial infarction, and data is emerging supporting the prognostic value of infarct size to predict left ventricular dysfunction and patient outcome [18, 37–39].

LGE-CMR has become an easy-to-use standard method of CMR imaging and is widely implemented in clinical patient care.

Myocardial Edema and the Myocardial Salvage Index

Edema is a non-specific response to any cellular insult, be it mechanical stress, toxins, or ischemia. It may therefore be a very useful marker for the acuity and extent of myocardial injury [40].

No-flow ischemia-induced myocardial injury develops after acute coronary occlusion and follows a distinct pattern: After a few minutes, water is released from its binding to intracellular proteins [41]. Furthermore, dysfunctional cell membranes cause water inflow from the interstitial space following sodium translocation into the intracellular compartments. Both may not be associated with a relevant increase of total tissue water content (cellular edema). Ongoing myocardial ischemia leads to death and necrotic disintegration of cardiomyocytes and, after about 60 min, to endothelial leakage with subsequent interstitial edema, generally associated with a net inflow of water into the injured tissue. While the immediate effects of ischemia affect the entire perfusion bed ("area at risk"), edema is a very early feature of ischemic injury, while the spatial extent of cardiomyocyte necrosis spreads from an initially subendocardial to a typically transmural distribution. The expansion of the irreversible injury is known as the "wave front phenomenon" [42].

Consequently, coronary revascularization before completion of this expansion within the area at risk will leave the affected myocardial territory with different tissue characteristics:

1. A central area with irreversible injury (necrosis, including possible microvascular obstruction and hemorrhage),
2. An area with reperfused, reversibly injured tissue

The extent of myocardial salvage, i.e., the amount of myocardium where irreversible injury could be prevented by early revascularization, directly reflects the success of the interventional therapy in acute myocardial infarction. The proportional amount of myocardial salvage within the area at risk (myocardial salvage index, MSI) is independent of the size of the area at risk, which is determined by the size of the perfusion bed and thus by the size of the vessel and the location of the occlusion. The MSI is calculated as follows:

$$\left(\text{volume}_{\text{area at risk}} - \text{volume}_{\text{myocardial salvage}}\right) / \text{volume}_{\text{area at risk}} \times 100$$

Because the MSI is independent from the size of the area at risk and therefore also from the location of the coronary occlusion, it is less sensitive to these confounders than infarct size or absolute myocardial salvage. It therefore should be considered the most suitable marker for assessing the success of reperfusion therapy.

Data obtained by nuclear and CMR techniques indicate a prognostic value for hard outcome [43, 44].

Although nuclear cardiology techniques have been well validated [45] and applied in clinical trials [46, 47], their clinical utility has been limited by time-consuming protocols, low spatial resolution, and radioactive tracers.

CMR of Myocardial Edema

Among other techniques, T2-weighted CMR of myocardial edema has rapidly attracted the interest of both researchers and clinicians. The technique does not require contrast agents or any periprocedural interventions. It simply utilizes the fact that protons bound in free water have a significant longer transversal (T2) relaxation time than those protons in other molecules. Importantly, a rapid increase of free water is an early consequence of ischemic injury [48] and leads to an early increase of T2 relaxation in ischemic tissue [49]. Therefore, MRI protocols sensitive for protons with long T2 ("T2-weighted" sequences) can be used to highlight tissue with high content of free water.

The diagnostic and prognostic value of T2-weighted imaging of myocardial edema has been demonstrated in acute myocardial infarction, acute myocarditis, stress-induced cardiomyopathy, hypertrophic cardiomyopathy, and transplant rejection. Similar to other injuries, the salvaged area at risk as a reversible tissue injury is characterized by edema in the absence of necrosis, i.e., the infarcted core of the affected perfusion bed. Since CMR can visualize both edema and necrosis, it may be viewed, in combination with late Gd enhancement CMR, as the modality of choice for the assessment of myocardial salvage after revascularization.

The assessment of the myocardial salvage index requires the acquisition of T2-weighted images (edema/reversible injury) and contrast-enhanced "late Gd enhancement" images (necrosis/irreversible injury) and a subsequent subtraction of the volume of irreversible injury from that of the edema, which includes both reversibly and irreversibly injured myocardium (Fig. 9.1).

This approach appears sufficiently robust to be used in animal models [50] and in clinical scenarios [51–53] of acute myocardial infarction. It compares very well with nuclear cardiology data [54] and has also shown prognostic potential value [44, 55].

Limitations of Assessing the Myocardial Salvage Index by CMR

Some technical difficulties have to be kept in mind: First, T2-weighted imaging is often hampered by its inherently low signal-to-noise ratio. Second, currently used CMR techniques often are sensitive to motion and flow artifacts. Third, most currently used approaches normalize signal intensity values to remote myocardium and therefore may be subject to artifacts and misregistration of apparently normal

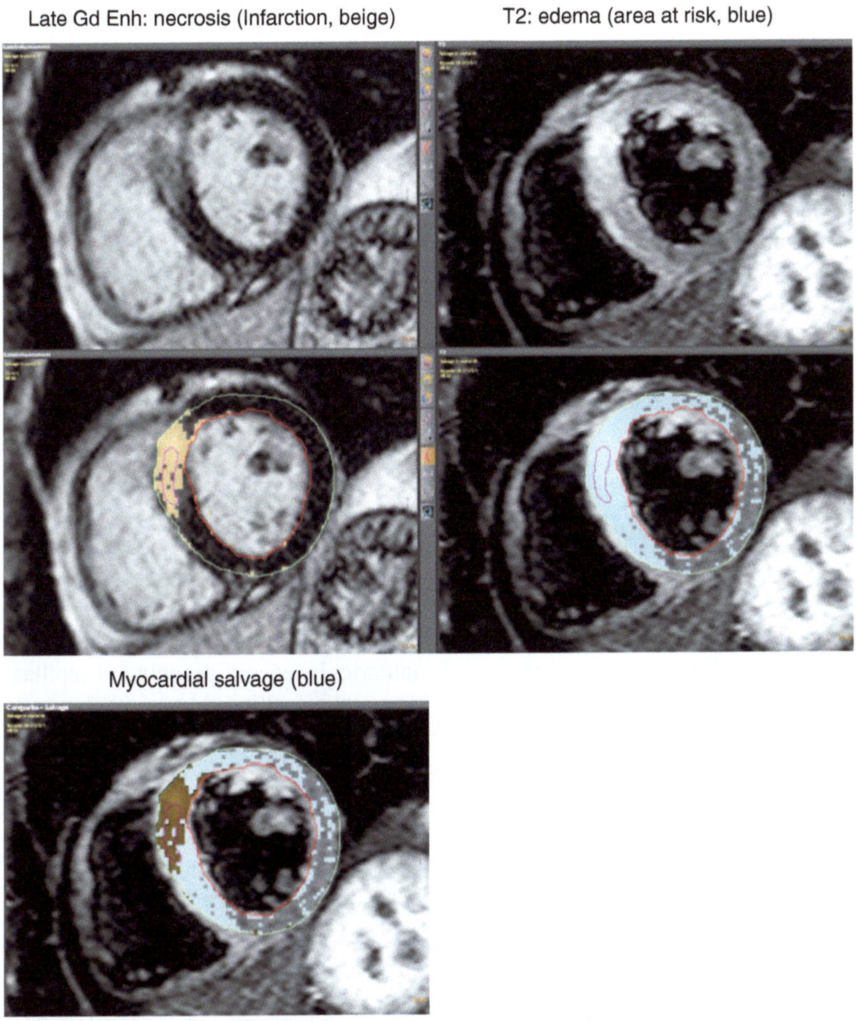

Fig. 9.1 Mid-ventricular short-axis views in a patient with reperfused myocardial infarction of the LAD territory. *Upper left quadrant*: Late Gd Enhancement (LGE) images showing a bright signal intensity of the midanteroseptal segment. *Lower left quadrant*: Color-coded visualization of an automated signal intensity analysis, showing the infarcted region as beige. *Upper right quadrant*: T2-weighted (water-sensitive) images showing bright signal intensity of the LAD territory as a marker for the area at risk. *Lower right quadrant*: Color-coded visualization of an automated signal intensity analysis, showing the injured region as *blue*. *Lower image*: Composite image showing both, infarcted myocardium (*brown*) and salvaged (*blue*) myocardium

myocardium. Furthermore, there is debate about suitable cutoff values to define significant myocardial edema [56].

Recent advances of T2 CMR technology include an improvement of the image quality and the introduction of T2 quantification ("mapping") [57], both overcoming such limitations.

Furthermore, the timing of CMR after revascularization is important, because postinfarct inflammation will reach its peak about 72 h after the insult, and therefore, infarct-related edema at this time may overestimate myocardial salvage. This may explain the observed "plateau" of salvage index values despite late reperfusion [44].

Even with these limitations, available data already indicate that the myocardial salvage index as determined by CMR should be used in clinical trials.

If concerns regarding its robustness can be sufficiently well addressed, it should also be integrated into the diagnostic work-up of patients after early revascularization. It is important to emphasize that this would happen as part of a comprehensive CMR exam, which also comprises the quantitative assessment of volumes, mass, function, and necrosis within scanner times of <20 min. It is to be expected that, in centers with access to CMR, such approach will be used as a standard tool in patients after myocardial infarction.

Microvascular Obstruction

In severe ischemic injury, the damage can involve the microvascular endothelium. Ischemic microvascular injury is characterized by a multitude of factors, including endothelial cell swelling, compression of capillaries by edema, plugging of capillaries by fibrin deposits, platelets, and white blood cells, facilitated by upregulation of cell adhesion molecules on the endothelial cell surface. This leads to microvascular obstruction, and the injury may be further exacerbated by embolization of plaque material and of epicardial artery thrombus during angioplasty of acute STEMI.

The phenomenon of microvascular obstruction was recognized in the heart as early as the 1970s [58] and has been assessed by different imaging methods, including coronary angiography with epicardial flow measurements, contrast-enhanced echocardiography, and SPECT imaging. Using coronary angiography-based flow measurements such as TIMI flow or TIMI frame count, microvascular obstruction can be indirectly assessed as "slow reflow" or "no reflow," and has been shown to be associated with impaired functional recovery and adverse outcome [59–64]. Contrast-enhanced CMR has been applied to display microvascular obstruction, without depending on epicardial flow measurements. Examples of myocardial infarction with and without microvascular obstruction are shown in Figs. 9.2 and 9.3. The approach uses the lack of contrast agent uptake as a marker for microvascular obstruction on a tissue level with high spatial resolution up to 1.3 × 1.5 mm in

Fig. 9.2 Mid-ventricular short-axis views in a patient with reperfused acute myocardial infarction of the LAD territory. *Upper row*: Diastolic (*left*) and systolic still frame showing hypokinesis of the midanterior segment. *Middle row, left*: Late Gd Enhancement (LGE) image with bright signal intensity indicating near-transmural infarction of the midanterior segment (*arrows*). *Middle row, right*: T2-weighted (water-sensitive) image with bright signal intensity indicating transmural edema of the midanterior segment (*arrows*). *Lower row*: Early Gd Enhancement image (acquired within <2 min after Gd injection) with homogeneously bright signal intensity indicating absence of microvascular obstruction (*arrows*)

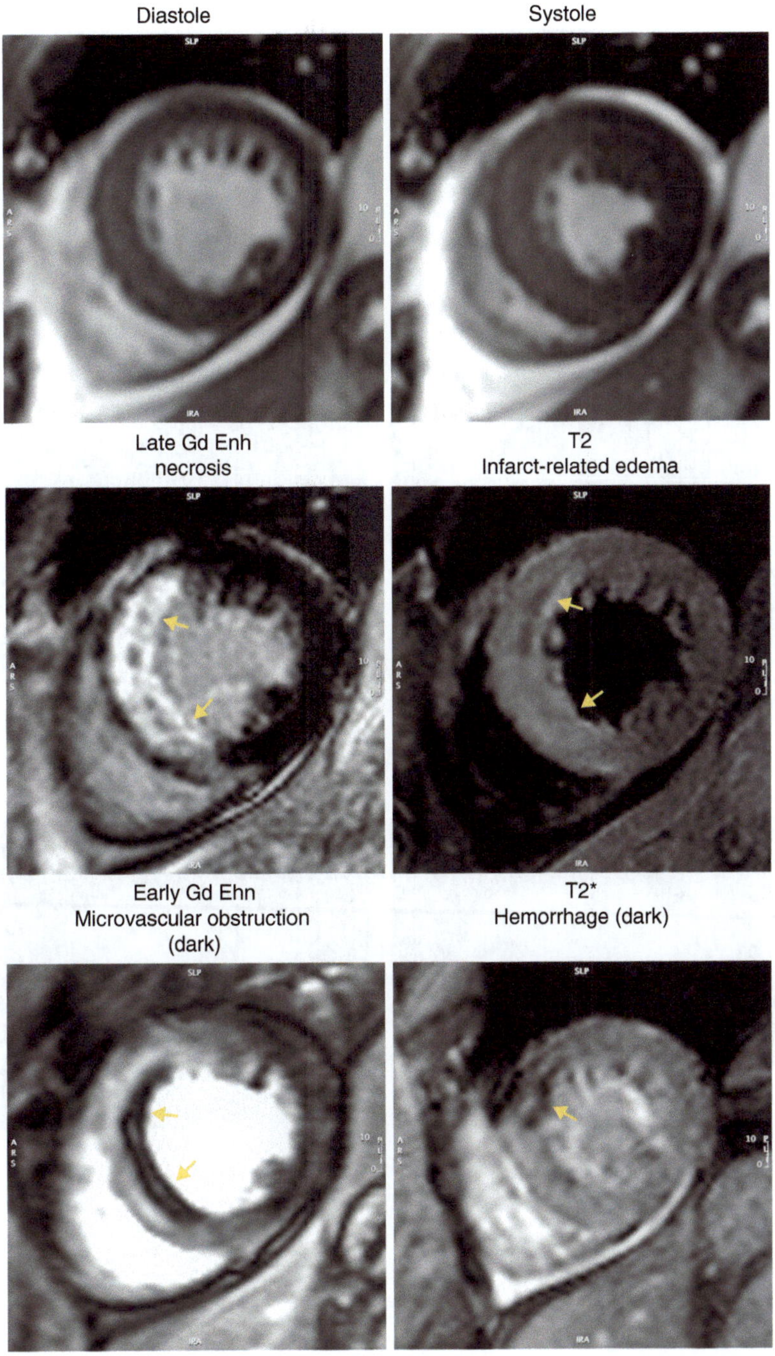
Diastole
Systole
Late Gd Enh
necrosis
T2
Infarct-related edema
Early Gd Ehn
Microvascular obstruction
(dark)
T2*
Hemorrhage (dark)

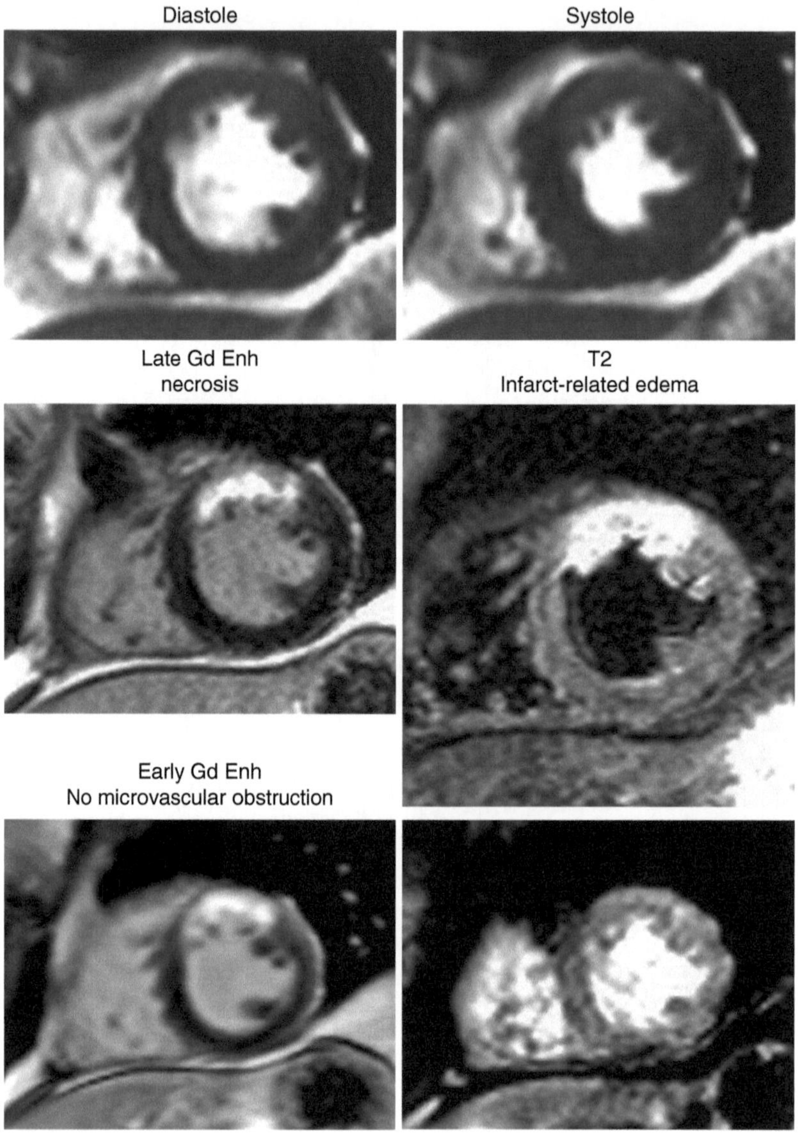
Diastole
Systole
Late Gd Enh
necrosis
T2
Infarct-related edema
Early Gd Enh
No microvascular obstruction

plane at a slice thickness of 5–10 mm. This yields a voxel size of as small as 0.2 g of tissue. One may therefore argue that CMR, due to this high spatial resolution, is a more sensitive method to detect microvascular obstruction in vivo, and it may detect microvascular obstruction before this results in hemodynamic consequences detectable as reduced epicardial coronary artery flow. In fact, some studies have demonstrated that in up to 40% of patients with microvascular obstruction detected by CMR, epicardial flow may still be normal [65–67]. The assessment of microvascular obstruction with contrast-enhanced CMR was validated in animal models of ischemia-reperfusion injury to microsphere flow [68] and ex vivo using Thioflavin S staining [69, 70].

The failure of myocardium to enhance after contrast injection, in the setting of an open epicardial coronary artery, is interpreted as microvascular obstruction and correlates with ex vivo Thioflavin S hypoenhancement [70]. Another animal study demonstrated that CMR hypoenhancement closely matches zones of myocardial blood flow <40% of remote, non-damaged tissue [69].

CMR Imaging Techniques for Microvascular Obstruction

After contrast injection, on CMR, microvascular obstruction appears as a zone of hypoenhancement surrounded by the hyperenhancement of cardiomyocyte necrosis in the infarction zone without microvascular injury. Specific contrast kinetics [71] allow for the assessment of microvascular obstruction in patients, and there is ongoing debate about the optimal approach, especially since there is no in vivo/ex vivo validation data available in humans.

First-pass perfusion shows an area of hypoperfused core in the center of cardiomyocyte necrosis, which may overestimate the zone of microvascular obstruction zone if there is a significant epicardial coronary artery stenosis distal to the culprit lesion. Therefore, this imaging approach may be very sensitive but less specific for microvascular obstruction.

Closest to the technique which was used earlier to validate contrast-enhanced CMR against Thioflavin S staining as an ex vivo gold standard in an animal model [69],

Fig. 9.3 Mid-ventricular short-axis views in a patient with late reperfusion of acute myocardial infarction of the LAD territory. *Upper row*: Diastolic (*left*) and systolic still frame showing hypokinesis of the midanterior (partial), anteroseptal, and inferoseptal segments. *Middle row, left*: Late Gd Enhancement (LGE) image with bright signal intensity indicating transmural infarction of the midanterior segment. *Middle row, right*: T2-weighted (water-sensitive) image with bright signal intensity indicating transmural edema of the midanterior segment. Note that the size of the edema is very similar to the size of the infarction, indicating the absence of significant salvage. *Lower row, left*: Early Gd Enhancement image (acquired within <2 min after Gd injection) with a low signal intensity core within the bright signal intensity of the infarction, indicating microvascular obstruction. *Right*: T2*-weighted (hemorrhage-sensitive) image showing regional signal intensity drop within the same region, indicating myocardial hemorrhage as a complication of late reperfusion

the late gadolinium technique applied early (around 2 min after contrast injection), also called "early enhancement," but not to be confused with a synonymous imaging approach for myocarditis [72], is commonly assumed to be more accurate and more robust to delineate areas of microvascular obstruction. The hypoenhanced infarct core visualized here is a result of hypoperfusion plus a very early stage of contrast diffusion into the microvascular obstruction territory. While current commercially available imaging techniques for first-pass perfusion only cover three or four short-axis slices across the left ventricle, but not the whole left ventricle, early gadolinium enhancement can cover the entire left ventricle in around three breath-hold acquisitions within 2 min or even in one breath-hold acquisition using a 3D imaging sequence for early enhancement [73].

Cores of larger areas of microvascular obstruction will still be visible on late gadolinium enhancement (LGE), i.e., ≥10 min after iv injection of gadolinium, giving the agent less time to diffuse into the obstructed area. Since this imaging technique is very commonly applied to assess infarct size, and it is easy to use and highly reproducible [74, 75], many investigators use LGE as a surrogate imaging approach to assess microvascular obstruction. The time delay of around 10 min between contrast injection and image acquisition leads to significant diffusion of contrast into the microvascular obstruction zone and therefore to a theoretical underestimation of the amount of microvascular obstruction. Thus, it is more specific but less sensitive for microvascular obstruction, and it may miss microvascular obstruction in patients who are positive by first-pass perfusion or early enhancement [76]. Recent data, however, indicate that this approach has a stronger prognostic value than first-pass or early application for late enhancement [77].

There is currently no consensus in the CMR community and no societal recommendation to use a specific imaging approach, and the quantified amount of microvascular obstruction varies significantly from one technique to the other. For example, in a study of 34 patients with acute reperfused STEMI, when the techniques were compared, using approach 1, CMR yielded an amount of microvascular obstruction of median 4.7 g; with technique 2, it was 2.3 g; and with technique 3, it was 0.2 g [77]; other studies have yielded similar results [73, 76, 78].

Clinical Significance of Imaging Microvascular Obstruction

The detrimental effect of microvascular obstruction has previously been demonstrated using angiographic measures of microvascular obstruction, associating no reflow or slow reflow with adverse patient outcome in large prospective studies [59, 62, 64].

The ability of CMR to comprehensively assess in one imaging session of around 30 min of scan time left ventricular regional and global function, myocardial edema and myocardial salvage, infarct size, and microvascular obstruction has led to studies investigating the effect of microvascular obstruction on functional and volumetric changes of the left ventricle as well as infarct remodeling in patients with myocardial infarction. Overall, this is at the moment an emerging field, and much of the data was obtained in studies with limited numbers of patients.

Microvascular obstruction on CMR is associated with residual ST segment elevation on the 12-lead electrocardiogram 1 h after reperfusion by angioplasty [79], as well as higher levels of troponin release as compared to myocardial infarction without microvascular obstruction [80].

In the acute phase, compared to myocardial infarction with unobstructed microvessels, the presence of microvascular obstruction on CMR is associated with larger myocardial infarcts, a larger transmural extent of cardiomyocyte necrosis as measured by LGE-CMR, larger end-diastolic and end-systolic volumes, and worse systolic function as reflected by a lower left ventricular ejection fraction [76]. Although at 4 months follow-up, after infarct remodeling, infarct size remains larger in the microvascular obstruction group, it has been observed that infarct involution (the compaction or shrinkage of scar secondary to shorter cross bridging between collagen fibers) is more pronounced in the microvascular obstruction group [76], leading to wall thinning in the chronic phase [81].

The consequences of microvascular obstruction have not been studied systematically, but recent data suggest that MVO may disappear in up to 38% of cases between day 2 and 1 week and is not observed after several months of follow-up [76, 82].

Prognostic Impact of Microvascular Obstruction

Several studies have assessed the prognostic effect of microvascular obstruction using CMR with different conclusions. MVO as assessed by first-pass perfusion at 1 week after infarction predicted infarct size at 1 year follow-up [82]. However, a recent study yielded infarct size by late enhancement as the only independent predictor of left ventricular systolic dysfunction at 2 years follow-up, independent of microvascular obstruction, infarct transmurality, and myocardial salvage [39]. Theoretically, an explanation to reconcile these studies would be that microvascular obstruction may be a marker of short-term and midterm functional recovery, but long term (>1 year), infarct size may prevail as the only independent predictor of left ventricular function and patient outcome.

The methodological advances in CMR tissue characterization have led to microvascular obstruction being used as an endpoint to measure treatment effects of interventions targeting microvascular protection.

Myocardial Reperfusion Hemorrhage

Hemorrhage has been described as a contributor to reperfusion injury in early studies using animal models. Microhemorrhage, characterized by occasional erythrocyte extravasation, is seen regularly with microvascular obstruction [58] and has to be separated from macroscopic reperfusion hemorrhage, which constitutes a gross bleeding into the myocardial tissue secondary to severe ischemic microvascular injury [83, 84].

In this situation, the vascular bed is no longer able to maintain its structure when exposed to a sudden increase of the perfusion pressure associated with myocardial reperfusion, and vascular disruption leads to significant amounts of blood extravasating into the necrotic tissue. While microhemorrhage can only be diagnosed with microscopic methods, gross hemorrhage is visible on macroscopic tissue stains. Reperfusion after prolonged ischemia typically causes macrohemorrhage [85] which is located in the subendocardial core of the ischemic zone, where tissue injury is most severe [84, 86].

CMR Imaging Techniques for Reperfusion Macrohemorrhage

Two imaging techniques are currently being applied to assess reperfusion macrohemorrhage using cardiovascular magnetic resonance: T2*-weighted CMR and T2-weighted CMR.

T2*-weighted CMR, applied as a gradient-echo pulse sequence with echo-planar imaging readout, is sensitive to small magnetic field inhomogeneities caused by free unpaired electrons on hemoglobin degradation products [87, 88]. The method is therefore highly specific for hemorrhage and as such used for intracerebral hemorrhage (see Fig. 9.3) [89, 90]. A study performed in our lab demonstrated that T2*-weighted gradient-echo imaging accurately reflects myocardial macrohemorrhage in vivo, compared to ex vivo TTC staining as a reference standard [91]. While current T2*-weighted GE-EPI imaging techniques are limited by image artifacts in around 5% of segments, especially at the myocardium-lung interface, T2* mapping techniques have lately been applied and may be more robust [92, 93]. A first patient study assessing reperfusion hemorrhage using T2*-weighted CMR was already published in 1999 and linked hemorrhage to larger infarct size, compared to nonhemorrhagic infarction [94].

Some authors have assumed a low subendocardial signal on T2-weighted may also be reflective of hemorrhage [95–97]. T2-weighted imaging, however, may be less specific, since the contrast is subject to several confounders such as regional blood volume.

Experimental studies assessing hemorrhage using T2-weighted methods have not investigated the role of microvascular obstruction and edema as confounders [96, 98, 99], and an expected discrepancy between T2- and T2*-weighted imaging signal has been described in clinical patient studies [92, 100]. Therefore, T2*-weighted imaging may be preferable over T2-weighted imaging for the assessment of reperfusion macrohemorrhage.

Clinical CMR Studies on Reperfusion Macrohemorrhage

Data in this field are still emerging. A recently published pilot study using T2* mapping in 50 patients with acute reperfused myocardial infarction found hemorrhage in 58% of patients. Hemorrhage was closely associated with microvascular obstruction; of note, hemorrhagic infarcts had larger infarct size and worse left ventricular ejection fraction (as a result of larger end-diastolic and end-systolic volumes); however, in a regression model, infarct size remained the only independent predictor of left ventricular systolic dysfunction, and neither hemorrhage nor microvascular obstruction was of independent predictive value. The close correlation of hemorrhage and microvascular obstruction suggests that there is a pathophysiological link between reperfusion macrohemorrhage and microvascular obstruction [93]. Another study in 48 patients found hemorrhage using T2*-weighted CMR in 63%, and hemorrhage was associated with larger end-systolic volumes and prolonged QRS complexes at 3 months follow-up [100].

Further, adequately powered prospective studies are needed to shed light on the differential effects of microvascular obstruction and reperfusion macrohemorrhage on left ventricular remodeling and patient outcome.

Limitations of CMR

Limitations of MRI include noncompatibility of certain metallic implants, claustrophobia, and limited access. While most orthopedic implants are MRI compatible, electronic implants like nerve stimulators and cochlear implants are considered not; patients with intracerebral vascular stents are usually non-eligible unless cleared by a neurosurgeon or neuroradiologist. Most patients with cardiac pacemakers and cardioverter-defibrillators cannot be examined by MRI. Although some studies have suggested that pacemakers may be safe, the magnetic field gradients applied during an MRI exam may induce currents in the electrodes, leading to significant heating of the tip of the lead, resulting in myocardial tissue damage and a change in pacing and detection thresholds; however, industry is making continued efforts to develop MR-compatible devices, and newer generation pacemakers and cardioverter-defibrillators will be MR compatible in the years to come. The American Heart Association recently endorsed CMR scanning of patients with pacemakers in situations where the benefits outweigh the risks [101]. Virtually all implanted mechanical heart valves are MR safe. Studies of coronary artery stents have shown that it is safe to scan patients with commonly available coronary stents, even early after the procedure [102].

The MR compatibility of most metal implants is summarized in reference manuals that should be available in every MRI suite and that can be consulted before a CMR to ensure patient safety. The Institute for Magnetic Resonance safety, Education, and Research provides an internet resource where devices are listed and can be researched for their MRI safety rating (http://www.mrisafety.com).

The complete examination of the patient with acute myocardial infarction requires the application of a Gadolinium-based contrast agent. While allergies against gadolinium are very rare and occur hardly more often than allergy-like reactions to placebo, patients should be questioned for allergic reactions, and patients with a documented history of allergy against Gadolinium should not be examined using a gadolinium-based contrast agent.

More recently, advanced renal insufficiency has emerged as a contraindication to gadolinium-based contrast agents. The retrospective analysis of large patient databases demonstrated an association of gadolinium-based studies in patients with renal failure and the occurrence of nephrogenic systemic sclerosis, a disorder resembling systemic sclerosis, that is based on an immune reaction against gadolinium molecules deposited primarily in the skin. The Food and Drug Administration has since issued a controversially discussed black-box warning for a number of gadolinium-based contrast agents. It is current consensus that patients with advanced renal insufficiency should not be scanned using those contrast agents [103]. The risk, however, is extremely low, even in patients with chronic kidney disease [104], and the safety profile of gadolinium agents is to be considered better than that of other compounds typically used in cardiovascular imaging.

Summary

CMR is an exceptionally powerful diagnostic tool in patients with acute myocardial infarction, especially because of its capability of providing a comprehensive assessment of myocardial tissue characteristics. These include edema/area at risk/myocardial salvage, necrosis/fibrosis, no reflow, and hemorrhage, all of which can be directly compared to regional and global ventricular morphology, volumes, and function. Although some of the approaches require additional in-depth validation data and is limited by its still growing availability, CMR can be very valuable for assessing the indication for acute interventions and quantify the success of revascularization procedures, both during the acute stage and at follow-up. The safety profile and reproducibility of CMR make it especially useful for clinical research.

References

1. Bruder O, Schneider S, Nothnagel D, Dill T, Hombach V, Schulz-Menger J, Nagel E, Lombardi M, Van Rossum AC, Wagner A, Schwitter J, Senges J, Sabin GV, Sechtem U, Mahrholdt H. EuroCMR (European Cardiovascular Magnetic Resonance) registry: results of the German pilot phase. J Am Coll Cardiol. 2009;54:1457–66.
2. Larose E, Cote J, Rodes-Cabau J, Noel B, Barbeau G, Bordeleau E, Miro S, Brochu B, Delarochelliere R, Bertrand OF. Contrast-enhanced cardiovascular magnetic resonance in the hyperacute phase of ST-elevation myocardial infarction. Int J Cardiovasc Imaging. 2009;25:519–27.
3. Atar D, Petzelbauer P, Schwitter J, Huber K, Rensing B, Kasprzak JD, Butter C, Grip L, Hansen PR, Süselbeck T. Effect of intravenous FX06 as an adjunct to primary percutaneous coronary intervention for acute ST-segment elevation myocardial infarction results of the F.I.R.E. (Efficacy of FX06 in the prevention of myocardial reperfusion injury) trial. J Am Coll Cardiol. 2009;53:720–9.
4. Bodi V, Sanchis J, Nunez J, Mainar L, Lopez-Lereu MP, Monmeneu JV, Rumiz E, Chaustre F, Trapero I, Husser O, Forteza MJ, Chorro FJ, Llacer A. Prognostic value of a comprehensive

cardiac magnetic resonance assessment soon after a first ST-segment elevation myocardial infarction. JACC Cardiovasc Imaging. 2009;2:835–42.
5. Cochet AA, Lorgis L, Lalande A, Zeller M, Beer JC, Walker PM, Touzery C, Wolf JE, Brunotte F, Cottin Y. Major prognostic impact of persistent microvascular obstruction as assessed by contrast-enhanced cardiac magnetic resonance in reperfused acute myocardial infarction. Eur Radiol. 2009;19:2117–26.
6. Friedrich M, Abdelaty H, Taylor A, Schulzmenger J, Messroghli D, Dietz R. The salvaged area at risk in reperfused acute myocardial infarction as visualized by cardiovascular magnetic resonance. J Am Coll Cardiol. 2008;51:1581–7.
7. Hombach V, Grebe O, Merkle N, Waldenmaier S, Höher M, Kochs M, Wöhrle J, Kestler HA. The prognostic significance of microvascular obstruction after myocardial infarction as defined by cardiovascular magnetic resonance. Eur Heart J. 2005;26:532–3.
8. Kim RJ, Albert TSE, Wible JH, Elliott MD, Allen JC, Lee JC, Parker M, Napoli A, Judd RM. Performance of delayed-enhancement magnetic resonance imaging with gadoversetamide contrast for the detection and assessment of myocardial infarction: an international, multicenter, double-blinded, randomized trial. Circulation. 2008;117:629–37.
9. Kwong RY. Detecting acute coronary syndrome in the emergency department with cardiac magnetic resonance imaging. Circulation. 2003;107:531–7.
10. Plein S, Greenwood J, Ridgway J, Cranny G, Ball S, Sivananthan M. Assessment of non-ST-segment elevation acute coronary syndromes with cardiac magnetic resonance imaging. J Am Coll Cardiol. 2004;44:2173–81.
11. Cury RC, Shash K, Nagurney JT, Rosito G, Shapiro MD, Nomura CH, Abbara S, Bamberg F, Ferencik M, Schmidt EJ, Brown DF, Hoffmann U, Brady TJ. Cardiac magnetic resonance with T2-weighted imaging improves detection of patients with acute coronary syndrome in the emergency department. Circulation. 2008;118:837–44.
12. Barkhausen J, Ruehm SG, Goyen M, Buck T, Laub G, Debatin JF. MR evaluation of ventricular function: true fast imaging with steady-state precession versus fast low-angle shot cine MR imaging: feasibility study. Radiology. 2001;219:264–9.
13. Ichikawa Y, Sakuma H, Kitagawa K, Ishida N, Takeda K, Uemura S, Motoyasu M, Nakano T, Nozaki A. Evaluation of left ventricular volumes and ejection fraction using fast steady-state cine MR imaging: comparison with left ventricular angiography. J Cardiovasc Magn Reson. 2003;5:333–42.
14. Grothues F, Smith GC, Moon JC, Bellenger NG, Collins P, Klein HU, Pennell DJ. Comparison of interstudy reproducibility of cardiovascular magnetic resonance with two-dimensional echocardiography in normal subjects and in patients with heart failure or left ventricular hypertrophy. Am J Cardiol. 2002;90:29–34.
15. Hatle L. How to diagnose diastolic heart failure a consensus statement. Eur Heart J. 2007;28:2421–3.
16. Rubenstein JC, Ortiz JT, Wu E, Kadish A, Passman R, Bonow RO, Goldberger JJ. The use of periinfarct contrast-enhanced cardiac magnetic resonance imaging for the prediction of late postmyocardial infarction ventricular dysfunction. Am Heart J. 2008;156:498–505.
17. Wu E, Ortiz JT, Tejedor P, Lee DC, Bucciarelli-Ducci C, Kansal P, Carr JC, Holly TA, Lloyd-Jones D, Klocke FJ, Bonow RO. Infarct size by contrast enhanced cardiac magnetic resonance is a stronger predictor of outcomes than left ventricular ejection fraction or end-systolic volume index: prospective cohort study. Heart. 2008;94:730–6.
18. Kim RJ, Fieno DS, Parrish TB, Harris K, Chen EL, Simonetti O, Bundy J, Finn JP, Klocke FJ, Judd RM. Relationship of MRI delayed contrast enhancement to irreversible injury, infarct age, and contractile function. Circulation. 1999;100:1992–2002.
19. Simonetti OP, Kim RJ, Fieno DS, Hillenbrand HB, Wu E, Bundy JM, Finn JP, Judd RM. An improved MR imaging technique for the visualization of myocardial infarction. Radiology. 2001;218:215–23.
20. Thygesen K, Alpert JS, White HD. Universal definition of myocardial infarction. Circulation. 2007;116:2634–53.

21. Ricciardi MJ, Wu E, Davidson CJ, Choi KM, Klocke FJ, Bonow RO, Judd RM, Kim RJ. Visualization of discrete microinfarction after percutaneous coronary intervention associated with mild creatine kinase-MB elevation. Circulation. 2001;103:2780–3.
22. Rehwald WG, Fieno DS, Chen E-L, Kim RJ, Judd RM. Myocardial magnetic resonance imaging contrast agent concentrations after reversible and irreversible ischemic injury. Circulation. 2002;105:224–9.
23. Barkhausen J, Ebert W, Debatin JF, Weinmann HJ. Imaging of myocardial infarction: comparison of magnevist and gadophrin-3 in rabbits. J Am Coll Cardiol. 2002;39:1392–8.
24. Fieno DS, Kim RJ, Chen EL, Lomasney JW, Klocke FJ, Judd RM. Contrast-enhanced magnetic resonance imaging of myocardium at risk: distinction between reversible and irreversible injury throughout infarct healing. J Am Coll Cardiol. 2000;36:1985–91.
25. Amado LC, Gerber BL, Gupta SN, Rettmann DW, Szarf G, Schock R, Nasir K, Kraitchman DL, Lima JA. Accurate and objective infarct sizing by contrast-enhanced magnetic resonance imaging in a canine myocardial infarction model. J Am Coll Cardiol. 2004;44:2383–9.
26. Wagner A, Mahrholdt H, Holly TA, Elliott MD, Regenfus M, Parker M, Klocke FJ, Bonow RO, Kim RJ, Judd RM. Contrast-enhanced MRI and routine single photon emission computed tomography (SPECT) perfusion imaging for detection of subendocardial myocardial infarcts: an imaging study. Lancet. 2003;361:374–9.
27. Selvanayagam JB, Porto I, Channon K, Petersen SE, Francis JM, Neubauer S, Banning AP. Troponin elevation after percutaneous coronary intervention directly represents the extent of irreversible myocardial injury: insights from cardiovascular magnetic resonance imaging. Circulation. 2005;111:1027–32.
28. Ingkanisorn WP, Rhoads KL, Aletras AH, Kellman P, Arai AE. Gadolinium delayed enhancement cardiovascular magnetic resonance correlates with clinical measures of myocardial infarction. J Am Coll Cardiol. 2004;43:2253–9.
29. Giannitsis E, Steen H, Kurz K, Ivandic B, Simon AC, Futterer S, Schild C, Isfort P, Jaffe AS, Katus HA. Cardiac magnetic resonance imaging study for quantification of infarct size comparing directly serial versus single time-point measurements of cardiac troponin T. J Am Coll Cardiol. 2008;51:307–14.
30. Klein C, Nekolla SG, Bengel FM, Momose M, Sammer A, Haas F, Schnackenburg B, Delius W, Mudra H, Wolfram D, Schwaiger M. Assessment of myocardial viability with contrast-enhanced magnetic resonance imaging: comparison with positron emission tomography. Circulation. 2002;105:162–7.
31. Abdel-Aty H, Zagrosek A, Schulz-Menger J, Taylor AJ, Messroghli D, Kumar A, Gross M, Dietz R, Friedrich MG. Delayed enhancement and T2-weighted cardiovascular magnetic resonance imaging differentiate acute from chronic myocardial infarction. Circulation. 2004;109:2411–6.
32. Aletras AH, Tilak GS, Natanzon A, Hsu LY, Gonzalez FM, Hoyt Jr RF, Arai AE. Retrospective determination of the area at risk for reperfused acute myocardial infarction with T2-weighted cardiac magnetic resonance imaging: histopathological and displacement encoding with stimulated echoes (DENSE) functional validations. Circulation. 2006;113:1865–70.
33. Mccrohon JA. Differentiation of heart failure related to dilated cardiomyopathy and coronary artery disease using gadolinium-enhanced cardiovascular magnetic resonance. Circulation. 2003;108:54–9.
34. Kumar A, Patton DJ, Friedrich MG. The emerging clinical role of cardiovascular magnetic resonance imaging. Can J Cardiol. 2010;26:313–22.
35. Assomull RG, Lyne JC, Keenan N, Gulati A, Bunce NH, Davies SW, Pennell DJ, Prasad SK. The role of cardiovascular magnetic resonance in patients presenting with chest pain, raised troponin, and unobstructed coronary arteries. Eur Heart J. 2007;28:1242–9.
36. Francois CJ, Schiebler ML, Reeder SB. Cardiac MRI evaluation of nonischemic cardiomyopathies. J Magn Reson Imaging. 2010;31:518–30; quiz 517.
37. Hombach V, Grebe O, Merkle N, Waldenmaier S, Hoher M, Kochs M, Wohrle J, Kestler HA. Sequelae of acute myocardial infarction regarding cardiac structure and function and their

prognostic significance as assessed by magnetic resonance imaging. Eur Heart J. 2005;26:549–57.
38. Kim RJ, Wu E, Rafael A, Chen EL, Parker MA, Simonetti O, Klocke FJ, Bonow RO, Judd RM. The use of contrast-enhanced magnetic resonance imaging to identify reversible myocardial dysfunction. N Engl J Med. 2000;343:1445–53.
39. Larose E, Rodes-Cabau J, Pibarot P, Rinfret S, Proulx G, Nguyen CM, Dery JP, Gleeton O, Roy L, Noel B, Barbeau G, Rouleau J, Boudreault JR, Amyot M, De Larochelliere R, Bertrand OF. Predicting late myocardial recovery and outcomes in the early hours of ST-segment elevation myocardial infarction traditional measures compared with microvascular obstruction, salvaged myocardium, and necrosis characteristics by cardiovascular magnetic resonance. J Am Coll Cardiol. 2010;55:2459–69.
40. Friedrich MG. Myocardial edema – a new clinical entity? Nat Rev Cardiol. 2010;7:292–6.
41. Landis EM. Micro-injection studies of capillary permeability: III. The effect of lack of oxygen on the permeability of the capillary wall to fluid and to the plasma protein. Am J Physiol. 1927;83:528–42.
42. Reimer KA, Jennings RB. The "wavefront phenomenon" of myocardial ischemic cell death. II. Transmural progression of necrosis within the framework of ischemic bed size (myocardium at risk) and collateral flow. Lab Invest. 1979;40:633–44.
43. Ndrepepa G, Mehilli J, Schwaiger M, Schuhlen H, Nekolla S, Martinoff S, Schmitt C, Dirschinger J, Schomig A, Kastrati A. Prognostic value of myocardial salvage achieved by reperfusion therapy in patients with acute myocardial infarction. J Nucl Med. 2004;45:725–9.
44. Eitel I, Desch S, Fuernau G, Hildebrand L, Gutberlet M, Schuler G, Thiele H. Prognostic significance and determinants of myocardial salvage assessed by cardiovascular magnetic resonance in acute reperfused myocardial infarction. J Am Coll Cardiol. 2010;55:2470–9.
45. Sinusas AJ, Trautman KA, Bergin JD, Watson DD, Ruiz M, Smith WH, Beller GA. Quantification of area at risk during coronary occlusion and degree of myocardial salvage after reperfusion with technetium-99m methoxyisobutyl isonitrile. Circulation. 1990;82:1424–37.
46. Christian TF, Gibbons RJ, Gersh BJ. Effect of infarct location on myocardial salvage assessed by technetium-99m isonitrile. J Am Coll Cardiol. 1991;17:1303–8.
47. Gibbons RJ, Valeti US, Araoz PA, Jaffe AS. The quantification of infarct size. J Am Coll Cardiol. 2004;44:1533–42.
48. Kuntz Jr ID, Brassfield TS, Law GD, Purcell GV. Hydration of macromolecules. Science. 1969;163:1329–31.
49. Tscholakoff D, Higgins CB, McNamara MT, Derugin N. Early-phase myocardial infarction: evaluation by MR imaging. Radiology. 1986;159:667–72.
50. Hedstrom E, Engblom H, Frogner F, Astrom-Olsson K, Ohlin H, Jovinge S, Arheden H. Infarct evolution in man studied in patients with first-time coronary occlusion in comparison to different species - implications for assessment of myocardial salvage. J Cardiovasc Magn Reson. 2009;11:38.
51. Friedrich MG, Abdel-Aty H, Taylor A, Schulz-Menger J, Messroghli D, Dietz R. The salvaged area at risk in reperfused acute myocardial infarction as visualized by cardiovascular magnetic resonance. J Am Coll Cardiol. 2008;51:1581–7.
52. Francone M, Bucciarelli-Ducci C, Carbone I, Canali E, Scardala R, Calabrese FA, Sardella G, Mancone M, Catalano C, Fedele F, Passariello R, Bogaert J, Agati L. Impact of primary coronary angioplasty delay on myocardial salvage, infarct size, and microvascular damage in patients with ST-segment elevation myocardial infarction: insight from cardiovascular magnetic resonance. J Am Coll Cardiol. 2009;54:2145–53.
53. Phrommintikul A, Abdel-Aty H, Schulz-Menger J, Friedrich MG, Taylor AJ. Acute oedema in the evaluation of microvascular reperfusion and myocardial salvage in reperfused myocardial infarction with cardiac magnetic resonance imaging. Eur J Radiol. 2010;74:e12–7.
54. Berry C, Kellman P, Mancini C, Chen MY, Bandettini WP, Lowrey T, Hsu LY, Aletras AH, Arai AE. Magnetic resonance imaging delineates the ischemic area at risk and myocardial salvage in patients with acute myocardial infarction. Circ Cardiovasc Imaging. 2010;3:527–35.

55. Eitel I, Desch S, Sareban M, Fuernau G, Gutberlet M, Schuler G, Thiele H. Prognostic significance and magnetic resonance imaging findings in aborted myocardial infarction after primary angioplasty. Am Heart J. 2009;158:806–13.
56. Wince WB, Kim RJ. Molecular imaging: T2-weighted CMR of the area at risk – a risky business? Nat Rev Cardiol. 2010;7:547–9.
57. Giri S, Chung YC, Merchant A, Mihai G, Rajagopalan S, Raman SV, Simonetti OP. T2 quantification for improved detection of myocardial edema. J Cardiovasc Magn Reson. 2009;11:56.
58. Kloner RA, Ganote CE, Jennings RB. The "no-reflow" phenomenon after temporary coronary occlusion in the dog. J Clin Invest. 1974;54:1496–508.
59. The GUSTO Angiographic Investigators. The effects of tissue plasminogen activator, streptokinase, or both on coronary-artery patency, ventricular function, and survival after acute myocardial infarction. N Engl J Med. 1993;329:1615–22.
60. Simes RJ, Topol EJ, Holmes Jr DR, White HD, Rutsch WR, Vahanian A, Simoons ML, Morris D, Betriu A, Califf RM, et al. Link between the angiographic substudy and mortality outcomes in a large randomized trial of myocardial reperfusion. Importance of early and complete infarct artery reperfusion. GUSTO-I investigators. Circulation. 1995;91:1923–8.
61. Ito H. No-reflow phenomenon and prognosis in patients with acute myocardial infarction. Nat Clin Pract Cardiovasc Med. 2006;3:499–506.
62. Gibson CM, Cannon CP, Murphy SA, Ryan KA, Mesley R, Marble SJ, McCabe CH, Van De Werf F, Braunwald E. Relationship of TIMI myocardial perfusion grade to mortality after administration of thrombolytic drugs. Circulation. 2000;101:125–30.
63. Gibson CM, Murphy SA, Rizzo MJ, Ryan KA, Marble SJ, McCabe CH, Cannon CP, Van de Werf F, Braunwald E. Relationship between TIMI frame count and clinical outcomes after thrombolytic administration. Thrombolysis in myocardial infarction (TIMI) study group. Circulation. 1999;99:1945–50.
64. Morishima I, Sone T, Okumura K, Tsuboi H, Kondo J, Mukawa H, Matsui H, Toki Y, Ito T, Hayakawa T. Angiographic no-reflow phenomenon as a predictor of adverse long-term outcome in patients treated with percutaneous transluminal coronary angioplasty for first acute myocardial infarction. J Am Coll Cardiol. 2000;36:1202–9.
65. Wu KC, Zerhouni EA, Judd RM, Lugo-Olivieri CH, Barouch LA, Schulman SP, Blumenthal RS, Lima JA. Prognostic significance of microvascular obstruction by magnetic resonance imaging in patients with acute myocardial infarction. Circulation. 1998;97:765–72.
66. Nijveldt R, Beek AM, Hirsch A, Stoel MG, Hofman MB, Umans VA, Algra PR, Twisk JW, van Rossum AC. Functional recovery after acute myocardial infarction: comparison between angiography, electrocardiography, and cardiovascular magnetic resonance measures of microvascular injury. J Am Coll Cardiol. 2008;52:181–9.
67. Appelbaum E, Kirtane AJ, Clark A, Pride YB, Gelfand EV, Harrigan CJ, Kissinger KV, Manning WJ, Gibson CM. Association of TIMI myocardial perfusion grade and ST-segment resolution with cardiovascular magnetic resonance measures of microvascular obstruction and infarct size following ST-segment elevation myocardial infarction. J Thromb Thrombolysis. 2009;27:123–9.
68. Kim RJ, Chen EL, Lima JA, Judd RM. Myocardial Gd-DTPA kinetics determine MRI contrast enhancement and reflect the extent and severity of myocardial injury after acute reperfused infarction. Circulation. 1996;94:3318–26.
69. Wu KC, Kim RJ, Bluemke DA, Rochitte CE, Zerhouni EA, Becker LC, Lima JA. Quantification and time course of microvascular obstruction by contrast-enhanced echocardiography and magnetic resonance imaging following acute myocardial infarction and reperfusion. J Am Coll Cardiol. 1998;32:1756–64.
70. Rochitte CE, Lima JA, Bluemke DA, Reeder SB, McVeigh ER, Furuta T, Becker LC, Melin JA. Magnitude and time course of microvascular obstruction and tissue injury after acute myocardial infarction. Circulation. 1998;98:1006–14.
71. Lima JA, Judd RM, Bazille A, Schulman SP, Atalar E, Zerhouni EA. Regional heterogeneity of human myocardial infarcts demonstrated by contrast-enhanced MRI. Potential mechanisms. Circulation. 1995;92:1117–25.

72. Friedrich MG, Sechtem U, Schulz-Menger J, Holmvang G, Alakija P, Cooper LT, White JA, Abdel-Aty H, Gutberlet M, Prasad S, Aletras A, Laissy JP, Paterson I, Filipchuk NG, Kumar A, Pauschinger M, Liu P. Cardiovascular magnetic resonance in myocarditis: a JACC white paper. J Am Coll Cardiol. 2009;53:1475–87.
73. Bekkers SC, Backes WH, Kim RJ, Snoep G, Gorgels AP, Passos VL, Waltenberger J, Crijns HJ, Schalla S. Detection and characteristics of microvascular obstruction in reperfused acute myocardial infarction using an optimized protocol for contrast-enhanced cardiovascular magnetic resonance imaging. Eur Radiol. 2009;19:2904–12.
74. Thiele H, Kappl MJ, Conradi S, Niebauer J, Hambrecht R, Schuler G. Reproducibility of chronic and acute infarct size measurement by delayed enhancement-magnetic resonance imaging. J Am Coll Cardiol. 2006;47:1641–5.
75. Wagner A, Mahrholdt H, Thomson L, Hager S, Meinhardt G, Rehwald W, Parker M, Shah D, Sechtem U, Kim RJ, Judd RM. Effects of time, dose, and inversion time for acute myocardial infarct size measurements based on magnetic resonance imaging-delayed contrast enhancement. J Am Coll Cardiol. 2006;47:2027–33.
76. Nijveldt R, Hofman MB, Hirsch A, Beek AM, Umans VA, Algra PR, Piek JJ, van Rossum AC. Assessment of microvascular obstruction and prediction of short-term remodeling after acute myocardial infarction: cardiac MR imaging study. Radiology. 2009;250:363–70.
77. Mather AN, Lockie T, Nagel E, Marber M, Perera D, Redwood S, Radjenovic A, Saha A, Greenwood JP, Plein S. Appearance of microvascular obstruction on high resolution first-pass perfusion, early and late gadolinium enhancement CMR in patients with acute myocardial infarction. J Cardiovasc Magn Reson. 2009;11:33.
78. Yan AT, Gibson CM, Larose E, Anavekar NS, Tsang S, Solomon SD, Reynolds G, Kwong RY. Characterization of microvascular dysfunction after acute myocardial infarction by cardiovascular magnetic resonance first-pass perfusion and late gadolinium enhancement imaging. J Cardiovasc Magn Reson. 2006;8:831–7.
79. Nijveldt R, van der Vleuten PA, Hirsch A, Beek AM, Tio RA, Tijssen JG, Piek JJ, van Rossum AC, Zijlstra F. Early electrocardiographic findings and MR imaging-verified microvascular injury and myocardial infarct size. JACC Cardiovasc Imaging. 2009;2:1187–94.
80. Neizel M, Futterer S, Steen H, Giannitsis E, Reinhardt L, Lossnitzer D, Lehrke S, Jaffe AS, Katus HA. Predicting microvascular obstruction with cardiac troponin T after acute myocardial infarction: a correlative study with contrast-enhanced magnetic resonance imaging. Clin Res Cardiol. 2009;98:555–62.
81. Baks T, van Geuns RJ, Biagini E, Wielopolski P, Mollet NR, Cademartiri F, van der Giessen WJ, Krestin GP, Serruys PW, Duncker DJ, de Feyter PJ. Effects of primary angioplasty for acute myocardial infarction on early and late infarct size and left ventricular wall characteristics. J Am Coll Cardiol. 2006;47:40–4.
82. Orn S, Manhenke C, Greve OJ, Larsen AI, Bonarjee VV, Edvardsen T, Dickstein K. Microvascular obstruction is a major determinant of infarct healing and subsequent left ventricular remodelling following primary percutaneous coronary intervention. Eur Heart J. 2009;30:1978–85.
83. Kloner RA, Ellis SG, Lange R, Braunwald E. Studies of experimental coronary artery reperfusion. Effects on infarct size, myocardial function, biochemistry, ultrastructure and microvascular damage. Circulation. 1983;68:I8–15.
84. Kloner RA, Alker KJ. The effect of streptokinase on intramyocardial hemorrhage, infarct size, and the no-reflow phenomenon during coronary reperfusion. Circulation. 1984;70: 513–21.
85. Capone RJ, Most AS. Myocardial hemorrhage after coronary reperfusion in pigs. Am J Cardiol. 1978;41:259–66.
86. Higginson LA, White F, Heggtveit HA, Sanders TM, Bloor CM, Covell JW. Determinants of myocardial hemorrhage after coronary reperfusion in the anesthetized dog. Circulation. 1982;65:62–9.
87. Bradley Jr WG. MR appearance of hemorrhage in the brain. Radiology. 1993;189:15–26.
88. Pauling L, Coryell CD. The magnetic properties and structure of the hemochromogens and related substances. Proc Natl Acad Sci USA. 1936;22:159–63.

89. Linfante I, Llinas RH, Caplan LR, Warach S. MRI features of intracerebral hemorrhage within 2 hours from symptom onset. Stroke. 1999;30:2263–7.
90. Hermier M, Nighoghossian N. Contribution of susceptibility-weighted imaging to acute stroke assessment. Stroke. 2004;35:1989–94.
91. Kumar A, Green JD, Sykes JM, Ephrat P, Carson JJ, Mitchell AJ, Wisenberg G, Friedrich MG. T2*-weighted cardiovascular magnetic resonance detects reperfusion hemorrhage in a dog model of myocardial infarction. Circulation. 2007;116:116 (abstract).
92. O'Regan DP, Ahmed R, Karunanithy N, Neuwirth C, Tan Y, Durighel G, Hajnal JV, Nadra I, Corbett SJ, Cook SA. Reperfusion hemorrhage following acute myocardial infarction: assessment with T2* mapping and effect on measuring the area at risk. Radiology. 2009;250:916–22.
93. O'Regan DP, Ariff B, Neuwirth C, Tan Y, Durighel G, Cook SA. Assessment of severe reperfusion injury with T2* cardiac MRI in patients with acute myocardial infarction. Heart. 2010;96:1885–91.
94. Ochiai K, Shimada T, Murakami Y, Ishibashi Y, Sano K, Kitamura J, Inoue S, Murakami R, Kawamitsu H, Sugimura K. Hemorrhagic myocardial infarction after coronary reperfusion detected in vivo by magnetic resonance imaging in humans: prevalence and clinical implications. J Cardiovasc Magn Reson. 1999;1:247–56.
95. Ganame J, Messalli G, Dymarkowski S, Rademakers FE, Desmet W, Van de Werf F, Bogaert J. Impact of myocardial haemorrhage on left ventricular function and remodelling in patients with reperfused acute myocardial infarction. Eur Heart J. 2009;30:1440–9.
96. Lotan CS, Bouchard A, Cranney GB, Bishop SP, Pohost GM. Assessment of postreperfusion myocardial hemorrhage using proton NMR imaging at 1.5 T. Circulation. 1992;86:1018–25.
97. Beek AM, Nijveldt R, van Rossum AC. Intramyocardial hemorrhage and microvascular obstruction after primary percutaneous coronary intervention. Int J Cardiovasc Imaging. 2010;26:49–55.
98. Basso C, Corbetti F, Silva C, Abudureheman A, Lacognata C, Cacciavillani L, Tarantini G, Marra MP, Ramondo A, Thiene G, Iliceto S. Morphologic validation of reperfused hemorrhagic myocardial infarction by cardiovascular magnetic resonance. Am J Cardiol. 2007;100:1322–7.
99. Lotan CS, Miller SK, Cranney GB, Pohost GM, Elgavish GA. The effect of postinfarction intramyocardial hemorrhage on transverse relaxation time. Magn Reson Med. 1992;23:346–55.
100. Mather AN, Fairbairn TA, Ball SG, Greenwood JP, Plein S. Reperfusion haemorrhage as determined by cardiovascular MRI is a predictor of adverse left ventricular remodelling and markers of late arrhythmic risk. Heart. 2011;97:453–9.
101. Levine GN, Gomes AS, Arai AE, Bluemke DA, Flamm SD, Kanal E, Manning WJ, Martin ET, Smith JM, Wilke N, Shellock FS. Safety of magnetic resonance imaging in patients with cardiovascular devices: an American Heart Association scientific statement from the Committee on Diagnostic and Interventional Cardiac Catheterization, Council on Clinical Cardiology, and the Council on Cardiovascular Radiology and Intervention: endorsed by the American College of Cardiology Foundation, the North American Society for Cardiac Imaging, and the Society for Cardiovascular Magnetic Resonance. Circulation. 2007;116:-2878–91.
102. Syed MA, Carlson K, Murphy M, Ingkanisorn WP, Rhoads KL, Arai AE. Long-term safety of cardiac magnetic resonance imaging performed in the first few days after bare-metal stent implantation. J Magn Reson Imaging. 2006;24:1056–61.
103. Kribben A, Witzke O, Hillen U, Barkhausen J, Daul AE, Erbel R. Nephrogenic systemic fibrosis: pathogenesis, diagnosis, and therapy. J Am Coll Cardiol. 2009;53:1621–8.
104. Pietsch H, Raschke M, Ellinger-Ziegelbauer H, Jost G, Walter J, Frenzel T, Lenhard D, Hutter J, Sieber MA. The role of residual gadolinium in the induction of nephrogenic systemic fibrosis-like skin lesions in rats. Invest Radiol. 2011;46:48–56.

Part IV
Management of Myocardial Reperfusion Injury

Chapter 10
Current Approaches to Prevention and Management of Reperfusion Injury

Wichert J. Kuijt, Judson Williams, Christopher B. Granger, Mitchell W. Krucoff, and Matthew T. Roe

Abstract As our understanding of the pathophysiological underpinnings of reperfusion injury has increased, many therapies directed at preventing the detrimental effects of this phenomenon have been tested. For primary PCI, this has ranged from mechanical protection from distal embolization of plaque material, preventing calcium overload after reperfusion, to the inhibition of specific inflammatory mediators. Although most have shown promise in smaller mechanistic clinical trials, only mechanical thrombectomy has thus far been shown to be of clinical benefit in larger investigations.

W.J. Kuijt, M.D.
Department of Cardiology, Academic Medical Center – University of Amsterdam, Room B2-213, Meibergdreef 9, Amsterdam 1105 AZ, The Netherlands
e-mail: wichert.kuijt@duke.edu

J. Williams, M.D., MHS
Department of Surgery, Division of Cardiac Surgery, Duke University, 2405 Englewood Ave., Durham 27705, NC, USA
e-mail: judsonw@alumni.princeton.edu

C.B. Granger, M.D.
Department of Cardiology, Division of Cardiovascular Medicine, Duke University Medical Center, Duke Clinical Research Institute, 2400 Pratt St., 27705, Durham, NC, USA
e-mail: christopher.granger@duke.edu

M.W. Krucoff, M.D., FACC, FAHA
Department of Medicine, Division of Cardiology, Duke University Medical Center, 508 Fulton Street, Room A3006 Cardiology, Durham, NC 27705, USA
e-mail: kruco001@mc.duke.edu

M.T. Roe, M.D., MHS (✉)
Division of Cardiovascular Medicine, Duke University Medical Center, Duke Clinical Research Institute, 2400 Pratt St., Room 7035, Durham, NC 27705, USA
e-mail: matthew.roe@duke.edu

J.C. Kaski et al. (eds.), *Management of Myocardial Reperfusion Injury*, DOI 10.1007/978-1-84996-019-9_10, © Springer-Verlag London 2012

Additionally, the occurrence of ventricular arrhythmias poses a threat not only due to (1) electrical failure and subsequent asystole but also because (2) bursts of ventricular activity around the time of reperfusion signify a larger infarct size and subsequent long-term risk of pump failure. Prophylactic treatment with antiarrhythmic drugs has thus far been shown to increase mortality, and investigations are ongoing to improve our understanding of these arrhythmias and to identify patients at high risk that may benefit from treatment.

For the prevention of reperfusion injury in coronary artery bypass grafting, the optimum combination of cardioplegic solutions and temperature has not yet been determined. No regimen has been shown to confer superior myocardial salvage over another, with cold blood crystalloid infusion having become the most used worldwide. As in primary PCI, the search continuous for specific cardioprotective compounds and identifying patients at high risk to optimize treatment strategies.

Keywords Prevention and management • Embolic events • Thrombectomy Aspiration catheter • Reperfusion arrhythmias • Pharmacological management Cardiac surgery • Myocardial reperfusion injury • Microvascular obstruction Coronary microembolization

Introduction

Since the first descriptions of the potentially detrimental effects of reperfusion of a previously occluded artery and subsequent myocellular damage due to the release of thrombogenic emboli from the disrupted plaque to influx of vasoactive and immunogenic compounds, there has been an ongoing search for effective interventions to protect against these harmful processes. Outside of the direct effects on the viability of the cells, these processes have been shown to potentially result in the electromechanical uncoupling of the ischemic cells and thus give rise to hemodynamically significant and potentially lethal arrhythmias around the time of revascularization and the immediate period after. This chapter will largely focus on three distinct entities that have been identified to contribute significantly to poor outcomes even in those patients that receive rapid and successful primary percutaneous coronary intervention (PCI): (1) distal embolization of micro- and macroscopic thrombus material at the culprit lesion, (2) the influx of vasoactive and thrombogenic compounds to the distal vasculature after opening of the vessel, and (3) the induction of reperfusion arrhythmias.

Embolic Protection and Thrombectomy

The occurrence of distal embolization at the time coronary intervention has been consistently correlated with poor outcome and impaired microvascular flow, even in patients achieving thrombolysis in myocardial infarction (TIMI) – flow grade III after primary PCI [1, 2]. As such, there has been a keen interest in developing treatment strategies to reduce and prevent the dislodging of thrombus material to the distal vasculature. However, the approaches taken to this end have differed widely in both their working mechanism and success.

Distal Embolic Protection

The goal of embolic protection is to protect the distal vasculature from the debris carried by the reestablished coronary flow. The predominant approach has been to place a filter or balloon downstream from the culprit lesion and as such block the emboli from descending further down into the microvasculature. This approach has been shown to be highly successful in the prevention of distal embolization and limiting periprocedural myocardial damage in procedures involving occluded saphenous venous grafts (SVG) [3, 4].

Of the distal embolic protection devices, the Guardwire has been most extensively investigated. The device deploys a balloon distal to the culprit lesion to be inflated after lesion crossing but before balloon inflation and stenting of the culprit artery. It is intended to be used in conjunction with the Export catheter, discussed below, to facilitate the removal of plaque during the PCI procedure. A number of clinical trials have investigated the efficacy of this device in patients presenting with a STEMI [5–8]. The device was successful in retrieving thrombotic material in ~70% of patients treated with this technique [7]. However, apart from a signal of more frequent TIMI-flow III in a small mechanistic trial, there were no indications that this device led to improved markers of reperfusion or clinical benefit. Essentially, the same observations apply to the devices that deploy a distal filter to retrieve liberated emboli, such as the FilterWire [9, 10] and the SpideRX [11]. Although they were successful in retrieving thrombotic material, there was virtually no improvement across a range of biomarkers. Of note, none of the devices proved to significantly alter the rate of distal embolization observed on the post-procedural angiogram, suggesting that processes before and during lesion crossing may be more important than manipulation of the thrombus after minimal flow has been reestablished by the guidewire.

Proximal Embolic Protection

Conceptually, proximal embolic protection, such as that provided by the Proxis device, may be more successful in preventing distal embolic protection during every phase of the PCI procedure. As the device is simultaneously capable of aspiration, the patient could benefit from both the lessening of thrombotic burden and protection of the distal vasculature. In the PREPARE trial, more robust ST segment resolution (STR, indicating successful reperfusion) was observed directly after primary PCI, suggesting that this approach may protect the myocardium in the immediate time frame after the procedure [12]. However, it was also observed that this difference dissipated quickly over time and was not accompanied by improved myocardial blush, less frequent occurrence of distal embolization, or smaller infarct size as measured by serum cardiac enzymes. This was confirmed in the large cardiac magnetic resonance imaging substudy, showing no significant differences in myocardial infarct size or functional measurements of the left ventricle [13].

Thrombectomy

The use of thrombectomy to reduce the thrombotic burden in the culprit artery prior to balloon inflation and stent placement has become increasingly more accepted as an option to improve the result of primary PCI. It has several potential benefits over the use of an occlusive device, such as the possibility to use the catheter before crossing the lesion, less dependence on favorable anatomy due to superior maneuverability and ease of use. As with previously described methods, several different types of technologies have been developed to free and extract the thrombus, and as with the other modalities, it seems there are diverging results in clinical trials [14].

Mechanical Thrombectomy and Aspiration

One of the approaches to thrombus removal is using a mechanical device to break up the thrombus and subsequently extract it, such as the X-Sizer. The device uses a helical cutter at the tip of the catheter to liberate debris and includes aspiration capability in the same catheter. Use of the X-Sizer was consistently shown to lead to better epicardial flow, improved myocardial blush grade, and more robust STR [15–17]. However, the clinical benefits are as of yet unknown due to the lack of larger trials in which clinical outcome can be ascertained or used in meta-analysis.

Rheolytic Thrombectomy and Aspiration

A different technique is used by the AngioJet. It utilizes high-pressure saline fluid streams to break up the thrombus and create a vacuum through which the debris is removed. Results of clinical trials have proven to be ambivalent, with one small trial suggesting benefit on angiographic and ECG biomarkers [18] and another larger trial suggesting possible harm with decreased epicardial flow and larger infarct size [19].

Aspiration Catheters

The most frequently used devices to reduce thrombotic burden are the various aspiration catheters, such as the Export [20–22], Diver [23, 24], Rescue [25, 26], TVAC

[27], and Pronto [28]. Although slightly different in design, they share the use of an external source of vacuum to aspirate the thrombus and blood in the coronary artery. Its main benefits are the ease of use of a simple over the wire catheter that is easily maneuverable and as such able to fit more diverse coronary anatomies than some of the other devices. Although a consistent improvement in various markers of reperfusion is seen with the various devices, there has been some hesitation over the effects of thrombosuction after Kaltoft and colleagues published a study showing that thrombosuction using the Rescue catheter may be associated with a larger infarct size. Subsequently, several additional smaller studies and a comprehensive meta-analysis have alleviated these concerns, and both the Export (EXPIRA) and TVAC (VAMPIRE) showed significant reductions in infarct size in the patients treated with thrombus aspiration. More importantly, the TAPAS trial randomized patients to either primary PCI with routine thrombectomy or primary PCI without routine thrombectomy and showed a reduction in impaired microvascular flow, improved STR, and rather surprisingly a significant reduction in 30-day and 1-year mortality in an all-comers population at a single center [22, 29]. This confirms the results of the meta-analysis by Burzotta [30] and suggests that routine simple thrombus aspiration may be of considerable benefit. However, none of these investigations were powered for clinical events and require confirmation in a larger, multicenter trial before thrombectomy can conclusively be recommended for all STEMI patients undergoing primary PCI.

Conclusions for Prevention and Treatment

At this time, it seems that the routine application of thrombectomy using an aspiration catheter may be indicated in patients who present with suitable coronary anatomy. The use of embolic protection devices does not seem to lead to clinical benefit, and the use of mechanical means of thrombus breakup need to be further investigated to warrant widespread use at this time (Table 10.1).

Pharmacological Treatment of Microvascular Obstruction and "No-Reflow"

The no-reflow phenomenon is a frequently encountered adverse reaction of the myocardial vasculature to ischemia and subsequent reperfusion. It was first identified in patients in whom, in spite of removal of the obstruction in the epicardial vessel, optimal flow was not reestablished. This gradually shifted as it was understood that in patients who did have satisfactory flow, the microvascular perfusion could still remain inhibited as evidenced by impaired myocardial blush grade and slow, incomplete normalization of the ST segment, shifting the targets of treatment downstream of the acute occlusion [33]. In the era of primary PCI, this entity has been well

Table 10.1 Methods of device interventions to reduce thrombus burden, distal embolization, and microvascular obstruction

Method	Number of patients	Results	Author
Aspiration thrombectomy			
Rescue	215	Improved STR in treatment group	Dudek et al. [25]
	72	No improvement in early surrogate markers and increased CMR IS	Kaltoft et al. [26]
Diver	99	Improved STR and MBG with thrombectomy	Burzotta et al. [23]
	76	Improved STR and MBG in treatment group	De Luca et al. [24]
Export	1,072	Improved STR and MBG in treatment group	Svilaas et al. [22]
	249	Lower 1-year cardiac mortality (3.6% vs. 6.7%) in treatment group	Vlaar et al. [29]
	175	No significant improvement in surrogate markers or clinical endpoints	Chevalier et al. [20]
		Improved MBG and reduced CMR IS with thrombectomy	Sardella et al. [21]
Pronto	148	Better STR, cTFC, and MBG in treatment group	Silva-Orrego et al. [28]
TVAC	355	Higher rate of MBG grade 3 in treatment group	Ikari et al. [27]
Mechanical/rheolytic thrombectomy			
AngioJet	501	Improved STR and lower 1 year with thrombectomy	Migliorini et al. [31]
	480	Worse TIMI-flow, larger SPECT IS and higher 30-day mortality in treatment arm (4.6% vs. 0.8%)	Ali et al. [19]
	100	Better STR, lower cTFC, and smaller SPECT IS in treatment group	Antoniucci et al. [18]
X-Sizer	201	Improved STR in thrombectomy group	Lefevre et al. [16]
	92	Improved STR and MBG with thrombectomy	Napodano et al. [32]
	61	Improved STR and cTFC in device group	Beran et al. [15]
Distal embolic protection			
Guardwire	501	No significant improvement in surrogate markers or clinical outcomes	Stone et al. [7]
	341	No significant improvement in surrogate markers or clinical outcomes	Muramatsu et al. [6]
	154	No significant improvement in surrogate markers or clinical outcomes	Matsuo et al. [5]
	116	Improvement in rate of TIMI-3 flow	Tahk et al. [8]
FilterWire	326	No significant improvement in surrogate markers or clinical outcomes	Kelbaeck et al. [10]
	200	Improvement in rate of TIMI-3 flow	Gick et al. [9]
SpideRX	140	No significant improvement in surrogate markers or clinical outcomes	Cura et al. [11]
Proximal embolic protection			
Proxis	284	Improved STR at end of PCI, no improvement in CMR IS	Haeck et al. [12, 13]

STR ST segment recovery, *CMR* cardiac magnetic resonance imaging, *IS* infarct size, *MBG* myocardial blush grade, *cTFC* corrected TIMI frame count, *TIMI* thrombolysis in myocardial infarction, *PCI* percutaneous coronary intervention

described and has become a target for adjuvant therapies, aimed at the presumed underlying causes. A multifactorial process, microvascular obstruction appears to be an interplay between vasoconstriction and cell swelling due to depletion of ATP and rapid influx of calcium, the influx of inflammatory compounds, and the detrimental effects of sudden pH shifts and free radicals causing reperfusion injury.

Calcium Channel Inhibitors

Verapamil

Calcium channel inhibitors have long been used in patients with angina due to coronary vasospasm as well as in hypertension due to the negative chronotropic and vasodilating properties of these drugs. Additionally, they may also inhibit the calcium overload of the sarcolemma after reperfusion and have benefits in the reduction of platelet aggregation, thus aiding with the treatment and prevention of reperfusion injury on multiple levels. Verapamil has been investigated using an intracoronary bolus followed by oral treatment [34, 35] and was shown to improve left ventricular function and myocardial perfusion as assessed by echocardiography. Further investigations will need to show whether these benefits translate into improved clinical outcome.

Nicardipine

Like verapamil, nicardipine exacts its action through inhibition of the slow L-channels but is seemingly more cardiospecific and as such may exhibit less systemic side effects than would be encountered with verapamil [36]. However, this has not yet been evaluated in clinical trials.

Adenosine

Adenosine is a naturally occurring purine nucleoside and asserts its effects by reducing the arteriolar resistance in the coronary vasculature and by reducing the heart rate, thus reducing demand and improving diastolic filling times. In smaller mechanistic trials, adenosine appeared to present benefits on multiple biomarker modalities such as improved echocardiographic perfusion, reducing infarct size and suggesting clinical benefit through both intracoronary and intravenous routes. However, the large randomized AMISTAD-II trial failed to show improvement in outcomes after intravenous injection of adenosine before and during primary PCI [37]. In a subgroup analysis, it appeared that patients presenting within 3 h after symptom onset and with anterior location of the infarct had significantly smaller infarcts and better clinical outcome [38]. However, these results would need to be corroborated in a separate investigation.

Nitrous Oxide Donors

Nitroglycerine and Nitroprusside

The potential benefit of nitrates to relieve MVO is due to its powerful vasodilation through nitrous oxide donation as well as mild arteriolar relaxation through the same mechanism. Additionally, both drugs exert their effect almost immediately and are rapidly metabolized, making them easy to use and titrate for individual patients to their hemodynamic parameters. Although evidence is limited, intracoronary nitroprusside was associated with improved clinical outcome. Targeted trials in patients exhibiting signs of MVO should follow to corroborate and extend these observations [39].

Nicorandil

Nicorandil is also a nitrous oxide donor but additionally activates the potassium channels in coronary vascular smooth muscle cells and thus improves both arterial and venous relaxation. Results of trials evaluating this drug have been mixed, with one smaller trial showing improved ST segment resolution and clinical outcome [40], whereas a larger trial did not show benefit on myocardial infarct size [41]. As such, further data is needed to assess the place of this drug in the interventional armamentarium.

Antithrombotics

GP IIb/IIIa Inhibition

Intensifying the antithrombotic treatment in patients with STEMI has long been a target of improved treatment in primary PCI. The use of GPIIb/IIIa inhibitors was thought to be especially attractive in this context due the virtually complete inhibition of platelet aggregation, combined with the potential benefit of downregulating the proliferation of endothelial and smooth muscle cells. The role of GPIIb/IIIa inhibitors as adjuvant treatment in primary PCI was established through multiple large clinical trials and significantly reduced reinfarction and in meta-analysis, appeared to improve mortality [42–46]. However, recent investigations into the use of these compounds on top of loading doses of clopidogrel have suggested that the routine early use of abciximab may not be indicated in all patients [47, 48]. Contrary to these results is the contemporary On-TIME 2 trial, which showed that in-ambulance administration of high-dose tirofiban was associated with a more rapid and complete normalization of the ST segment and improved 30-day and 1-year clinical outcome [49, 50]. A promising development is the renewed emphasis in increasing dosing and availability locally by injecting abciximab, and potentially small-molecule drugs such as tirofiban and eptifibatide, through an intracoronary route. Smaller mechanistic trials suggest that intracoronary administration may enhance myocardial salvage but minimize bleeding risks associated with systemic administration of GP IIb-IIIa inhibitors [51], but early these results will have to be confirmed in larger trials powered for clinical endpoints.

Intracoronary Streptokinase

The adjunctive use of thrombolytics in primary PCI has not been successful, and this approach appears to cause more harm with the increased risks of bleeding, exceeding the benefits of potential earlier breakup of the coronary thrombus [52, 53]. However, the use of thrombolytics may have the benefit of removing fibrinous microemboli that antiplatelet medications cannot break up. As such, the use of these drugs is now under investigation when provided through intracoronary injections to minimize systemic sequelae and maximize local efficacy. Although the first effort in for this was promising and improved coronary flow reserve and microvascular perfusion [54], the previous studies in this field warrant caution before adapting thrombolytic compounds again in the treatment of STEMI.

Conclusions for Prevention and Treatment

Although several drug types have shown promise in reducing the detrimental vascular and thrombotic complications of reperfusion, none so far has translated into long-term benefit in trials powered to assess clinical efficacy. However, there might be considerable benefit from these drugs in selected patients who show signs of "no-reflow" after primary PCI and have large areas at risk, something subgroup analysis of the various trials has frequently hinted at (Table 10.2). The judicious use of drugs such as adenosine and nitrates in those patients who are hemodynamically stable might be a reasonable treatment option for persistent microvascular obstruction.

Prevention and Treatment of Reperfusion Arrhythmias

Ventricular arrhythmias around STEMI are quite frequent [59, 60] and associated with considerable mortality during and after hospitalization. The ischemic and reperfused myocardium constitutes a potent source of decoupled cells to initiate arrhythmias and as such research has focused on the significance of these events as well as preventive measures. Additionally, more recent investigations have increased the realization that not only subacute substrate can act arrhythmogenic but also the acute influx of normal blood after recanalization of the infarct artery.

Table 10.2 Pharmacological interventions to reduce microvascular obstruction after primary PCI

Intervention	Mechanism of action	Number of patients	Trial design	Results	Author
Antithrombotics					
Abciximab	GP IIb/IIIa inhibition	2,082	IV vs. placebo	No significant improvement in STR, MBG, or outcome	Stone et al. [46]
		300	IV vs. placebo	Reduced no-reflow, improved LVEF and clinical outcome	Montalescot et al. [44]
		210	Early vs. late IV	Reduced angio-graphic reflow and improved LVEF	Maioli et al. [43]
		534	IC vs. IV	No difference in STR; better MBG and lower CK-MB IS in presence of better pre-procedural TIMI-flow	Gu et al. [55]
		200	IC vs. IV	Reduced no-reflow on Doppler and improved LVEF	Thiele et al. [51]
Tirofiban	GP IIb/IIIa inhibition	984	Prehospital vs. provisional	Improved STR and lower rate of 30 day MACE (5.8% vs. 8.6%)	van't Hof et al. [49] ten Berg et al. [50]
Streptokinase	Plasminogen activation	41	IC vs. placebo	Reduced no-reflow on Doppler and smaller CMR IS	Sezer et al. [54, 56]
Vasodilators					
Adenosine	Reduction of heart rate and arteriolar resistance	2,118	IV vs. placebo	Reduced SPECT IS and MACE in anterior MI in high dose	Ross et al. [37]
		54	IC vs. placebo	Reduced angio-graphic no-reflow and SPECT IS	Marzilli et al. [57]
		30	IV vs. placebo	Improved perfusion on contrast echocardiography and smaller SPECT IS	Micari et al. [58]
Verapamil	Negative chronotropic, vasodilating, reduction calcium overload	40	IC vs. placebo	Improved perfusion on contrast echocardiography and LVEF	Taniyama et al. [34]

Table 10.2 (continued)

Intervention	Mechanism of action	Number of patients	Trial design	Results	Author
Verapamil vs. adenosine		150	IC/IC vs. placebo	Both reduced angiographic no-reflow and improved LVEF compared to placebo	Vijayalakshmi et al. [35]
Nitroprusside/ nitroglyc-erin	Vasodilation through NO donation	98	IC vs. placebo	No significant differences in biomarkers	Amit et al. [39]
Nicorandil	Arterial and venous relaxation through NO donation and K-channel inhibition	1,216	IV vs. placebo	No improvement in biomarkers	Kitakaze et al. [41]
		368	IV vs. placebo	Reduced angio-graphic reflow and improved STR, lower rates of MACE (6.5% vs. 16.4%)	Ishii et al. [40]

GP glycoprotein, *IV* intravenous, *IC* intracoronary, *STR* ST segment recovery, *MBG* myocardial blush grade, *LVEF* left ventricular ejection fraction, *CMR* cardiac magnetic resonance imaging, *IS* infarct size, *TIMI* thrombolysis in myocardial infarction, *PCI* percutaneous coronary intervention

Ventricular Arrhythmias During Hospitalization

The incidence of ventricular arrhythmias is very frequent during the initial phase after primary PCI and is thought to be responsible for a large part of in-hospital and 30-day mortality [59]. Despite the considerable impact of these events, there has been a relative dearth of investigations as to what the optimal treatment is for these patients. Prior investigations have focused mainly on using antiarrhythmic drugs, such as amiodarone [61], lidocaine [62], and flecainide [63], in a prophylactic setting that do not show a clear signal of benefit but may actually increase mortality [64, 65]. As such, using these compounds in all patients with STEMI is contraindicated. In a regular clinical setting, treating these often hemodynamically unstable cardiac rhythms is evidently indicated, and the clinical recommendations in the ACC/AHA guidelines [66] are derivative of the investigations in other clinical settings complicated by ventricular arrhythmias such as out-of-hospital cardiac arrests, and it is unclear whether these findings can be translated indiscriminately to the in-hospital management. Normal ACLS protocols should be followed. Thus, guidelines recommend the use of amiodarone in the case of sustained/polymorphic ventricular arrhythmias as a IIa/I indication and lidocaine as IIb in both cases. However, both recommendations are level C due to the lack of clinical trial evidence. A recent analysis from the GUSTO IIb and III investigations suggests that in early survivors, the use of lidocaine may have more favorable results in these patients [67]. Further complicating the situation are suggestions that the beneficial effect of amiodarone may be limited to those who have received concomitant beta blockers, which is contraindicated in hemodynamically unstable STEMI patients, emphasizing the need for randomized comparisons to assess optimal treatment [68].

Ventricular Arrhythmias at Reperfusion

The occurrence of ventricular arrhythmias at the time of recanalization of the epicardial vessel has been described from the early phases of thrombolytic treatment [69] and frequently seen as an accelerated idioventricular rhythm with or without hemodynamic problems. While initially being hailed as a positive sign of coronary patency after confirmation with angiography [70, 71], it has been becoming increasingly clear that these "ventricular bursts" [72], while strongly associated with restored coronary flow, may be a harbinger of increased myocardial distress and necrosis, as evidenced by the significantly larger infarct size in patients in whom this phenomenon occurs [72] (Fig. 10.1). As of now, there are no therapies that specifically target this type of arrhythmia. The challenge with these patients is that the arrhythmia is likely an epiphenomenon of the underlying damage from the noxious consequences of reperfusion injury. As such, therapy for this as of yet poorly understood event should probably focus on treatment of both the symptoms (potentially hemodynamically significant arrhythmias) as well as the processes that lead to reperfusion injury such as calcium overload, influx of immune mediators, and microvascular vasoconstriction. However, as discussed earlier in this chapter, as of yet, there are no established successful options.

Conclusions for Prevention and Treatment

As of now, there are no specific treatments or regimens tailored to the occurrence of ventricular arrhythmias in the acute and subacute phases of STEMI. Guidelines recommended treatments involve the use of normal ACLS protocols. Amiodarone and lidocaine are the preferred compounds with which to treat the reperfusion arrhythmias. Future investigations should focus on identifying patients at high risk of developing severe ventricular arrhythmias in the early phase (<30 days), and interventional studies should focus on evaluating pharmacological treatment and/or treatment with an ICD or extracorporeal defibrillator.

For the separate phenomenon of reperfusion "ventricular burst," there are no treatments that have been specifically assessed in this setting. The specific pathophysiological causes of these reperfusion arrhythmias are as of yet poorly understood and are in need of further elucidation before treatment can be considered.

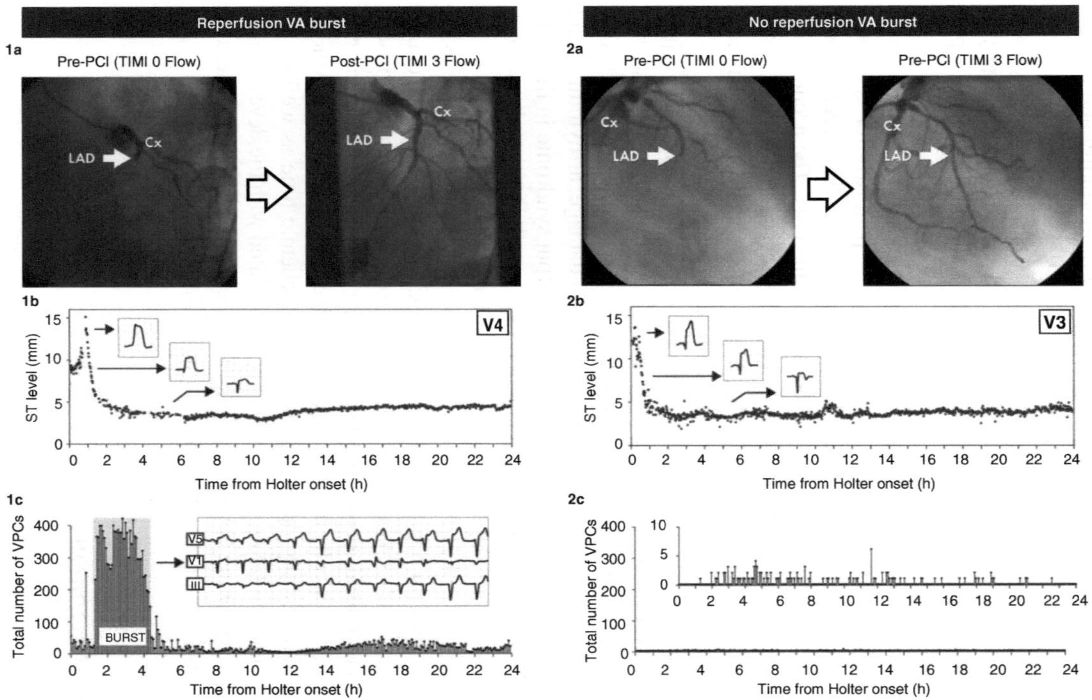

Fig. 10.1 Concomitantly acquired coronary angiography assessments of pre- and post-primary percutaneous coronary intervention TIMI flow grades in two study subjects (1**a**, 2**a**) with a total occlusion in the proximal left anterior descending artery (*LAD*), continuous digital 12-lead electrocardiography monitoring for ST segment recovery analysis with both subjects having ≥50% stable ST segment recovery (1**b**, 2**b**), and complete beat to beat Holter monitoring for quantitative rhythm analysis, identifying (1**c**) or not identifying (2**c**) patient-specific ventricular arrhythmia "bursts" by using independent statistical outlier detection methodology. *Cx* circumflex artery, *LMA* left marginal artery (From Majidi et al. [98], with permission from Oxford University Press)

Myocardial Reperfusion Injury in Cardiac Surgery

Manifestations

Ischemia-reperfusion injury remains an important source of morbidity and mortality following coronary artery bypass grafting (CABG) [73]. CABG involves a surgeon-induced temporary occlusion of coronary flow which is followed by a greater than preoperative restoration of blood flow. As such, CABG and cardiac surgery in general represents a unique model for understanding the pathophysiology of reperfusion injury.

The complex mechanisms underlying reperfusion injury following CABG remain to some degree uncertain. Among the described pathogenic pathways for ischemia-reperfusion injury is cellular apoptosis induced by the excess free radicals accumulated through anaerobic metabolism during the period of ischemia [74]. The accumulated free radicals activate apoptosis, potentially manifesting as myocardial dysfunction if enough cardiac myocytes are affected. The other leading mechanistic hypothesis centers around intracellular Ca^{2+} overload during ischemia and reperfusion [75].

The particular form of myocardial necrosis which may occur in reperfusion injury is known as contraction band necrosis, and this has been found to be present in 30–90% of CABG patients suffering early mortality [76, 77]. Clinically, reperfusion injury following CABG manifests as vascular endothelial damage, arrhythmias, and myocardial stunning, which may result in low cardiac output syndrome in the early postoperative period [78]. Myocardial stunning may last for only a few hours postoperatively or persist for several days despite the restoration of normal blood flow.

The clinical importance of ischemia-reperfusion injury continues to grow as an older, more comorbid patient population is undergoing CABG in the modern era. In these patients, the risk and consequences of adverse sequelae attributable to ischemia-reperfusion is increased. Few clinical studies exist with regard to clinical risk factors for developing a clinically important postoperative reperfusion injury. Among the limited data available, long operative myocardial ischemic time as well as the performance of coronary endarterectomy have been associated with the development of reperfusion injury following CABG [73, 77, 79]. Recent preoperative MI has also been proposed as a risk factor for reperfusion injury following CABG [73].

Prevention and Treatment

Pharmacological Adjuncts

No medical treatment has yet been shown to be effective in reducing the incidence of adverse outcomes attributable to postoperative ischemia-reperfusion injury. Aspirin therapy administered within 48 h of CABG has been shown to reduce the incidence of postoperative death and cardiovascular and cerebrovascular ischemic events [80]. Angiotensin converting enzyme inhibitors, beta blockers, and cholesterol-lowering medications are currently recommended as secondary prevention measures for most patients following CABG [81]; however, none have been proposed as modifying the pathogenesis of ischemia-reperfusion injury. Moreover, while nitrates, beta blockers, and calcium channel blockers are commonly used by anesthesiologists perioperatively, no pharmacologic intervention has been shown effective in reducing the incidence of perioperative myocardial infarction or death.

Experimental preclinical evidence suggests that administration of the nucleoside adenosine may reduce the rate of ATP depletion during ischemia, attenuate myocardial stunning, and enhance myocardial energetics following ischemia-reperfusion injury [82]. Adenosine receptor agonists represent a class of agents proposed to augment local endogenous adenosine levels during periods of ischemia [83]. Acadesine is one adenosine receptor agonist presently under study in a phase 3 multinational randomized controlled study. The trial, termed RED-CABG (Reduction in Cardiovascular Events by AcaDesine in Subjects Undergoing CABG) will evaluate the potential clinical benefit of this therapy in patients undergoing elective CABG [84].

Another class of agents believed to have promise in reducing reperfusion injury following CABG is the sodium-hydrogen exchangers (NHEs). These are a family of membrane proteins functioning in the transport of hydrogen ions in exchange for sodium ions [85]. The EXPEDITION trial (Na^+/H^+ Exchange Inhibition to Prevent Coronary Events in Acute Cardiac Conditions) was conducted to address the efficacy and safety of NHE inhibition by cariporide in the prevention of death or MI in patients undergoing CABG. Results indicated protection against cardiac events following CABG but an overall increase in mortality primarily due to a stroke [86]. Investigators have concluded that NHEs continue to hold promise as a class of agents that could reduce myocardial injury associated with ischemia-reperfusion injury significantly.

There is robust laboratory evidence for an important role of the signaling molecule nitric oxide (NO) in determining myocardial tolerance to ischemia. However, reports are conflicting, and NO has been reported to both exacerbate reperfusion injury as well as exert a cardioprotective effect [87, 88]. These conflicting data remain to be reconciled, and further studies are required to determine the role NO may play in protecting the heart following ischemia-reperfusion.

Cardioplegic Techniques

A variety of cardioplegic techniques have been proposed through the years, and many have been reported to confer superior myocardial protection and/or improve patient outcomes following CABG. However, no single technique has demonstrated clear superiority in protecting against reperfusion injury. Thus, a variety of solutions, temperatures, and methods for administering the solutions are presently in use around the world.

The optimal delivery method of a cardioplegic solution is an ongoing point of discussion [89]. Cardioplegia delivery methods (Table 10.3) include intermittent or

Table 10.3 Options for delivery of cardioplegic solutions

Infusion types	Infusion temperatures	Infusion intervals
Antegrade	Tepid	Continuous
Retrograde	Warm	Intermittent
Combined	Cold	

continuous antegrade via the coronary ostia or the aortocoronary graft, continuous or intermittent retrograde via the coronary sinus, antegrade followed by retrograde, and simultaneous antegrade and retrograde infusions. While continuous techniques have the theoretical advantage of improved perfusion and reduced ischemia, intermittent techniques allow for a drier operative field. Retrograde techniques have the theoretical advantage of a more homogeneous distribution of the cardioplegic solution to poorly collateralized regions of the heart.

The introduction of cold cardioplegic techniques has been reported to result in a decrease in the rate of contraction band necrosis, the pattern observed in reperfusion injury among CABG patients suffering early mortality [77]. Cold crystalloid techniques began in the 1980s in many centers before becoming widely adopted. Continuous warm cardioplegia was subsequently developed with hopes of preventing deleterious effects of hypothermic ischemia [90]. However, warm or normothermic cardioplegia has not been shown to reduce myocardial cell damage compared to cold crystalloid cardioplegia [91]. The use of blood instead of crystalloid centers on the theoretical advantage of providing some degree of reoxygenation of the myocardium intraoperatively [80]. Blood also has excellent osmotic and buffering properties and contains antioxidants and free-radical scavengers. In clinical studies, cold blood cardioplegia has been shown to provide excellent myocardial protection. However, crystalloid cardioplegia has been shown to also provide good results and at a lower cost with a more clear operative field.

The bretschneider HTK (histidine-tryptophan-ketoglutarate) solution is used most commonly for organ preservation for transplantation but has recently gained traction as a cardioplegic agent that allows single-dose administration [92]. The single-dose property is of particular interest with minimally invasive operative techniques for valvular, coronary, and aortic disease. Single-dose HTK cardioplegia has yet to be rigorously tested against repeated-dose blood cardioplegia, although an initial study has not shown improved outcomes [93].

The myocardial protection technique used most frequently in current practice throughout the world is cold blood cardioplegia. Cold blood solutions are typically prepared by combining autologous blood from the cardiopulmonary bypass circuit with a crystalloid solution. The ratio of blood to crystalloid is variable depending on the center and surgeon preference, with the most common ratios being 8:1, 4:1, and 2:1. The crystalloid solution consists of a combination of citrate-phosphate-dextrose, tris-hydroxymethyl-aminomethane, or bicarbonate as a buffer, and potassium chloride. The citrate-phosphate-dextrose is used to lower the ionic calcium, a potentially critical mechanistic component of reperfusion injury. The buffer agent is added to maintain an alkaline pH of approximately 7.8, and potassium is used to arrest the heart. The temperature of the solution is typically lowered to between 12°C and 4°C.

Ischemic Preconditioning and Other Techniques

While hypothermia and cardioplegic infusions remain the cornerstone of myocardial protection during on-pump heart surgery, other cardioprotective techniques are available, including intermittent cross-clamping techniques [94]. Ischemic preconditioning represents a process in which adaptation by the myocardium to brief transient ischemia may induce tolerance against a subsequent ischemic insult such as that encountered during CABG. Suggested mechanisms for this phenomenon include the stimulation of adenosine receptors by adenosine released during ischemia, enhanced expression of heat shock proteins, and involvement of protein kinase C and ATP-dependent potassium channels [95]. An active area of investigation, termed pharmacologic preconditioning, centers on development of pharmacologic stimulation of the proposed ischemic preconditioning mechanistic pathways.

CABG may also be performed without arresting the heart for cardiopulmonary bypass, using off-pump CABG (OPCAB) techniques. During OPCAB, blood circulation is disrupted in each bypassed area only during the time in which the distal anastomosis is performed. As such, OPCAB has been proposed as a technique for reducing the impact of ischemia-reperfusion injury following operative revascularization [96]. At present, there exists limited pathological data regarding the extent to which the myocardium is reversibly damaged after OPCAB, and the role and indications for this technique are still being determined.

Intermittent aortic cross-clamping with fibrillation and moderate hypothermic perfusion (30–32°C) is infrequently in use today but is another non-cardioplegic technique worth mentioning. With this approach, ascending aortic cannulation is achieved, and CABG is performed without arresting the heart. Instead, the heart is in ventricular fibrillation during the distal anastomoses. After completion of the distal anastomoses, the heart is defibrillated, and any proximal aortic-based anastomoses are performed on the beating heart using a partial aortic occlusion clamp [97].

Conclusions

CABG represents a unique model for understanding the pathophysiology, prevention, and treatment of ischemia-reperfusion injury. Several promising pharmacologic adjuncts are underdevelopment and investigation. The administration of cardioplegic solutions for myocardial protection remains the mainstay for prevention of reperfusion injury during arrest for cardiopulmonary bypass; however, the ideal solution, technique, and delivery method remain to be determined.

References

1. Henriques JP, Zijlstra F, Ottervanger JP, de Boer MJ, van't Hof AW, Hoorntje JC, Suryapranata H. Incidence and clinical significance of distal embolization during primary angioplasty for acute myocardial infarction. Eur Heart J. 2002;23:1112–7.
2. Henriques JPS, Zijlstra F. Frequency and sequelae of ST elevation acute myocardial infarction caused by spontaneous distal embolization from unstable coronary lesions. Am J Cardiol. 2003;91:708–11.
3. Mauri L, Cox D, Hermiller J, Massaro J, Wahr J, Tay SW, Jonas M, Popma JJ, Pavliska J, Wahr D, Rogers C. The proximal trial: proximal protection during saphenous vein graft intervention using the proxis embolic protection system: a randomized, prospective, multicenter clinical trial. J Am Coll Cardiol. 2007;50:1442–9.
4. Stone GW, Rogers C, Hermiller J, Feldman R, Hall P, Haber R, Masud A, Cambier P, Caputo RP, Turco M, Kovach R, Brodie B, Herrmann HC, Kuntz RE, Popma JJ, Ramee S, Cox DA. Randomized comparison of distal protection with a filter-based catheter and a balloon occlusion and aspiration system during percutaneous intervention of diseased saphenous vein aorto-coronary bypass Grafts. Circulation. 2003;108:548–53.
5. Matsuo A, Inoue N, Suzuki K, Nakamura R, Fujita H, Miki S, Yokoi Y. Limitations of using a guardwire temporary occlusion and aspiration system in patients with acute myocardial infarction: multicenter investigation of coronary artery protection with a distal occlusion device in acute myocardial infarction (MICADO). J Invasive Cardiol. 2007;19:132–8.
6. Muramatsu T, Kozuma K, Tsukahara R, Ito Y, Fujita N, Suwa S, Koyama S, Saitoh M, Kamiya H, Nakamura M. Comparison of myocardial perfusion by distal protection before and after primary stenting for acute myocardial infarction: angiographic and clinical results of a randomized controlled trial. Catheter Cardiovasc Interv. 2007;70:677–82.
7. Stone GW, Webb J, Cox DA, Brodie BR, Qureshi M, Kalynych A, Turco M, Schultheiss HP, Dulas D, Rutherford BD, Antoniucci D, Krucoff MW, Gibbons RJ, Jones D, Lansky AJ, Mehran R. Distal microcirculatory protection during percutaneous coronary intervention in acute ST-segment elevation myocardial infarction: a randomized controlled trial. JAMA. 2005;293:1063–72.
8. Tahk SJ, Choi BJ, Choi SY, Yoon MH, Gwon HC, Hong GR, Kim YJ, Hur SH, Kim KB, Koo BK, Lee SH, Yoon J. Distal protection device protects microvascular integrity during primary percutaneous intervention in acute myocardial infarction: a prospective, randomized, multicenter trial. Int J Cardiol. 2008;123(2):162–8. Epub 2007 May 8.
9. Gick M, Jander N, Bestehorn HP, Kienzle RP, Ferenc M, Werner K, Comberg T, Peitz K, Zohlnhofer D, Bassignana V, Buettner HJ, Neumann FJ. Randomized evaluation of the effects of filter-based distal protection on myocardial perfusion and infarct size after primary percutaneous catheter intervention in myocardial infarction with and without ST-segment elevation. Circulation. 2005;112:1462–9.
10. Kelbaek H, Terkelsen CJ, Helqvist S, Lassen JF, Clemmensen P, Klovgaard L, Kaltoft A, Engstrom T, Botker HE, Saunamaki K, Krusell LR, Jorgensen E, Hansen HH, Christiansen EH, Ravkilde J, Kober L, Kofoed KF, Thuesen L. Randomized comparison of distal protection versus conventional treatment in primary percutaneous coronary intervention: the drug elution and distal protection in ST-elevation myocardial infarction (DEDICATION) trial. J Am Coll Cardiol. 2008;51:899–905.
11. Cura FA, Escudero AG, Berrocal D, Mendiz O, Trivi MS, Fernandez J, Palacios A, Albertal M, Piraino R, Riccitelli MA, Gruberg L, Ballarino M, Milei J, Baeza R, Thierer J, Grinfeld L, Krucoff M, O'Neill W, Belardi J. Protection of distal embolization in high-risk patients with acute ST-segment elevation myocardial infarction (PREMIAR). Am J Cardiol. 2007;99: 357–63.
12. Haeck JDE, Koch KT, Bilodeau L, Van der Schaaf RJ, Henriques JPS, Vis MM, Baan Jr J, Van der Wal AC, Piek JJ, Tijssen JGP, Krucoff MW, De Winter RJ. Randomized comparison of primary percutaneous coronary intervention with combined proximal embolic protection and

thrombus aspiration versus primary percutaneous coronary intervention alone in ST-segment elevation myocardial infarction: the (PRoximal Embolic Protection in Acute myocardial infarction and Resolution of ST-Elevation) study. JACC Cardiovasc Interv. 2009;2:934–43.
13. Haeck JD, Kuijt WJ, Koch KT, Bilodeau L, Henriques JP, Rohling WJ, Baan J, Vis MM, Nijveldt R, van Geloven N, Groenink M, Piek JJ, Tijssen JG, Krucoff MW, De Winter RJ. Infarct size and left ventricular function in the PRoximal Embolic Protection in Acute myocardial infarction and Resolution of ST-segment Elevation (PREPARE) trial: ancillary cardiovascular magnetic resonance study. Heart. 2010;96:190–5.
14. Burzotta F, Testa L, Giannico F, Biondi-Zoccai GGL, Trani C, Romagnoli E, Mazzari M, Mongiardo R, Siviglia M, Niccoli G, De Vita M, Porto I, Schiavoni G, Crea F. Adjunctive devices in primary or rescue PCI: a meta-analysis of randomized trials. Int J Cardiol. 2008;123:313–21.
15. Beran G, Lang I, Schreiber W, Denk S, Stefenelli T, Syeda B, Maurer G, Glogar D, Siostrzonek P. Intracoronary thrombectomy with the X-sizer catheter system improves epicardial flow and accelerates ST-segment resolution in patients with acute coronary syndrome: a prospective, randomized, controlled study. Circulation. 2002;105:2355–60.
16. Lefevre T, Garcia E, Reimers B, Lang I, Di MC, Colombo A, Neumann FJ, Chavarri MV, Brunel P, Grube E, Thomas M, Glatt B, Ludwig J. X-sizer for thrombectomy in acute myocardial infarction improves ST-segment resolution: results of the X-sizer in AMI for negligible embolization and optimal ST resolution (X AMINE ST) trial. J Am Coll Cardiol. 2005;46:246–52.
17. Napodano M, Pasquetto G, Sacca S, Cernetti C, Scarabeo V, Pascotto P, Reimers B. Intracoronary thrombectomy improves myocardial reperfusion in patients undergoing direct angioplasty for acute myocardial infarction. J Am Coll Cardiol. 2003;42:1395–402.
18. Antoniucci D, Valenti R, Migliorini A, Parodi G, Memisha G, Santoro GM, Sciagra R. Comparison of rheolytic thrombectomy before direct infarct artery stenting versus direct stenting alone in patients undergoing percutaneous coronary intervention for acute myocardial infarction. Am J Cardiol. 2004;93:1033–5.
19. Ali A, Cox D, Dib N, Brodie B, Berman D, Gupta N, Browne K, Iwaoka R, Azrin M, Stapleton D, Setum C, Popma J. Rheolytic thrombectomy with percutaneous coronary intervention for infarct size reduction in acute myocardial infarction: 30-day results from a multicenter randomized study. J Am Coll Cardiol. 2006;48:244–52.
20. Chevalier B, Gilard M, Lang I, Commeau P, Roosen J, Hanssen M, Lefevre T, Carrie D, Bartorelli A, Montalescot G, Parikh K. Systematic primary aspiration in acute myocardial percutaneous intervention: a multicentre randomised controlled trial of the export aspiration catheter. EuroIntervention. 2008;4:222–8.
21. Sardella G, Mancone M, Bucciarelli-Ducci C, Agati L, Scardala R, Carbone I, Francone M, Di RA, Benedetti G, Conti G, Fedele F. Thrombus aspiration during primary percutaneous coronary intervention improves myocardial reperfusion and reduces infarct size: the EXPIRA (thrombectomy with export catheter in infarct-related artery during primary percutaneous coronary intervention) prospective, randomized trial. J Am Coll Cardiol. 2009;53:309–15.
22. Svilaas T, Vlaar PJ, van der Horst I, Diercks GF, de Smet BJ, van den Heuvel AF, Anthonio RL, Jessurun GA, Tan ES, Suurmeijer AJ, Zijlstra F. Thrombus aspiration during primary percutaneous coronary intervention. N Engl J Med. 2008;358:557–67.
23. Burzotta F, Trani C, Romagnoli E, Mazzari MA, Rebuzzi AG, De VM, Garramone B, Giannico F, Niccoli G, Biondi-Zoccai GG, Schiavoni G, Mongiardo R, Crea F. Manual thrombus-aspiration improves myocardial reperfusion: the randomized evaluation of the effect of mechanical reduction of distal embolization by thrombus-aspiration in primary and rescue angioplasty (REMEDIA) trial. J Am Coll Cardiol. 2005;46:371–6.
24. De Luca L, Sardella G, Davidson CJ, De Persio PG, Beraldi M, Tommasone T, Mancone M, Nguyen BL, Agati L, Gheorghiade M, Fedele F. Impact of intracoronary aspiration thrombectomy during primary angioplasty on left ventricular remodelling in patients with anterior ST elevation myocardial infarction. Heart. 2006;92:951–7.
25. Dudek D, Mielecki W, Legutko J, Chyrchel M, Sorysz D, Bartus S, Rzeszutko L, Dubiel JS. Percutaneous thrombectomy with the rescue system in acute myocardial infarction. Kardiol Pol. 2004;61:523–33.

26. Kaltoft A, Bottcher M, Nielsen SS, Hansen HH, Terkelsen C, Maeng M, Kristensen J, Thuesen L, Krusell LR, Kristensen SD, Andersen HR, Lassen JF, Rasmussen K, Rehling M, Nielsen TT, Botker HE. Routine thrombectomy in percutaneous coronary intervention for acute ST-segment-elevation myocardial infarction: a randomized, controlled trial. Circulation. 2006; 114:40–7.
27. Ikari Y, Sakurada M, Kozuma K, Kawano S, Katsuki T, Kimura K, Suzuki T, Yamashita T, Takizawa A, Misumi K, Hashimoto H, Isshiki T. Upfront thrombus aspiration in primary coronary intervention for patients with ST-segment elevation acute myocardial infarction: report of the VAMPIRE (VAcuuM asPIration thrombus REmoval) trial. JACC Cardiovasc Interv. 2008;1:424–31.
28. Silva-Orrego P, Colombo P, Bigi R, Gregori D, Delgado A, Salvade P, Oreglia J, Orrico P, de Biase A, Piccalo G, Bossi I, Klugmann S. Thrombus aspiration before primary angioplasty improves myocardial reperfusion in acute myocardial infarction: the DEAR-MI (Dethrombosis to Enhance Acute Reperfusion in Myocardial Infarction) study. J Am Coll Cardiol. 2006;48:1552–9.
29. Vlaar PJ, Svilaas T, van der Horst IC, Diercks GFH, Fokkema ML, de Smet BJGL, van den Heuvel AFM, Anthonio RL, Jessurun GA, Tan E-S, Suurmeijer AJH, Zijlstra F. Cardiac death and reinfarction after 1 year in the Thrombus Aspiration during Percutaneous coronary intervention in Acute myocardial infarction Study (TAPAS): a 1-year follow-up study. Lancet. 2008;371:1915–20.
30. Burzotta F, De Vita M, Gu YL, Isshiki T, Lefèvre T, Kaltoft A, Dudek D, Sardella G, Orrego PS, Antoniucci D, De Luca L, Biondi-Zoccai GGL, Crea F, Zijlstra F. Clinical impact of thrombectomy in acute ST-elevation myocardial infarction: an individual patient-data pooled analysis of 11 trials. Eur Heart J. 2009;30:2193–203.
31. Migliorini A, Stabile A, Rodriguez AE, Gandolfo C, Rodriguez Granillo AM, Valenti R, Parodi G, Neumann F-J, Colombo A, Antoniucci D. Comparison of AngioJet rheolytic thrombectomy before direct infarct artery stenting with direct stenting alone in patients with acute myocardial infarction: the JETSTENT trial. J Am Coll Cardiol. 2010;56:1298–306.
32. Napodano M, Ramondo A, Tarantini G, Peluso D, Compagno S, Fraccaro C, Frigo AC, Razzolini R, Iliceto S. Predictors and time-related impact of distal embolization during primary angioplasty. Eur Heart J. 2009;30:305–13.
33. Roe MT, Ohman EM, Maas ACP, Christenson RH, Mahaffey KW, Granger CB, Harrington RA, Califf RM, Krucoff MW. Shifting the open-artery hypothesis downstream: the quest for optimal reperfusion. J Am Coll Cardiol. 2001;37:9–18.
34. Taniyama Y, Ito H, Iwakura K, Masuyama T, Hori M, Takiuchi S, Nishikawa N, Higashino Y, Fujii K, Minamino T. Beneficial effect of intracoronary verapamil on microvascular and myocardial salvage in patients with acute myocardial infarction. J Am Coll Cardiol. 1997;30:1193–9.
35. Vijayalakshmi K, Whittaker VJ, Kunadian B, Graham J, Wright RA, Hall JA, Sutton A, de Belder MA. Prospective, randomised, controlled trial to study the effect of intracoronary injection of verapamil and adenosine on coronary blood flow during percutaneous coronary intervention in patients with acute coronary syndromes. Heart. 2006;92:1278–84.
36. Fugit MD, Rubal BJ, Donovan DJ. Effects of intracoronary nicardipine, diltiazem and verapamil on coronary blood flow. J Invasive Cardiol. 2000;12:80–5.
37. Ross AM, Gibbons RJ, Stone GW, Kloner RA, Alexander RW. A randomized, double-blinded, placebo-controlled multicenter trial of adenosine as an adjunct to reperfusion in the treatment of acute myocardial infarction (AMISTAD-II). J Am Coll Cardiol. 2005;45:1775–80.
38. Kloner RA, Forman MB, Gibbons RJ, Ross AM, Alexander RW, Stone GW. Impact of time to therapy and reperfusion modality on the efficacy of adenosine in acute myocardial infarction: the AMISTAD-2 trial. Eur Heart J. 2006;27:2400–5.
39. Amit G, Cafri C, Yaroslavtsev S, Fuchs S, Paltiel O, Abu-Ful A, Weinstein JM, Wolak A, Ilia R, Zahger D. Intracoronary nitroprusside for the prevention of the no-reflow phenomenon after primary percutaneous coronary intervention in acute myocardial infarction. A randomized, double-blind, placebo-controlled clinical trial. Am Heart J. 2006;152:887.e9–14.

40. Ishii H, Ichimiya S, Kanashiro M, Amano T, Imai K, Murohara T, Matsubara T. Impact of a single intravenous administration of nicorandil before reperfusion in patients with ST-segment-elevation myocardial infarction. Circulation. 2005;112:1284–8.
41. Kitakaze M, Asakura M, Kim J, Shintani Y, Asanuma H, Hamasaki T, Seguchi O, Myoishi M, Minamino T, Ohara T, Nagai Y, Nanto S, Watanabe K, Fukuzawa S, Hirayama A, Nakamura N, Kimura K, Fujii K, Ishihara M, Saito Y, Tomoike H, Kitamura S. Human atrial natriuretic peptide and nicorandil as adjuncts to reperfusion treatment for acute myocardial infarction (J-WIND): two randomised trials. Lancet. 2007;370:1483–93.
42. Kandzari DE, Hasselblad V, Tcheng JE, Stone GW, Califf RM, Kastrati A, Neumann F-J, Brener SJ, Montalescot G, Kong DF, Harrington RA. Improved clinical outcomes with abciximab therapy in acute myocardial infarction: a systematic overview of randomized clinical trials. Am Heart J. 2004;147:457–62.
43. Maioli M, Bellandi F, Leoncini M, Toso A, Dabizzi RP. Randomized early versus late abciximab in acute myocardial infarction treated with primary coronary intervention (RELAx-AMI trial). J Am Coll Cardiol. 2007;49:1517–24.
44. Montalescot G, Barragan P, Wittenberg O, Ecollan P, Elhadad S, Villain P, Boulenc J-M, Morice M-C, Maillard L, Pansiéri M, Choussat R, Pinton P. Platelet glycoprotein IIb/IIIa inhibition with coronary stenting for acute myocardial infarction. N Engl J Med. 2001;344: 1895–903.
45. Neumann F-J, Blasini R, Schmitt C, Alt E, Dirschinger J, Gawaz M, Kastrati A, Schomig A. Effect of glycoprotein IIb/IIIa receptor blockade on recovery of coronary flow and left ventricular function after the placement of coronary-artery stents in acute myocardial infarction. Circulation. 1998;98:2695–701.
46. Stone GW, Grines CL, Cox DA, Garcia E, Tcheng JE, Griffin JJ, Guagliumi G, Stuckey T, Turco M, Carroll JD, Rutherford BD, Lansky AJ. Comparison of angioplasty with stenting, with or without abciximab, in acute myocardial infarction. N Engl J Med. 2002;346:957–66.
47. Stone GW, Witzenbichler B, Guagliumi G, Peruga JZ, Brodie BR, Dudek D, Kornowski R, Hartmann F, Gersh BJ, Pocock SJ, Dangas G, Wong SC, Kirtane AJ, Parise H, Mehran R. Bivalirudin during primary PCI in acute myocardial infarction. N Engl J Med. 2008; 358:2218–30.
48. Mehilli J, Kastrati A, Schulz S, Frungel S, Nekolla SG, Moshage W, Dotzer F, Huber K, Pache J, Dirschinger J, Seyfarth M, Martinoff S, Schwaiger M, Schomig A, for the Bavarian Reperfusion Alternatives Evaluation-3 Study I. Abciximab in patients with acute ST-segment-elevation myocardial infarction undergoing primary percutaneous coronary intervention after clopidogrel loading: a randomized double-blind trial. Circulation. 2009;119:1933–40.
49. van't Hof AWJ, ten Berg J, Heestermans T, Dill T, Funck RC, van Werkum W, Dambrink J-HE, Suryapranata H, van Houwelingen G, Ottervanger JP, Stella P, Giannitsis E, Hamm C. Prehospital initiation of tirofiban in patients with ST-elevation myocardial infarction undergoing primary angioplasty (On-TIME 2): a multicentre, double-blind, randomised controlled trial. Lancet. 2008;372:537–46.
50. ten Berg JM, van't Hof AWJ, Dill T, Heestermans T, van Werkum JW, Mosterd A, van Houwelingen G, Koopmans PC, Stella PR, Boersma E, Hamm C. Effect of early, pre-hospital initiation of high bolus dose tirofiban in patients with ST-segment elevation myocardial infarction on short- and long-term clinical outcome. J Am Coll Cardiol. 2010;55:2446–55.
51. Thiele H, Schindler K, Friedenberger J, Eitel I, Furnau G, Grebe E, Erbs S, Linke A, Mobius-Winkler S, Kivelitz D, Schuler G. Intracoronary compared with intravenous bolus abciximab application in patients with ST-elevation myocardial infarction undergoing primary percutaneous coronary intervention: the randomized Leipzig immediate percutaneous coronary intervention abciximab IV versus IC in ST-elevation myocardial infarction trial. Circulation. 2008;118:49–57.
52. Assessment of the Safety and Efficacy of a New Treatment Strategy with Percutaneous Coronary Intervention (ASSENT-4 PCI) investigators. Primary versus tenecteplase-facilitated percutaneous coronary intervention in patients with ST-segment elevation acute myocardial infarction (ASSENT-4 PCI): randomised trial. Lancet. 2006;367:569–78.

53. Ellis SG, Tendera M, de Belder MA, van Boven AJ, Widimsky P, Janssens L, Andersen HR, Betriu A, Savonitto S, Adamus J, Peruga JZ, Kosmider M, Katz O, Neunteufl T, Jorgova J, Dorobantu M, Grinfeld L, Armstrong P, Brodie BR, Herrmann HC, Montalescot G, Neumann F-J, Effron MB, Barnathan ES, Topol EJ. Facilitated PCI in patients with ST-elevation myocardial infarction. N Engl J Med. 2008;358:2205–17.
54. Sezer M, Çimen A, Aslanger E, Elitok A, Umman B, Bugra Z, Yormaz E, Türkmen C, Adalet I, Nisanci Y, Umman S. Effect of intracoronary streptokinase administered immediately after primary percutaneous coronary intervention on long-term left ventricular infarct size, volumes, and function. J Am Coll Cardiol. 2009;54:1065–71.
55. Gu YL, Kampinga MA, Wieringa WG, Fokkema ML, Nijsten MW, Hillege HL, van den Heuvel AFM, Tan E-S, Pundziute G, van der Werf R, Hoseyni Guyomi S, van der Horst ICC, Zijlstra F, de Smet BJGL. Intracoronary versus intravenous administration of abciximab in patients with ST-segment elevation myocardial infarction undergoing primary percutaneous coronary intervention with thrombus aspiration: the comparison of intracoronary versus intravenous abciximab administration during emergency reperfusion of ST-segment elevation myocardial infarction (CICERO) trial. Circulation. 2010;122:2709–17.
56. Sezer M, Oflaz H, Gören T, Okçular İ, Umman B, Nişanci Y, Bilge AK, Şanli Y, Meriç M, Umman S. Intracoronary streptokinase after primary percutaneous coronary intervention. N Engl J Med. 2007;356:1823–34.
57. Marzilli M, Orsini E, Marraccini P, Testa R. Beneficial effects of intracoronary adenosine as an adjunct to primary angioplasty in acute myocardial infarction. Circulation. 2000;101:2154–9.
58. Micari A, Belcik TA, Balcells EA, Powers E, Wei K, Kaul S, Lindner JR. Improvement in microvascular reflow and reduction of infarct size with adenosine in patients undergoing primary coronary stenting. Am J Cardiol. 2005;96:1410–5.
59. Mehta RH, Starr AZ, Lopes RD, Hochman JS, Widimsky P, Pieper KS, Armstrong PW, Granger CB, for the AAMII. Incidence of and outcomes associated with ventricular tachycardia or fibrillation in patients undergoing primary percutaneous coronary intervention. JAMA. 2009;301:1779–89.
60. Al-Khatib SM, Stebbins AL, Califf RM, Lee KL, Granger CB, White HD, Armstrong PW, Topol EJ, Ohman EM. Sustained ventricular arrhythmias and mortality among patients with acute myocardial infarction: results from the GUSTO-III trial. Am Heart J. 2003;145:515–21.
61. Dorian P, Cass D, Schwartz B, Cooper R, Gelaznikas R, Barr A. Amiodarone as compared with lidocaine for shock-resistant ventricular fibrillation. N Engl J Med. 2002;346:884–90.
62. Zygmunt PS, John HA, Bogdan S, Andrzej D, Jerzy K, Edmund N, Grazyna S, David FK, Christopher BG. Multicenter randomized trial and a systematic overview of lidocaine in acute myocardial infarction. Am Heart J. 1999;137:792–8.
63. Echt DS, Liebson PR, Mitchell LB, Peters RW, Obias-Manno D, Barker AH, Arensberg D, Baker A, Friedman L, Greene HL, Huther ML, Richardson DW. Mortality and morbidity in patients receiving encainide, flecainide, or placebo. N Engl J Med. 1991;324:781–8.
64. Hine LK, Laird N, Hewitt P, Chalmers TC. Meta-analytic evidence against prophylactic use of lidocaine in acute myocardial infarction. Arch Intern Med. 1989;149:2694–8.
65. Piccini JP, Berger JS, O'Connor CM. Amiodarone for the prevention of sudden cardiac death: a meta-analysis of randomized controlled trials. Eur Heart J. 2009;30:1245–53.
66. Zipes DP, Camm AJ, Borggrefe M, Buxton AE, Chaitman B, Fromer M, Gregoratos G, Klein G, Moss AJ, Myerburg RJ, Priori SG, Quinones MA, Roden DM, Silka MJ, Tracy C, Smith Jr SC, Jacobs AK, Adams CD, Antman EM, Anderson JL, Hunt SA, Halperin JL, Nishimura R, Ornato JP, Page RL, Riegel B, Blanc J-J, Budaj A, Dean V, Deckers JW, Despres C, Dickstein K, Lekakis J, McGregor K, Metra M, Morais J, Osterspey A, Tamargo JL, Zamorano JL. ACC/AHA/ESC 2006 guidelines for management of patients with ventricular arrhythmias and the prevention of sudden cardiac death: a report of the American College of Cardiology/American Heart Association Task Force and the European Society of Cardiology Committee for Practice Guidelines (Writing Committee to develop guidelines for management of patients with ventricular arrhythmias and the prevention of sudden cardiac death). J Am Coll Cardiol. 2006;48:e247–346.

67. Piccini JP, Schulte PJ, Pieper KS, Mehta RH, White HD, Van de Werf F, Ardissino D, Califf RM, Granger CB, Ohman EM, Alexander JH. Antiarrhythmic drug therapy for sustained ventricular arrhythmias complicating acute myocardial infarction. Crit Care Med. 2011;39(1): 78–83. doi:10.1097/CCM.1090b1013e3181fd1096ad1097.
68. Boutitie F, Boissel J-P, Connolly SJ, Camm AJ, Cairns JA, Julian DG, Gent M, Janse MJ, Dorian P, Frangin G. Amiodarone interaction with ß-blockers: analysis of the merged EMIAT (European Myocardial Infarct Amiodarone Trial) and CAMIAT (Canadian Amiodarone Myocardial Infarction Trial) databases. Circulation. 1999;99:2268–75.
69. Goldberg S, Greenspon AJ, Urban PL, Muza B, Berger B, Walinsky P, Maroko PR. Reperfusion arrhythmia: a marker of restoration of antegrade flow during intracoronary thrombolysis for acute myocardial infarction. Am Heart J. 1983;105:26–32.
70. Gorgels APM, Vos MA, Letsch IS, Verschuuren EA, Bär FWHM, Janssen JHA, Wellens HJJ. Usefulness of the accelerated idioventricular rhythm as a marker for myocardial necrosis and reperfusion during thrombolytic therapy in acute myocardial infarction. Am J Cardiol. 1988;61:231–5.
71. Gressin V, Louvard Y, Pezzano M, Lardoux H. Holter recording of ventricular arrhythmias during intravenous thrombolysis for acute myocardial infarction. Am J Cardiol. 1992;69:152–9.
72. Majidi M, Kosinski AS, Al-Khatib SM, Lemmert ME, Smolders L, van Weert A, Reiber JHC, Tzivoni D, Bär FWHM, Wellens HJJ, Gorgels APM, Krucoff MW. Reperfusion ventricular arrhythmia 'bursts' in TIMI 3 flow restoration with primary angioplasty for anterior ST-elevation myocardial infarction: a more precise definition of reperfusion arrhythmias. Europace. 2008;10:988–97.
73. Weman SM, Karhunen PJ, Penttila A, Jarvinen AA, Salminen US. Reperfusion injury associated with one-fourth of deaths after coronary artery bypass grafting. Ann Thorac Surg. 2000;70:807–12.
74. Bolli R, Marban E. Molecular and cellular mechanisms of myocardial stunning. Physiol Rev. 1999;79:609–34.
75. Piper HM, Garcia-Dorado D. Prime causes of rapid cardiomyocyte death during reperfusion. Ann Thorac Surg. 1999;68:1913–9.
76. Bulkely BH, Hutchins GM. Myocardial consequences of coronary artery bypass graft surgery. The paradox of necrosis in areas of revascularization. Circulation. 1977;56:906–13.
77. Moore GW, Hutchins GM. Coronary artery bypass grafts in 109 autopsied patients. Statistical analysis of graft and anastomosis patency and regional myocardial injury. JAMA. 1981; 246:1785–9.
78. Vaage J, Valen G. Pathophysiology and mediators of ischemia-reperfusion injury with special reference to cardiac surgery. A review. Scand J Thorac Cardiovasc Surg Suppl. 1993;41:1–18.
79. Buckberg GD. A proposed "solution" to the cardioplegic controversy. J Thorac Cardiovasc Surg. 1979;77:803–15.
80. Ferraris VA, Ferraris SP, Moliterno DJ, Camp P, Walenga JM, Messmore HL, Jeske WP, Edwards FH, Royston D, Shahian DM, Peterson E, Bridges CR, Despotis G. The society of thoracic surgeons practice guideline series: aspirin and other antiplatelet agents during operative coronary revascularization (executive summary). Ann Thorac Surg. 2005;79:1454–61.
81. Eagle KA, Guyton RA, Davidoff R, Edwards FH, Ewy GA, Gardner TJ, Hart JC, Herrmann HC, Hillis LD, Hutter Jr AM, Lytle BW, Marlow RA, Nugent WC, Orszulak TA. ACC/AHA 2004 guideline update for coronary artery bypass graft surgery: a report of the American College of Cardiology/American Heart Association Task Force on practice guidelines (Committee to update the 1999 guidelines for coronary artery bypass graft surgery). Circulation. 2004;110:e340–437.
82. Teoh LK, Grant R, Hulf JA, Pugsley WB, Yellon DM. The effect of preconditioning (ischemic and pharmacological) on myocardial necrosis following coronary artery bypass graft surgery. Cardiovasc Res. 2002;53:175–80.
83. Mangano DT. Effects of acadesine on myocardial infarction, stroke, and death following surgery. A meta-analysis of the 5 international randomized trials. The Multicenter Study of Perioperative Ischemia (McSPI) Research Group. JAMA. 1997;277:325–32.

84. Mangano DT, Miao Y, Tudor IC, Dietzel C. Post-reperfusion myocardial infarction: long-term survival improvement using adenosine regulation with acadesine. J Am Coll Cardiol. 2006;48: 206–14.
85. Boyce SW, Bartels C, Bolli R, Chaitman B, Chen JC, Chi E, Jessel A, Kereiakes D, Knight J, Thulin L, Theroux P. Impact of sodium-hydrogen exchange inhibition by cariporide on death or myocardial infarction in high-risk CABG surgery patients: results of the CABG surgery cohort of the GUARDIAN study. J Thorac Cardiovasc Surg. 2003;126:420–7.
86. Mentzer Jr RM, Bartels C, Bolli R, Boyce S, Buckberg GD, Chaitman B, Haverich A, Knight J, Menasche P, Myers ML, Nicolau J, Simoons M, Thulin L, Weisel RD. Sodium-hydrogen exchange inhibition by cariporide to reduce the risk of ischemic cardiac events in patients undergoing coronary artery bypass grafting: results of the expedition study. Ann Thorac Surg. 2008;85:1261–70.
87. Feng Q, Lu X, Jones DL, Shen J, Arnold JM. Increased inducible nitric oxide synthase expression contributes to myocardial dysfunction and higher mortality after myocardial infarction in mice. Circulation. 2001;104:700–4.
88. Belge C, Massion PB, Pelat M, Balligand JL. Nitric oxide and the heart: update on new paradigms. Ann N Y Acad Sci. 2005;1047:173–82.
89. Cohen G, Borger MA, Weisel RD, Rao V. Intraoperative myocardial protection: current trends and future perspectives. Ann Thorac Surg. 1999;68:1995–2001.
90. Ikonomidis JS, Rao V, Weisel RD, Hayashida N, Shirai T. Myocardial protection for coronary bypass grafting: the Toronto Hospital perspective. Ann Thorac Surg. 1995;60:824–32.
91. Jacquet LM, Noirhomme PH, Van Dyck MJ, El Khoury GA, Matta AJ, Goenen MJ, Dion RA. Randomized trial of intermittent antegrade warm blood versus cold crystalloid cardioplegia. Ann Thorac Surg. 1999;67:471–7.
92. Arslan A, Sezgin A, Gultekin B, Ozkan S, Akay T, Uguz E, Tasdelen A, Aslamaci S. Low-dose histidine-tryptophan-ketoglutarate solution for myocardial protection. Transplant Proc. 2005;37:3219–22.
93. Fannelop T, Dahle GO, Salminen PR, Moen CA, Matre K, Mongstad A, Eliassen F, Segadal L, Grong K. Multidose cold oxygenated blood is superior to a single dose of bretschneider HTK-cardioplegia in the pig. Ann Thorac Surg. 2009;87:1205–13.
94. Abd-Elfattah AS, Ding M, Wechsler AS. Intermittent aortic crossclamping prevents cumulative adenosine triphosphate depletion, ventricular fibrillation, and dysfunction (stunning): is it preconditioning? J Thorac Cardiovasc Surg. 1995;110:328–39.
95. Miller MJ. Preconditioning for cardioprotection against ischemia reperfusion injury: the roles of nitric oxide, reactive oxygen species, heat shock proteins, reactive hyperemia and antioxidants – a mini review. Can J Cardiol. 2001;17:1075–82.
96. Menon AK, Albes JM, Oberhoff M, Karsch KR, Ziemer G. Occlusion versus shunting during midcab: effects on left ventricular function and quality of anastomosis. Ann Thorac Surg. 2002;73:1418–23.
97. Casthely PA, Shah C, Mekhjian H, Swistel D, Yoganathan T, Komer C, Miguelino RA, Rosales R. Left ventricular diastolic function after coronary artery bypass grafting: a correlative study with three different myocardial protection techniques. J Thorac Cardiovasc Surg. 1997; 114:254–60.
98. Majidi M, Kosinski AJ, Al-Khatib SM, Lemmert ME, et al. Reperfusion ventricular arrhythmia 'bursts' predict larger infarct size despite TIMI 3 flow restoration with primary angioplasty for anterior ST-elevation myocardial infarction. Eur Heart J. 2009;30(7):759.

Chapter 11
Endogenous Cardioprotective Strategies

Abhiram Prasad and Bernard John Gersh

Abstract The field of cardioprotection to reduce reperfusion injury has been characterized by a plethora of experimental studies with multiple pharmacological agents that have shown great promise in the laboratory, but have lacked clinical efficacy. This has led to diminishing enthusiasm for the translation of cardioprotection into clinical practice. In contrast, the field of endogenous cardiac protection is particularly appealing given that early clinical studies have documented feasibility and efficacy. Strategies for endogenous cardioprotection include ischemic preconditioning, ischemic postconditioning, and remote ischemic conditioning. However, the clinical trials performed to date have been small, used surrogate endpoints, and had strict inclusion and exclusion criteria. Larger trials are needed that will allow assessment of the applicability to a wider patient population with prior infarcts, prior revascularization, reduced ejection fraction, history of congestive heart failure, use of multiple pharmacological agents, and presence of multiple coexisting diseases. Moreover, understanding the mechanisms for the apparent benefit may lead to the development of new drugs and molecules that could target the fundamental processes of ischemia–reperfusion injury.

Keywords Reperfusion Injury • Preconditioning • Postconditioning

A. Prasad, M.D., FRCP, FACC (✉)
Department of Medicine, Division of Cardiovascular Diseases, Mayo Clinic,
200 First Street, Rochester, MN 55905, USA
e-mail: prasad.abhiram@mayo.edu

B.J. Gersh, MBChB, D.Phil., FRCP, Ph.D. (Hon Causa)
Division of Cardiovascular Diseases, Mayo Clinic,
200 First Street SW, Rochester 55905, MN, USA

Department of Medicine, Mayo Clinic College of Medicine,
Rochester, MN, USA
e-mail: gersh.bernard@mayo.edu

J.C. Kaski et al. (eds.), *Management of Myocardial Reperfusion Injury*,
DOI 10.1007/978-1-84996-019-9_11,

Introduction

Activation of endogenous cardioprotective mechanisms against myocardial reperfusion injury using a mechanical stimulus, as opposed to a pharmacological approach, is emerging as an attractive possibility for clinical application. In this chapter, we present the evidence for such strategies, focusing on the concepts of ischemic preconditioning, ischemic postconditioning, and remote ischemic conditioning. The data are derived from studies conducted in animal models of myocardial ischemia–reperfusion injury, observational studies, and clinical trials in patients undergoing cardiovascular surgery or percutaneous coronary intervention (PCI).

Ischemic Preconditioning

Preclinical Studies

Ischemic preconditioning (IPC) was originally described by Murry and colleagues in 1986 [1]. In their landmark experiment, they demonstrated that four cycles of 5 min of sublethal ischemia interrupted by 5 min of reperfusion had protective effects against myocardial necrosis during subsequent prolonged infarct-inducing ischemia. In this canine model, there was a 75% reduction in infarct size. The phenomenon has subsequently been replicated in other animal species, such as rats, rabbits, and pigs, and in multiple organs such as the brain, kidney, skeletal muscle, skin, and the liver [2]. In animal studies, IPC reduces not only infarct size but diminishes reperfusion arrhythmias, cardiomyocyte energy requirements, and endothelial injury, and accelerates myocardial functional recovery [3]. There appear to be two time windows of protection, one that follows immediately after the IPC stimulus and lasts for 3–4 h (early or classical preconditioning) and a second window that occurs approximately 24 h after the IPC stimulus and may last for up to 72 h (delayed or late preconditioning or "second window of protection") [4, 5].

The precise mechanisms involved in IPC are unknown, but they appear to involve multiple triggers, mediators, and end-effectors (Fig. 11.1) [3]. Receptor-dependent triggers, such as endogenous adenosine, bradykinin, and opioids, and nonreceptor-dependent triggers such as nitric oxide and reactive oxygen species have been proposed. The current hypothesis is that these triggers activate mediators such as G protein–coupled receptors, phosphoinositide-3 kinase, Akt, guanylate cyclase, and other protein kinases which promote the opening of ATP-dependent mitochondrial potassium (mKATP) channels that ultimately inhibit the opening of mitochondrial permeability transition pore (mPTP) during reperfusion. The mPTP is a nonspecific pore of the inner mitochondrial membrane which opens in the first few minutes of myocardial reperfusion. Its opening leads to cell death by uncoupling oxidative phosphorylation and inducing mitochondrial swelling [6], and it is postulated that

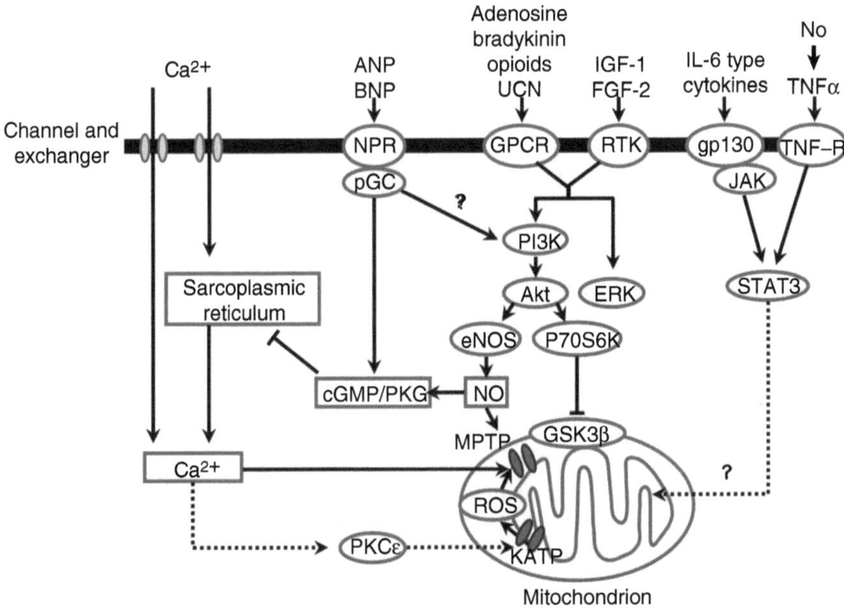

Fig. 11.1 Signaling mechanisms in pre-/postconditioning. Several extracellular factors produced endogenously are known to play an essential role in ischemic postconditioning (adenosine, bradykinin, and opioid peptides). However, other additional autacoids could play a role since their exogenous administration at reperfusion mimics the effect of ischemic postconditioning. These include natriuretic peptides (ANP and BNP), peptide growth factors (IGF-1 and FGF-2), and TNF-a. After binding to cell surface receptors, these autacoids promote the activation of kinase signaling pathways. The precise sequence of elements in these pathways and the extent of interaction between different pathways are unclear. However, evidence from some models implicates the activation of PI3K/Akt and p42/p44 ERKs. This pathway, known as the RISK pathway, is proposed to result in inhibition of mPTP opening at reperfusion, via distal components of the cascade which include NO and inhibition of GSK3β(beta). The extent to which cGMP accumulation and PKG activation contribute to ischemic postconditioning is not clearly defined at present, but several pieces of evidence support the hypothesis that the activation of cGMP/PKG, either by NO or by other factors such as natriuretic peptides, is protective during reperfusion by attenuating Ca^{2+} cycling which may be a stimulus for mPTP opening. Furthermore, it has been proposed that the activation of an intramitochondrial pool of PKC1 might cause opening of the mitochondrial KATP channel (mitoKATP), resulting in a slight increase in reactive oxygen species (ROS) formation which eventually causes MPTP inhibition. An alternative pathway, the so-called SAFE pathway, has been proposed to play a role in ischemic postconditioning. The major components of the SAFE pathway are TNF-a, the kinase JAK which phosphorylates the transcription factor STAT3. It is proposed that after translocation to the nucleus, STAT3 controls the transcription of factors that confer cardioprotection. Also, a mitochondrial localization of STAT3 has been suggested; however, both actions of STAT3 need to be finally proven. *eNOS* endothelial nitric oxide synthase, *GPCR* G protein–coupled receptor, *GSK3β(beta)* glycogen synthase kinase-3β(beta), *MPTP* mitochondrial permeability transition pore, *ERK* p42/p44 extracellular regulated kinase, *NPR* natriuretic peptide receptor, *Pgc* particulate guanylyl cyclase, *PKG* cGMP-dependent protein kinase, *RTK* receptor tyrosine kinase, *SR* sarcoplasmic reticulum, *TNF-R* TNF receptor, ? unclear at present (From Ovize et al. [49]. Reprinted with kind permission from Oxford University Press)

this may be a final common pathway resulting in reperfusion injury following prolonged ischemia. Additional mechanisms that appear to be recruited by IPC during the first few minutes of reperfusion include the activation of the reperfusion injury salvage kinase (RISK) pathway, which are a family of protein kinases (e.g., protein kinase C, Akt, and Erk1/2) that appear to prevent cardiomyocyte calcium overload, inhibit mPTP opening, and recruit antiapoptotic pathways [7].

"Warm-Up" and Preinfarction Angina

Despite the large body of experimental studies, until recently, there has been a paucity of evidence to support the hypothesis that IPC can be induced in humans. However, in vitro studies using human myocardial tissue [8], the occurrence of "warm-up" angina in some patients, and the possible cardioprotective effects of preinfarction angina in subset analyses of clinical studies provide circumstantial evidence for IPC in humans. "Warm-up" angina is the phenomenon in which an initial period of physical exertion in some patients with coronary artery disease leads to a reduction in the severity of anginal symptoms during subsequent activity [9]. The intensity of exercise must be sufficient to induce myocardial ischemia in order to improve the anginal threshold or else the warm-up effect does not seem to occur. The mechanism by which "warm-up" angina reduces subsequent ischemia is not known, but it has been suggested that myocardial metabolic adaptation which resembles IPC may be responsible [10].

Similarly, a history of preinfarction angina appears to be associated with a smaller myocardial infarct size, greater myocardial viability and contractile function, lower incidence of life-threatening ventricular arrhythmias, lower in-hospital, and long-term mortality compared to patients who suffer an acute myocardial infarction without preceding angina [11–15]. This effect may be absent in diabetics [16] and older patients [17], although in the elderly, high level of physical activity may preserve the cardioprotective effect of preinfarction angina [18]. The mechanisms by which preinfarction angina confers cardioprotection are unknown, and some have suggested that coronary collateral recruitment rather than IPC may be responsible for the beneficial effects. However, there are data to suggest that the benefits of preinfarction angina are independent of the coronary collateral circulation, cardiovascular risk factors, and antianginal drug therapy [11]. In contrast, the fact that prodromal angina confers cardioprotection in a time-dependent fashion supports a role for preconditioning since it is similar to the time frame in which IPC has been observed to occur in animal models [12]. For example, in a study of patients with unstable angina requiring PCI, the frequency of an ischemic response during the first balloon inflation was 50%, 65%, 77%, and 96% among patients with their last episode of chest pain 0–6, 6–12, 12–24, and >24 h before PCI [19]. In contrast, patients whose last episode of angina was more than 24 h before PCI showed the greatest amount of PCI-related preconditioning during the second balloon inflation, suggesting a diminished effect of preceding angina. Finally, another mechanism that has been proposed is that preinfarction angina leads to more rapid thrombolysis and earlier reperfusion of the infarct-related artery following thrombolysis [20].

Experimental Clinical Studies of IPC

Several studies using exercise stress testing have attempted to quantify and replicate the phenomenon of warm-up angina. Kelion and colleagues demonstrated among patients with multivessel coronary artery disease that the onset of angina and electrocardiographic evidence of myocardial ischemia was delayed and occurred at a higher rate-pressure product, and the extent of left ventricular regional wall motion abnormality was reduced during a second stress performed 30 min after the first [21]. In another study, patients with stable angina and a significant stenosis of the left anterior descending coronary artery were randomly assigned to one of two stress test protocols designed to invoke either the early phase or delayed phase of IPC [22]. The early IPC protocol subjects underwent three sequential stress tests at least 2 weeks before PCI, while the delayed IPC group had five sequential stress tests within 24 h prior to PCI. During PCI, there was no significant difference in intracoronary pressure-derived collateral flow index between the groups. In the delayed IPC group, compared with the initial stress test, there was an increase in the ischemic threshold on the test performed 24 h later. Moreover, during the first balloon inflation, the magnitude of ST segment elevation was less in the delayed IPC group compared to those who received early IPC only. However, there was a significant attenuation in the amount of ST segment elevation seen at the time of the second balloon inflation in the early IPC patients that did not occur in the delayed IPC group. The findings support the concept of the two cardioprotective windows of IPC and also that ischemia during PCI is attenuated in humans by a delayed cardioprotective effects of exercise.

Perhaps the most direct evidence for IPC in the human heart has been demonstrated in patients undergoing PCI in whom an initial balloon inflation for duration of at least 60–90 s reduces myocardial ischemia during subsequent balloon inflations, measured as the severity of angina, ST segment elevation, QT interval dispersion, ventricular ectopic activity, creatine kinase levels, lactate production, and left ventricular dysfunction [23–29]. However, there are data to suggest that IPC during PCI cannot be elicited in the elderly and that this may be due to impaired activity of the KATP channels [30]. Experimental studies during PCI have also shed light on the potential mechanisms for the cardioprotective effects of the initial balloon inflation in humans. Measurement of cardiac vein blood flow and angiographic quantification of the collateral circulation have shown that mechanisms in addition to collateral recruitment are responsible [31]. As in the animal studies, these studies suggest a role for KATP channels [32], adenosine receptors [33], opioid receptors [34], nitric oxide [35], and the bradykinin pathway [36].

Animal experiments have demonstrated that, in addition to cardiomyocyte injury, ischemia–reperfusion leads to coronary endothelial dysfunction [37]. This concept was evaluated in humans by Kharbanda and colleagues. In their study, the forearm of healthy volunteers was rendered ischemic for 20 min. Endothelial function of the ipsilateral radial artery was assessed by measuring flow-mediated dilation and in the microcirculation by the blood flow response to an intra-arterial infusion of acetylcholine. Ischemia–reperfusion reduced flow-mediated dilation (7.7 ± 1.5–$3.5 \pm 0.9\%$) and the vasodilation in response to acetylcholine, but not the responses to an endothelium-independent vasodilator. However, if IPC (three 5-min cycles) was performed prior to the ischemia–reperfusion, endothelial dysfunction did not develop [38]. Recent evidence suggests that pharmacological preconditioning with rosuvastatin may also confer similar effects. Pretreatment with the drug has been shown to protect against endothelial injury caused by ischemia and reperfusion, via activation of the cyclooxygenase-2 pathway [39].

Clinical Studies in Patients Undergoing Coronary Artery Bypass Graft Surgery

Cardiac surgical procedures such as coronary artery bypass graft (CABG) surgery are another clinical setting, in which ischemia–reperfusion injury occurs, and provide a clinical model to investigate the potential impact of IPC. Unlike PCI, since the ischemia is global during cardiopulmonary bypass, the impact of coronary collateral circulation does not act as a confounding factor.

IPC during cardiac surgery has been performed by intermittent cross clamping of the aorta to produce repetitive transient ischemia of the heart. In patients with normothermic cardiopulmonary bypass, this has been shown to significantly lower serum troponin T concentrations at 72 h after surgery compared to patients who were not preconditioned suggesting that there was less myonecrosis [40, 41]. However, efforts to study IPC during hypothermic and/or cardioplegic arrest have produced variable results with some studies showing a lack of efficacy [42, 43]. In a systematic review of 22 randomized trials during cardiac surgery consisting of 933 patients, IPC was associated with significant reductions in ventricular arrhythmias, inotrope requirements, and intensive care unit stay with a nonsignificant trend toward a reduction in mortality [44]. In these studies, IPC was generally performed after the initiation of cardiopulmonary bypass, but before any additional myocardial protection was initiated. All patients undergoing on-pump surgery also received cardioplegia or intermittent cross clamp fibrillation with or without adjunctive cooling. The benefits were present in the subgroup receiving cardioplegia, but no benefit was detected in patients receiving intermittent cross clamp fibrillation.

Overall, at this time, there is no consensus on the routine role of IPC in cardiac surgery, in part, because of the evolution of differing cardioprotection techniques, the confounding cardioprotective effects of some anesthetics agents, and changes in surgical techniques. Large clinical trials will be required to definitively investigate the impact of IPC on hard clinical endpoints. Potential disadvantages of IPC performed during cardiac surgery are that it can prolong the duration of cardiopulmonary bypass with its associated risks and the potential risk for atheroembolism due to the repeated manipulation of the aorta. Pharmacological preconditioning, using agents such as opioids and isoflurane, has also shown potential for cardioprotection during surgery in preliminary studies and may offer an alternative strategy to IPC [45, 46].

Ischemic Postconditioning

Preclinical Studies of Ischemic Postconditioning

A major limitation to the translation of IPC into clinical practice for conditions where it would be most desirable, for example, ST-segment elevation myocardial infarction, is the unpredictable nature of acute plaque rupture and coronary artery occlusion. The interest in the field has recently been rekindled by the work of Zhao and colleagues because they have demonstrated in a canine model that three 30-s alternating cycles of ischemia and reperfusion, at the onset of myocardial reperfusion, can also reduce myocardial infarct size [47]. This concept has been named ischemic postconditioning (IPost). Although IPost is a distinct protocol, it shares many of the underlying signaling pathways that have been proposed for IPC. Subsequent studies have reproduced IPost in several animal species and in organs other than heart (e.g., brain and kidney). IPost appears to confer cardioprotection by reducing cardiomyocyte apoptosis and contracture, organelle dysfunction, coronary endothelial dysfunction, microvascular injury, and tissue edema. In addition to reducing infarct size, IPost reduces reperfusion arrhythmias, neutrophil adherence to the endothelium, and accumulation in the ischemic myocardium [48]. The mechanistic paradigm that has been proposed resembles that described previously for IPC and likely involves multiple triggers and mediators that ultimately inhibit the opening of the mPTP [49].

As with IPC, the beneficial effects of IPost appear to be dependent on the index ischemic time and the actual protocol itself. Figure 11.2 illustrates a theoretical construct of the potential relationships between ischemia duration and the impact of IPost. In rats, IPost applied after 30–45 min of infarct inducing ischemia appears to be effective, but not when the duration of lethal ischemia is ≥60 min [50]. Of note, IPost also does not appear to reduce infarct size if the duration of index ischemia is very short and may even be harmful [51]. There is a paucity of data regarding the optimal protocol with respect to the delay after which the first reocclusion should be performed, the duration and number of reocclusions, and the duration of the intermittent reperfusion. Experimental data suggests that IPost must be initiated very soon, probably within 1 min, after establishing reperfusion into the occluded circulation [50, 52–54]. The frequency and duration of the cycles of reocclusion and reperfusion during IPost also impact on the ability to confer cardioprotection. Indeed, Zhao and Vinten-Johansen have reported that in their initial studies conducted in 1992 in an anesthetized rabbit model of coronary artery occlusion–reperfusion, 5 min of ischemia followed by 5 min of reperfusion repeated over several cycles did not reduce infarct size [48]. The current evidence suggests that there is significant variability in animal models with somewhere

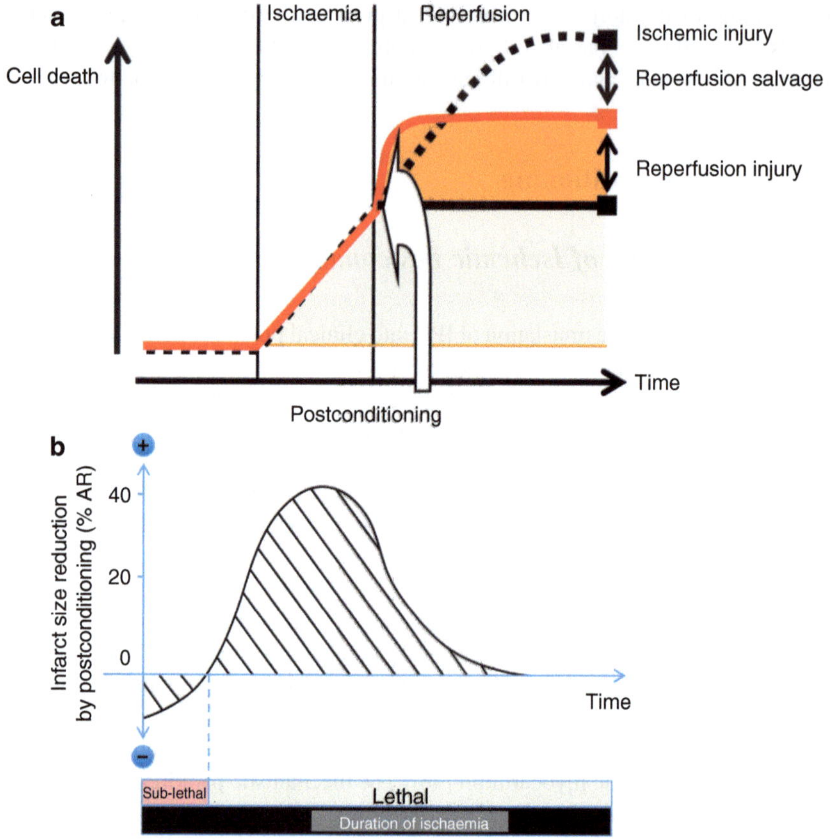

Fig. 11.2 (**a**) The concept of lethal reperfusion injury. During ischemia, irreversible cell injury leading to cell death occurs within the ischemic risk zone in a time-dependent manner. In the absence of reperfusion, ischemic injury would progressively kill more and more cells, eventually accounting for near total cell death (*broken line*). Reperfusion halts the process of ischemic cell death but in its early stages imposes injury that results in further cell death, beyond that due to the ischemic period: this is lethal reperfusion injury. The net result, however, is that the reperfused tissue sustains less cell death than would occur in ischemic tissue without reperfusion. Hence, targeting cell death due to reperfusion has the potential to maximize cell salvage. Postconditioning applied at the onset of reperfusion limits the extent of reperfusion injury and maximizes reperfusion salvage. (**b**) Attenuation of lethal reperfusion injury as a function of the duration of the preceding index ischemia. Infarct size reduction by protective interventions performed after reperfusion (e.g., ischemic postconditioning) may vary according to the duration of the preceding ischemia. Experimental studies show that with prolonged periods of index ischemia, the potential to minimize tissue salvage (infarct size reduction) may be limited probably because the extent of lethal ischemic injury is so severe. With briefer lethal periods of ischemia, interventions at reperfusion are able to confer marked reduction in infarct size. When the index ischemic event is so brief that no infarction occurs (sublethal ischemia), the application of ischemic postconditioning at the onset of reperfusion may prove injurious and cause a small degree of infarction (From Ovize et al. [49]. Reprinted with kind permission from Oxford University Press)

between 3 and 8 cycles of ischemia–reperfusion needed with cycle durations of approximately 30 s to produce IPost [50, 51, 55].

Potential reasons that are often mentioned for the failure to translate the preclinical evidence for cardiac conditioning into clinical practice include the fact that unlike most animal studies that are conducted in young healthy animals, patients with acute myocardial infarction are typically elderly with an atherothrombotic vasculature, have multiple comorbidities, and are concomitantly treated with drugs, all of which are factors that may interfere with cardioprotection [56]. Therefore, there is increasing focus on designing animal studies to address these issues. Several studies suggest that IPost may be less or not effective in reducing infarct size in older mice [57, 58], but there is intriguing data that this may be restored by modifying the IPost algorithm in older animals [59]. In contrast, the age of the animals did not appear to impact IPost in a rat model [60]. Similarly, whatever little data that are available regarding the impact of comorbid conditions on IPost are conflicting. For example, there are animal studies showing that hypercholesterolemia inhibits IPost in rabbits [61], while others have shown conflicting results [62]. Potential explanations for the discordant findings may relate to the severity and duration of the disease state and extracardiac pathologies in the different models. Obese animals, as well as those with abnormal glucose metabolism or hypertension, also appear to be resistant to the cardioprotective effects of IPC [63, 64].

Clinical Studies of Ischemic Postconditioning

The potential clinical application of IPost during PCI for myocardial infarction has been well recognized, and several recent "proof of concept" studies have demonstrated efficacy (Table 11.1). The earliest reports were published in 2005 by Laskey and Staat and colleagues [65, 66]. Laskey randomized patients with ST elevation myocardial infarction to IPost or standard therapy *after* TIMI 2 or 3 antegrade epicardial flow was established in the infarct-related artery. This was accomplished in 18 instances by guidewire passage only and in 3 instances by a short (≤30 s) balloon inflation. He demonstrated that the magnitude of ST segment resolution and the coronary flow reserve in the culprit artery were greater in patients with adjunctive IPost, compared to the control group [65]. However, infarct size was not measured in this study. Staat and colleagues randomized patients with ST segment elevation myocardial infarction to IPost after reperfusion by direct stenting, while the control subjects received standard management [66]. Determinants of infarct size, such as ischemia duration, area at risk, and collateral flow, were comparable between the two groups. IPost was associated with a 36% reduction in infract size, measured as the area under the curve for creatine kinase release over the first 72 h after intervention. Myocardial blush grade, a marker of microvascular reperfusion, was also significantly better than in the control primary PCI patients. In another study, the same group of investigators reported a sustained benefit of IPost with smaller infarct size at 6 months and a 7% higher left ventricular ejection fraction [67]. Subsequently,

Table 11.1 Randomized trials of postconditioning in STEMI

Study	Year	*n*	Duration (h)	IPost protocol	Inclusion criteria	Exclusion criteria	Endpoints (with IPost)
Laskey et al. [65]	2005	Control $n = 7$	Control 5.7 ± 3.0	Two cycles of 90-s inflation/deflation each separated by 3–5 min	TIMI 0/1 flow	>12 h of symptoms	↑ Coronary flow reserve
		IPost $n = 10$	IPost 4.6 ± 2.2			>70% stenosis in a non-culprit artery	↑ ST segment resolution
						Angiographic evidence of collaterals to IRA	
						Hemodynamic instability	
						Electrical instability	
						Thrombolytic therapy	
Staat et al. [66]	2005	Control $n = 16$	Control 5.5 ± 0.7;	Four cycles of 60-s inflation/deflation	<6 h after onset of pain	Cardiac arrest, shock	↓CK-MB 72 h AUC
		IPost $n = 14$	IPost 5.3 ± 0.6		0.1 mv ST in 3 contiguous leads	Previous AMI	↑ Blush grade
					Culprit artery LAD or RCA (large)	TIMI < 2 or 3 flow post PCI	
					TIMI 0 flow grade	Rentrop ≥ 1 collateral flow to IRA	
Ma et al. [68]	2006	Control $n = 47$	Control 7.1 ± 2.5	Three cycles of 30-s inflation/deflation	≤12 h after symptom onset	Prior CABG/PCI/MI	↑ Coronary flow velocity
		IPost $n = 47$	IPost 6.6 ± 2.5		>0.1 mv ST in 2 contiguous leads		↓ CK-MB 72 h peak level
							↓ WMSI (8 weeks)
							↑ Brachial artery vasodilator response

Yang et al. [69]	2007	Control $n=18$ IPost $n=23$	Control 4.4 ± 0.7 IPost 5.2 ± 0.8	Three cycles of 30-s inflation/deflation	>0.1 mv ST ↑ in 2 contiguous leads	Cardiogenic shock Left main occlusion ≥TIMI 1 in IRA Prior MI Treatment with glycoprotein IIb/IIIa inhibitor prior to PCI	↓ Infarct size ↑ Ejection fraction (echo) ↓ CK-MB
Thibault et al. [67]	2008	Control $n=21$ IPost $n=17$	Control 5.0 ± 1.7 IPost 4.7 ± 1.4	Four cycles of 60-s inflation/deflation	<6 h after onset of pain >0.1 mv ST ↑ in 2 contiguous leads Culprit artery LAD or RCA TIMI 0 flow	Cardiac arrest, shock Preinfarction angina <48 h Rentrop grade ≥1 collateral flow to IRA	↓ Plasma CK/TnI at 72 h ↓ SPECT at 6 months ↑ Ejection fraction (echo) at 1 year
Laskey et al. [70]	2008	Control $n=12$ IPost $n=12$	Control 3.7 ± 0.9 IPost 3.8 ± 0.7	Two cycles of 90-s inflation/deflation	≤6 h after onset of pain ≥0.2 mv ST ↑ TIMI 0/1 flow LAD IRA	Age > 90 years Thrombolytic therapy Prior CABG, MI Nonculprit >70% stenosis; Hemodynamic instability; Electrical instability	Resolution of ST segment changes; Doppler velocimetry in infarct-related artery
Lonborg et al. [71]	2010	Control $n=59$ IPost $n=59$	Control 2.5 ± 3.3 IPost 4.0 ± 2.5	Four cycles of 30-s inflation/deflation	<12 h after onset of pain >0.1 mv ST ↑ in 2 contiguous leads	TIMI > 1 flow pre PCI TIMI < 2 flow post PCI Nonculprit >70% stenosis Shock, LBBB Prior CABG, MI Severe renal/liver failure	↓ Infarct size ↓ Heart failure

AUC area under the curve, *IRA* infarct-related artery, *LAD* left anterior descending, *RCA* right coronary artery, *TIMI* thrombolysis in myocardial infarction, *WMSI* wall score motion index

studies have also enrolled very small number of patients, but consistently reported a beneficial effect of IPost [68–70].

The largest clinical trial and one that used cardiac magnetic resonance imaging as the gold standard for assessing myocardial salvage and infarct size during IPost has recently been published by Lønborg and colleagues [71]. One hundred and eighteen patients with ST segment elevation myocardial infarction requiring primary PCI were randomized to either IPost or a control group. IPost was performed immediately after obtaining reperfusion with four balloon occlusions, each lasting 30 s, followed by 30 s of reperfusion. Postconditioning resulted in a 19% relative reduction in infarct size at 3 months, as judged by the presence of delayed enhancement. There was also a reduction in the incidence of heart failure in the conditioned group.

In addition, a retrospective study evaluated the number of balloon inflations used during primary PCI and reported that patients with four or more inflations had smaller infarcts compared to those in whom reperfusion was established with fewer inflations [72]. While one must bear in mind that there may be publication bias, the studies had restricted inclusion criteria, and the technique can only be applied to patients receiving mechanical reperfusion therapy; these preliminary studies clearly demonstrate the feasibility of performing IPost within the context of contemporary management of ST segment elevation myocardial infarction. It is encouraging that the protocols shown to be effective in the clinical studies so far would not unduly prolong the procedure duration in the catheterization laboratory and will not impact on the door-to-balloon time, a key quality measure. At this time, large clinical trials that have adequate power to explore clinical endpoints such as mortality, development of heart failure, and duration of hospitalization are needed in order to advance the field.

Remote Ischemic "Conditioning"

Preclinical Studies of Remote "Conditioning"

Despite the importance of the discovery and its potential for clinical applications, IPost is limited by the fact that it requires direct intervention on the target organ. A solution to this limitation is offered by the observation that remote ischemia in a distant organ or vascular bed may also confer cardioprotection during subsequent ischemia [73]. In their landmark experiment, Przyklenk and colleagues showed that short-lived ischemia in myocardium supplied by the circumflex coronary artery diminished the size of infarction in the territory of the left anterior descending artery during subsequent lethal ischemia, a concept that was termed intraorgan preconditioning [73]. The concept of remote preconditioning (RPC) was further developed in experimental studies showing that transient ischemia of a wide range of organs, such as the kidney and small bowel, induced protection against subsequent myocardial infarction (Fig. 11.3). Indeed, the protection may extend beyond the heart and

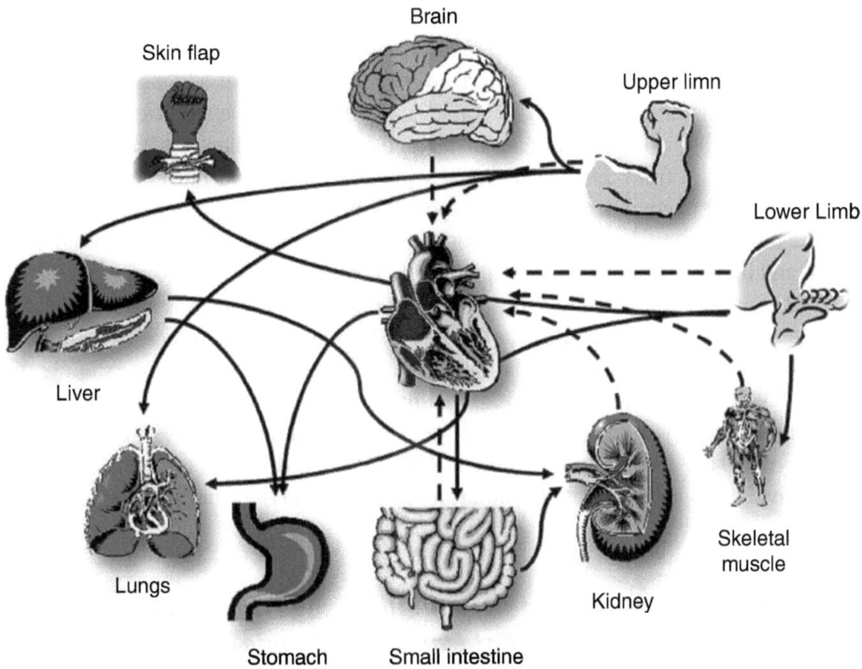

Fig. 11.3 Inter-organ protection against ischemia–reperfusion injury: this figure depicts the evolution of remote ischemic preconditioning from a concept that was initially used to denote an intramyocardial reduction in infarct size. Following this initial discovery, it was observed that brief ischemia and reperfusion of organs distant or remote from the heart had the ability to mediate a subsequent reduction in myocardial infarct size (see *dashed black arrows*). The concept has now been expanded between noncardiac organs and tissues such that it represents a general form of inter-organ protection against ischemia–reperfusion injury (*solid black arrows* depict the remote preconditioning organ "pointing" to the protected organ or tissue and emanating from the preconditioning organ or tissue) (From Hausenloy and Yellon [85]. Reprinted with kind permission from Oxford University Press)

may even be effective in protecting other organs such as the brain [74–83]. However, the potential for clinical application was most clearly demonstrated by the experiment in which the transient limb ischemia was effective in reducing myocardial infarct size in a rabbit [84].

The precise mechanisms responsible for the effects of RPC are not completely understood and are likely to vary depending on the site of the remote tissue and species studied [85]. However, evidence suggests that there may be a combination of neuronal, humoral, and systemic processes at play. Support for the neuronal hypothesis comes from experiments in which a ganglion blocker such as hexamethonium has been shown to abolish RPC in animals [75, 80] and humans [86]. It has been proposed that the neuronal pathways consist of an afferent limb from the remote ischemic organ to the central nervous system which in turn sends out an efferent limb to the distant target tissues. Signaling mediators in the afferent loop, potentially, include adenosine, bradykinin, and calcitonin gene-related peptide. The efferent signal has not been well characterized, but local release of adenosine may play a role. Support for the humoral hypothesis is derived from experiments in which RPC has been shown to occur in a transplanted (denervated) heart [87] and in which coronary effluent from an isolated, locally preconditioned heart has been shown to protect another ex vivo heart against myocardial infarction [88]. Potential mediators for the humoral signal include the renin–angiotensin, opioid, endocannabinoid systems, and ligands for G protein–coupled receptors [89, 90]. The intra-myocyte pathways that are activated by the neuronal and/or humoral mechanisms are likely to be similar to that proposed for classical IPC [85]. Finally, systemic processes that may contribute to RPC include modulation of inflammatory processes. For example, in healthy volunteers, transient limb ischemia suppresses neutrophil adhesion and phagocytic activity, as well as expression of proinflammatory genes in circulating leukocytes [91, 92]. In a murine model, RPC has been shown to upregulate cardioprotective genes and suppress proinflammatory genes in the heart [93].

Clinical Studies of Remote Preconditioning (Transient Limb Ischemia Prior to the Onset of Cardiac Ischemia)

Kharbanda and colleagues were among the first to demonstrate that transient limb ischemia could invoke RPC in humans [38]. Their protocol consisted of four cycles of 5 min of ischemia followed by 5 min of reperfusion of an arm which then protected against endothelial dysfunction induced by subsequent prolonged ischemia in the contralateral arm. This phenomenon appears to be modulated by the "dose" and timing of the limb ischemia in relation to whether RPC is performed in the lower or upper limb. For example, Loukogeorgakis and colleagues [94] have reported that two 5-min cycles of lower-limb ischemia–reperfusion protects against postischemic endothelial dysfunction, but the same protocol in the upper limb is ineffective. However, three cycles of upper-limb ischemia–reperfusion did protect against endothelial injury [94].

The impact of transient limb ischemia on cardiac troponin I release after elective PCI has recently been reported in 242 consecutive patients [95]. Patients were randomized to receive either three 5-min cycles of upper-limb ischemia (blood pressure cuff inflated to 200 mmHg around the upper arm) followed by 5 min of reperfusion or to a control group in which an un-inflated cuff was placed around the arm before arrival into the catheterization laboratory. RPC reduced PCI-related myonecrosis, and in addition it was associated with patients experiencing less chest discomfort and ST segment deviation compared to the control subjects. Somewhat surprisingly since the study was underpowered to detect differences in clinical endpoint, the composite endpoint of major adverse cardiac or cerebral event rate at 6 months was lower in the remote IPC group. This observation suggests that RPC, perhaps by modifying the inflammatory response to PCI, may have chronic beneficial effects beyond the acute effects at the time of the revascularization. However, these findings were not reproduced in a similar study conducted by Prasad and Colleagues from the Mayo Clinic published subsequently [105]. There are several potential reasons for the different findings between the two studies. With regards to the study by Prasad and Colleagues: i) the sample size was smaller raising the possibility of a false negative result; ii) ischemia-reperfusion was induced using 3 minute cycles as opposed to 5 minutes resulting in a shorter period of preconditioning; iii) cuff inflations were performed immediately preceding PCI as opposed to approximately one hour before; iv) one-third presented with an acute coronary syndrome requiring urgent procedures in the hospital as opposed to the CRISP Stent study in which all cases were elective.; v) cardiac troponin T was used to detect myonecrosis as opposed to troponin I; and vi) patients were older and had a higher frequency of diabetes mellitus, characteristics in which preconditioning has been shown to be less effective.

Several studies have examined the efficacy of transient limb ischemia in patients undergoing cardiac surgery. The earliest study was conducted in just eight male patients who were randomly allocated to either RPC or a control group. RPC was performed in the right upper limb with two cycles of 3 min of ischemia separated with 2 min of reperfusion. RPC did not reduce creatinine kinase, but did diminish lactate dehydrogenase release, suggesting a potential impact on myocardial metabolism [96]. A larger but nonetheless small randomized study during cardiac surgery was subsequently conducted in 17 RPC-treated and 20 control children with congenital heart disease. Remote ischemic preconditioning was induced by four 5-min cycles of lower-limb ischemia and reperfusion using a blood pressure cuff. Bypass and cross clamp times were similar in the two groups. RPC-treated patients had lower troponin I release, postoperative inotrope score, and airway resistance [97]. In another randomized controlled trial, adults ($n=27$) undergoing elective (on-pump) coronary bypass surgery received RPC with three 5-min cycles of right upper-limb ischemia (cuff inflated to 200 mmHg) with an intervening 5-min period of reperfusion [98]. Patients were not given inhalation anesthesia to avoid their confounding influence on cardioprotection. RPC reduced troponin T release by 43% over the first 48 h after surgery. In a follow-up study, the same investigators using an identical protocol also confirmed the efficacy of RPC in patients receiving inhaled anesthesia and cold blood cardioplegia for cardioprotection [99]. Thus, the aggregate data so far from small “proof of concept” studies indicates that RPC reduces myocardial injury in children and adults undergoing cardiac surgery. Larger clinical trials are currently being conducted that will hopefully provide important information to develop clinical practice.

Major vascular surgery in patients with peripheral vascular disease is frequently accompanied by cardiac ischemic complications due to the concomitant coronary artery disease. A recent intriguing study investigated the efficacy of lower limb ischemia for inducing RPC of the heart and kidneys in a randomized clinical trial of 82 patients undergoing elective aortic aneurysm repair [100]. RPC was performed by two cycles of intermittent cross clamping of the common iliac artery with 10-min ischemia followed by 10-min reperfusion. RPC reduced the incidence of postoperative myocardial infarction by 22%, renal impairment by 23%, and reduced the duration of postoperative critical care. These encouraging but highly preliminary data provide the basis for larger clinical trials in an arena in which preoperative interventions have, in general, failed to reduce cardiovascular complications.

Clinical and Experimental Studies of Remote Per-/Postconditioning (Transient Limb Ischemia After the Onset of Cardiac Ischemia)

RPC, as described above, is typically performed prior to the onset of target organ ischemia. However, this is not possible in certain circumstances such as during acute myocardial infarction or stroke. Animal experiments suggest that similar to IPost, "remote postconditioning" may also be feasible. Kerendi and colleagues have demonstrated in an animal model that a short period of renal ischemia reduces the extent of myocardial infarction when applied after the onset of coronary ischemia, but immediately before and during reperfusion [101]. Transient limb ischemia in an experimental study, performed after the onset of cardiac ischemia and before reperfusion, has also been shown to reduce infarct size [102]. This form of RPC is sometimes referred to as remote *per*conditioning. Similarly, remote postconditioning in which the transient limb ischemia is performed at the time of coronary reperfusion has also been shown to be effective in a porcine myocardial infarction model [103].

The first study to investigate remote *per*conditioning in humans has recently been published by Botker et al. [104]. They enrolled 333 consecutive patients with a suspected first ST-segment elevation myocardial infarction undergoing primary PCI. Patients were randomized to either remote conditioning performed during transport to hospital or a control group. The conditioning was performed by intermittent arm ischemia through four cycles of 5 min of cuff inflation and 5 min of deflation. The primary endpoint of myocardial salvage index at 30 days, measured by SPECT imaging, was increased in the remote-conditioning group (0.55 vs. 0.75, $p=0.03$). However, there was no improvement in secondary endpoints such as ST segment resolution, peak troponin levels, and left ventricular ejection fraction. This study provided the much needed feasibility and "proof of concept" data that will propel further investigation into the translation of RPC for acute coronary syndromes, especially ST-segment elevation myocardial infarction.

In conclusion, remote ischemic conditioning appears to be a simple, cost-effective, and readily applicable technique that may be performed in humans by transient limb ischemia using a blood pressure cuff. The studies so far have not reported any adverse effects. Early clinical trials have provided encouraging results both in the setting of elective procedures and during acute myocardial infarction. As with RPC and IPost, larger clinical trials are now needed to establish definitively whether or not this technique has a role in clinical practice.

Conclusions

After an initial inertia in translating IPC into clinical practice, the demonstration of IPost and RPC has expedited the process in the recent few years. The clinical trials performed to date have been small, used surrogate endpoints, and had strict inclusion and exclusion criteria. It remains to be established whether ischemic conditioning, whether direct or remote, performed before or after the onset of lethal ischemia, actually reduces clinical endpoints such as mortality. Moreover, larger trials will allow assessment of the applicability to a wider patient population with prior infarcts, prior revascularization, reduced ejection fraction, history of congestive heart failure, use of multiple pharmacological agents, and presence of multiple coexisting diseases. In addition, further study is required to evaluate whether delayed conditioning can be applied in humans. The major challenge for the future will be to find funding to conduct large multicenter trials given that there is no inherent intellectual property associated with IPC per se (which is otherwise an attractive aspect of this concept), limiting the interest from industry to develop the field. The field of cardioprotection to reduce reperfusion injury has been characterized by a plethora of experimental studies with multiple pharmacological agents that have shown great promise in the laboratory. This has led to a large clinical agenda with disappointing results and diminishing enthusiasm in many quarters. The field of endogenous cardiac protection is particularly appealing given the clinical trials that document feasibility and signals suggesting efficacy. The time is ripe for larger clinical trials. Moreover, understanding the mechanisms of apparent benefit may lead to the development of new drugs and molecules that could target the fundamental processes of ischemia–reperfusion injury.

References

1. Murry CE, Jennings RB, Reimer KA. Preconditioning with ischemia: a delay of lethal cell injury in ischemic myocardium. Circulation. 1986;74:1124.
2. Yellon DM, Downey JM. Preconditioning the myocardium: from cellular physiology to clinical cardiology. Physiol Rev. 2003;83:1113–51.
3. Eisen A, Fisman EZ, Rubenfire M, Freimark D, McKechnie R, Tenenbaum A, Motro M, Adler Y. Ischemic preconditioning: nearly two decades of research. A comprehensive review. Atherosclerosis. 2004;172:201–10.
4. Marber MS, Latchman DS, Walker JM, Yellon DM. Cardiac stress protein elevation 24 hours after brief ischemia or heat stress is associated with resistance to myocardial infarction. Circulation. 1993;88:1264–72.
5. Kuzuya T, Hoshida S, Yamashita N, et al. Delayed effects of sublethal ischemia on the acquisition of tolerance to ischemia. Circ Res. 1993;72:1293–9.
6. Hausenloy DJ, Yellon DM. The mitochondrial permeability transition pore: its fundamental role in mediating cell death during ischaemia and reperfusion. J Mol Cell Cardiol. 2003;35:339–41.
7. Hausenloy DJ, Yellon DM. New directions for protecting the heart against ischaemia-reperfusion injury: targeting the Reperfusion Injury Salvage Kinase (RISK)-pathway. Cardiovasc Res. 2004;61:448–60.

8. Walker DM, Walker JM, Pugsley WB, et al. Preconditioning in isolated superfused human muscle. J Mol Cell Cardiol. 1995;27:1349.
9. Bogaty P, Poirier P, Boyer L, et al. What induces the warm-up ischemia/angina phenomenon: exercise or myocardial ischemia? Circulation. 2003;107:1858.
10. Okazaki Y, Kodama K, Sato H, et al. Attenuation of increased regional myocardial oxygen consumption during exercise as a major cause of warm-up phenomenon. J Am Coll Cardiol. 1993;21:1597.
11. Kloner RA, Shook T, Przyklenk K, et al. Previous angina alters in-hospital outcome in TIMI 4. A clinical correlate to preconditioning? Circulation. 1995;91:37.
12. Kloner RA, Shook T, Antman EM, for the TIMI-9B Investigators, et al. Prospective temporal analysis of the onset of preinfarction angina versus outcome. An ancillary study in TIMI-9B. Circulation. 1998;97:1042.
13. Anzai T, Yoshikawa T, Asakura Y, et al. Preinfarction angina as a major predictor of left ventricular function and long-term prognosis after a first Q wave myocardial infarction. J Am Coll Cardiol. 1995;26:319.
14. Ottani F, Galvani M, Ferrini D, et al. Prodromal angina limits infarct size. A role for ischemic preconditioning. Circulation. 1995;91:291.
15. Shiraki H, Yoshikawa T, Anzai T, et al. Association between preinfarction angina and a lower risk of right ventricular infarction. N Engl J Med. 1998;338:941.
16. Ishihara M, Inoue I, Kawagoe T, et al. Diabetes mellitus prevents ischemic preconditioning in patients with a first acute anterior wall myocardial infarction. J Am Coll Cardiol. 2001;38:1007.
17. Abete T, Ferrara N, Cacciatore F. Angina-induced protection against myocardial infarction in adult and elderly patients: a loss of preconditioning mechanism in the aging heart? J Am Coll Cardiol. 1997;30:947.
18. Abete P, Ferrara N, Cacciatore F, et al. High level of physical activity preserves the cardioprotective effect of preinfarction angina in elderly patients. J Am Coll Cardiol. 2001;38:1357.
19. Lim R, Laskey WK. Ischemic preconditioning in unstable coronary syndromes: evidence for time dependence. J Am Coll Cardiol. 1997;30:1461.
20. Andreotti F, Pasceri V, Hackett DR, et al. Preinfarction angina as a predictor of more rapid coronary thrombolysis in patients with acute myocardial infarction. N Engl J Med. 1996;334:7.
21. Kelion AD, Webb TP, Gardner MA, et al. The warm-up effect protects against ischemic left ventricular dysfunction in patients with angina. J Am Coll Cardiol. 2001;37:705.
22. Lambiase PD, Edwards RJ, Cusack MR, et al. Exercise-induced ischemia initiates the second window of protection in humans independent of collateral recruitment. J Am Coll Cardiol. 2003;41:1174.
23. Deutsch E, Berger M, Kussmaul WG, et al. Adaptation to ischemia during percutaneous transluminal coronary angioplasty. Clinical, hemodynamic, and metabolic features. Circulation. 1990;82:2044.
24. Laskey WK. Beneficial impact of preconditioning during PTCA on creatine kinase release. Circulation. 1999;99:2085.
25. Cribier A, Korsatz L, Koning R, et al. Improved myocardial ischemic response and enhanced collateral circulation with long repetitive coronary occlusion during angioplasty: a prospective study. J Am Coll Cardiol. 1992;20:578.
26. Eltchaninoff H, Cribier A, Tron C, et al. Adaptation to myocardial ischemia during coronary angioplasty demonstrated by clinical, electrocardiographic, echocardiographic, and metabolic parameters. Am Heart J. 1997;133:490.
27. Okishige K, Yamashita K, Yoshinaga H, et al. Electrophysiological effects of ischemic preconditioning on QT dispersion during coronary angioplasty. J Am Coll Cardiol. 1996;28:70.
28. Airaksinen KE, Huikuri HV. Antiarrhythmic effect of repeated coronary occlusion during balloon angioplasty. J Am Coll Cardiol. 1997;29:1035.
29. Lindhardt TB, Kelbaek H, Madsen JK, et al. Continuous monitoring of global left ventricular ejection fraction during percutaneous transluminal coronary angioplasty. Am J Cardiol. 1998;81:853.

30. Lee TM, Su SF, Chou TF, et al. Loss of preconditioning by attenuated activation of myocardial ATP-sensitive potassium channels in elderly patients undergoing coronary angioplasty. Circulation. 2002;105:334.
31. Billinger M, Fleisch M, Eberli FR, et al. Is the development of myocardial tolerance to repeated ischemia in humans due to preconditioning or to collateral recruitment? J Am Coll Cardiol. 1999;33:1027.
32. Tomai F, Crea F, Gaspardone A, et al. Ischemic preconditioning during coronary angioplasty is prevented by glibenclamide, a selective ATP-sensitive K+ channel blocker. Circulation. 1994;90:700.
33. Leesar MA, Stoddard M, Ahmed M, et al. Preconditioning of human myocardium with adenosine during coronary angioplasty. Circulation. 1997;95:2500.
34. Tomai F, Crea F, Gaspardone A, et al. Effects of naloxone on myocardial ischemic preconditioning in humans. J Am Coll Cardiol. 1999;33:1863.
35. Leesar MA, Stoddard MF, Dawn B, et al. Delayed preconditioning-mimetic action of nitroglycerin in patients undergoing coronary angioplasty. Circulation. 2001;103:2935.
36. Leesar MA, Stoddard MF, Manchikalapudi S, Bolli R. Bradykinin-induced preconditioning in patients undergoing coronary angioplasty. J Am Coll Cardiol. 1999;34:639.
37. Richard V, Kaeffer N, Tron C, Thuillez C. Ischemic preconditioning protects against coronary endothelial dysfunction induced by ischemia and reperfusion. Circulation. 1994;89:1254–61.
38. Kharbanda RK, Mortensen UM, White PA, et al. Transient limb ischemia induces remote ischemic preconditioning in vivo. Circulation. 2002;106:2881–3.
39. Liuni A, Luca MC, Gori T, Parker JD. Rosuvastatin prevents conduit artery endothelial dysfunction induced by ischemia and reperfusion by a cyclooxygenase-2-dependent mechanism. J Am Coll Cardiol. 2010;55:1002–6.
40. Jenkins DP, Pugsley WB, Alkhulaifi AM, et al. Ischaemic preconditioning reduces troponin-T release in patients undergoing cardiac surgery. Heart. 1997;77:314.
41. Teoh LK, Grant R, Hulf JA, et al. The effect of preconditioning (ischemic and pharmacological) on myocardial necrosis following coronary artery bypass graft surgery. Cardiovasc Res. 2002;53:175.
42. Teoh LK, Grant R, Hulf JA, et al. A comparison between ischemic preconditioning, intermittent cross-clamp fibrillation and cold crystalloid cardioplegia for myocardial protection during coronary artery bypass graft surgery. Cardiovasc Surg. 2002;10:251.
43. Kaukoranta PK, Lepojarvi MP, Ylitalo KV, et al. Normothermic retrograde blood cardioplegia with or without preceding ischemic preconditioning. Ann Thorac Surg. 1997;63:1268.
44. Walsh SR, Tang TY, Kullar P, et al. Ischaemic preconditioning during cardiac surgery: systematic review and meta-analysis of perioperative outcomes in randomised clinical trials. Eur J Cardiothorac Surg. 2008;34:985.
45. Bell SP, Sack MN, Patel A, et al. Delta opioid receptor stimulation mimics ischemic preconditioning in human heart muscle. J Am Coll Cardiol. 2000;36:2296.
46. Belhomme D, Peynet J, Louzy M, et al. Evidence for preconditioning by isoflurane in coronary artery bypass graft surgery. Circulation. 1999;100:II340.
47. Zhao Z-Q, Corvera JS, Halkos ME, et al. Inhibition of myocardial injury by ischemic postconditioning during reperfusion: comparison with ischemic preconditioning. Am J Physiol Heart Circ Physiol. 2003;285:H579–88.
48. Granfeldt A, Lefer DJ, Vinten-Johansen J. Protective ischaemia in patients: preconditioning and postconditioning. Cardiovasc Res. 2009;83:234–46.
49. Ovize M, Baxter GF, Di Lisa F, Working Group of Cellular Biology of Heart of European Society of Cardiology, et al. Postconditioning and protection from reperfusion injury: where do we stand? Position paper from the Working Group of Cellular Biology of the Heart of the European Society of Cardiology. Cardiovasc Res. 2010;87:406–23.
50. Skyschally A, van Caster P, Iliodromitis EK, Schulz R, Kremastinos DT, Heusch G. Ischemic postconditioning – experimental models and protocol algorithms. Basic Res Cardiol. 2009; 104:469–83.

51. Manintveld OC, Te Lintel HM, van den Bos EJ, Suurenbroek GM, Dekkers DH, Verdouw PD, et al. Cardiac effects of postconditioning depend critically on the duration of index ischemia. Am J Physiol Heart Circ Physiol. 2007;292:H1551–60.
52. Kin H, Zhao Z-Q, Sun H-Y, Wang N-P, Corvera JS, Halkos ME, et al. Postconditioning attenuates myocardial ischemia/reperfusion injury by inhibiting events in the early minutes of reperfusion. Cardiovasc Res. 2004;62:74–85.
53. Philipp S, Downey JM, Cohen MV. Postconditioning must be initiated in less than 1 minute following reperfusion and is dependent on adenosine receptors and PI3-kinase. Circulation. 2004;110:III–168.
54. Yang X-M, Proctor JB, Cui L, Krieg T, Downey JM, Cohen MV. Multiple, brief coronary occlusions during early reperfusion protect hearts by targeting cell signaling pathways. J Am Coll Cardiol. 2004;44:1103–10.
55. Iliodromitis EK, Downey JM, Heusch G, Kremastinos DT. What is the optimal postconditioning algorithm? J Cardiovasc Pharmacol Ther. 2009;14:269–73.
56. Prasad A, Stone G, Holmes D, Gersh B. Reperfusion injury, microvascular dysfunction and cardioprotection: the "dark side" of reperfusion. Circulation. 2009;120:2105–12.
57. Boengler K, Schulz R, Heusch G. Loss of cardioprotection with ageing. Cardiovasc Res. 2009;83:247–61.
58. Przyklenk K, Maynard M, Darling CE, Whittaker P. Aging mouse hearts are refractory to infarct size reduction with post-conditioning. J Am Coll Cardiol. 2008;51:1393–8.
59. Boengler K, Buechert A, Heinen Y, Roeskes C, Hilfiker-Kleiner D, Heusch G, et al. Cardioprotection by ischemic postconditioning is lost in aged and STAT3-deficient mice. Circ Res. 2008;102:131–5.
60. Yin Z, Gao H, Wang H, Li L, Di C, Luan R, et al. Ischemic postconditioning protects both adult and aged Sprague Dawley rat hearts from ischemia/reperfusion injury through the PI3-K/Akt and GSK-3beta pathway. Clin Exp Pharmacol Physiol. 2009;36:756–63.
61. Iliodromitis EK, Zoga A, Vrettou A, et al. The effectiveness of postconditioning and preconditioning on infarct size in hypercholesterolemic and normal anesthetized rabbits. Atherosclerosis. 2006;188:356–62.
62. Donato M, D'Annunzio V, Berg G, Gonzalez G, Schreier L, Morales C, et al. Ischemic postconditioning reduces infarct size by activation of A1 receptors and K+ (ATP) channels in both normal and hypercholesterolemic rabbits. J Cardiovasc Pharmacol. 2007;49:287–92.
63. Bouhidel O, Pons S, Souktani R, Zini R, Berdeaux A, Ghaleh B. Myocardial ischemic postconditioning against ischemia/reperfusion is impaired in ob/ob mice. Am J Physiol Heart Circ Physiol. 2008;295:H1580–6.
64. Wagner C, Kloeting I, Strasser RH, Weinbrenner C. Cardioprotection by postconditioning is lost in WOKW rats with metabolic syndrome: role of glycogen synthase kinase 3beta. J Cardiovasc Pharmacol. 2008;52:430–7.
65. Laskey WK. Brief repetitive balloon occlusions enhance reperfusion during percutaneous coronary intervention for acute myocardial infarction: a pilot study. Catheter Cardiovasc Interv. 2005;65:361–7.
66. Staat P, Rioufol G, Piot C, et al. Postconditioning the human heart. Circulation. 2005;112:2143–8.
67. Thibault H, Piot C, Staat P, et al. Long-term benefit of postconditioning. Circulation. 2008;117:1037–44.
68. Ma XJ, Zhang XH, Li CM, Luo M. Effect of postconditioning on coronary blood flow velocity and endothelial function in patients with acute myocardial infarction. Scand Cardiovasc J. 2006;40:327–33.
69. Yang XC, Liu Y, Wang LF, et al. Reduction in myocardial infarct size by postconditioning in patients after percutaneous coronary intervention. J Invasive Cardiol. 2007;19:424–30.
70. Laskey WK, Yoon S, Calzada N, Ricciardi MJ. Concordant improvements in coronary flow reserve and ST-segment resolution during percutaneous coronary intervention for acute myocardial infarction: a benefit of postconditioning. Catheter Cardiovasc Interv. 2008;72:212–20.

71. Lonborg J, Kelbaek H, Vejlstrup N, et al. Cardioprotective effects of ischemic postconditioning in patients treated with primary percutaneous coronary intervention, evaluated by magnetic resonance. Circ Cardiovasc Interv. 2010;3:34–41.
72. Darling CE, Solari PB, Smith CS, Furman MI, Przyklenk K. "Postconditioning" the human heart: multiple balloon inflations during primary angioplasty may confer cardioprotection. Basic Res Cardiol. 2007;102:274–8.
73. Przyklenk K, Bauer B, Ovize M, Kloner RA, Whittaker P. Regional ischemic "preconditioning" protects remote virgin myocardium from subsequent sustained coronary occlusion. Circulation. 1993;87:893–9.
74. Lang SC, Elsasser A, Scheler C, et al. Myocardial preconditioning and remote renal preconditioning – identifying a protective factor using proteomic methods? Basic Res Cardiol. 2006;101:149–58.
75. Gho BC, Schoemaker RG, van den Doel MA, Duncker DJ, Verdouw PD. Myocardial protection by brief ischemia in noncardiac tissue. Circulation. 1996;94:2193–200.
76. Takaoka A, Nakae I, Mitsunami K, et al. Renal ischemia/reperfusion remotely improves myocardial energy metabolism during myocardial ischemia via adenosine receptors in rabbits: effects of "remote preconditioning". J Am Coll Cardiol. 1999;33:556–64.
77. Verdouw PD, Gho BC, Koning MM, Schoemaker RG, Duncker DJ. Cardioprotection by ischemic and nonischemic myocardial stress and ischemia in remote organs. Implications for the concept of ischemic preconditioning. Ann N Y Acad Sci. 1996;793:27–42.
78. Tokuno S, Hinokiyama K, Tokuno K, Lowbeer C, Hansson LO, Valen G. Spontaneous ischemic events in the brain and heart adapt the hearts of severely atherosclerotic mice to ischemia. Arterioscler Thromb Vasc Biol. 2002;22:995–1001.
79. Schoemaker RG, van Heijningen CL. Bradykinin mediates cardiac preconditioning at a distance. Am J Physiol Heart Circ Physiol. 2000;278:H1571–6.34.
80. Liem DA, Verdouw PD, Ploeg H, Kazim S, Duncker DJ. Sites of action of adenosine in interorgan preconditioning of the heart. Am J Physiol Heart Circ Physiol. 2002;283:H29–37.
81. Wolfrum S, Schneider K, Heidbreder M, Nienstedt J, Dominiak P, Dendorfer A. Remote preconditioning protects the heart by activating myocardial PKCepsilon-isoform. Cardiovasc Res. 2002;55:583–9.
82. Ates E, Genc E, Erkasap N, et al. Renal protection by brief liver ischemia in rats. Transplantation. 2002;74:1247–51.
83. Singh D, Chopra K. Evidence of the role of angiotensin AT(1) receptors in remote renal preconditioning of myocardium. Methods Find Exp Clin Pharmacol. 2004;26:117–22.
84. Birnbaum Y, Hale SL, Kloner RA. Ischemic preconditioning at a distance: reduction of myocardial infarct size by partial reduction of blood supply combined with rapid stimulation of the gastrocnemius muscle in the rabbit. Circulation. 1997;96:1641–6.
85. Hausenloy DJ, Yellon DM. Remote ischaemic preconditioning: underlying mechanisms and clinical application. Cardiovasc Res. 2008;79:377–86.
86. Loukogeorgakis SP, Panagiotidou AT, Broadhead MW, Donald A, Deanfield JE, MacAllister RJ. Remote ischemic preconditioning provides early and late protection against endothelial ischemia-reperfusion injury in humans: role of the autonomic nervous system. J Am Coll Cardiol. 2005;46:450–6.
87. Konstantinov IE, Li J, Cheung MM, et al. Remote ischemic preconditioning of the recipient reduces myocardial ischemia-reperfusion injury of the denervated donor heart via a Katp channel-dependent mechanism. Transplantation. 2005;79:1691–5.
88. Dickson EW, Lorbar M, Porcaro WA, et al. Rabbit heart can be "preconditioned" via transfer of coronary effluent. Am J Physiol. 1999;277:H2451–7.
89. Patel HH, Moore J, Hsu AK, Gross GJ. Cardioprotection at a distance: mesenteric artery occlusion protects the myocardium via an opioid sensitive mechanism. J Mol Cell Cardiol. 2002;34:1317–23.
90. Hajrasouliha AR, Tavakoli S, Ghasemi M, et al. Endogenous cannabinoids contribute to remote ischemic preconditioning via cannabinoid CB2 receptors in the rat heart. Eur J Pharmacol. 2008;579:246–52.

91. Shimizu M, Sexena P, Konstantinov IE, et al. Remote ischemic preconditioning decreases adhesion and selectively modifies functional responses of human neutrophils. J Surg Res. 2009;158:155–61.
92. Konstantinov IE, Arab S, Kharbanda RK, et al. The remote ischemic preconditioning stimulus modifies inflammatory gene expression in humans. Physiol Genomics. 2004;19:143–50.
93. Konstantinov IE, Arab S, Li J, et al. The remote ischemic preconditioning stimulus modifies gene expression in mouse myocardium. J Thorac Cardiovasc Surg. 2005;130:1326–32.
94. Loukogeorgakis SP, Williams R, Panagiotidou AT, et al. Transient limb ischemia induces remote preconditioning and remote postconditioning in humans by a K(ATP)-channel dependent mechanism. Circulation. 2007;116:1386–95.
95. Hoole SP, Heck PM, Sharples L, et al. Cardiac Remote Ischemic Preconditioning in Coronary Stenting (CRISP Stent) Study: a prospective, randomized control trial. Circulation. 2009;119: 820–7.
96. Gunaydin B, Cakici I, Soncul H, et al. Does remote organ ischaemia trigger cardiac preconditioning during coronary artery surgery? Pharmacol Res. 2000;41:493–6.
97. Cheung MM, Kharbanda RK, Konstantinov IE, et al. Randomized controlled trial of the effects of remote ischemic preconditioning on children undergoing cardiac surgery: first clinical application in humans. J Am Coll Cardiol. 2006;47:2277–82.
98. Hausenloy DJ, Mwamure PK, Venugopal V, et al. Effect of remote ischaemic preconditioning on myocardial injury in patients undergoing coronary artery bypass graft surgery: a randomized controlled trial. Lancet. 2007;370:575–9.
99. Venugopal V, Hausenloy DJ, Ludman A, et al. Remote ischaemic preconditioning reduces myocardial injury in patients undergoing cardiac surgery with cold blood cardioplegia: a randomised controlled trial. Heart. 2009;95(19):1567–71.
100. Ali ZA, Callaghan CJ, Lim E, et al. Remote ischemic preconditioning reduces myocardial and renal injury after elective abdominal aortic aneurysm repair: a randomized controlled trial. Circulation. 2007;116(11 suppl):I98–105.
101. Kerendi F, Kin H, Halkos ME, et al. Remote postconditioning. Brief renal ischemia and reperfusion applied before coronary artery reperfusion reduces myocardial infarct size via endogenous activation of adenosine receptors. Basic Res Cardiol. 2005;100:404–12.
102. Schmidt MR, Smerup M, Konstantinov IE, et al. Intermittent peripheral tissue ischemia during coronary ischemia reduces myocardial infarction through a KATP-dependentmechanism: first demonstration of remote ischemic perconditioning. Am J Physiol Heart Circ Physiol. 2007;292:H1883–90.
103. Andreka G, Vertesaljai M, Szantho G, et al. Remote ischaemic postconditioning protects the heart during acute myocardial infarction in pigs. Heart. 2007;93:749–52.
104. Botker HE, Kharbanda R, Schmidt MR, et al. Remote ischaemic conditioning before hospital admission, as a complement to angioplasty, and effect on myocardial salvage in patients with acute myocardial infarction: a randomised trial. Lancet. 2010;375:727–34.
105. Prasad A, Gossel M, Hoyt J, Lennon R, Polk L, Simari R, Holmes D, Rihal C, Lerman A. Remote ischemic preconditioning immediately before percutaneous coronary intervention does not impact myocardial necrosis, inflammatory response and circulating endothelial progenitor cell counts. Catheter Cardiovasc Interv. 2012 Apr 19. doi:10.1002/ccd.24443. [Epub ahead of print]

Chapter 12
Novel Treatment Strategies

Derek J. Hausenloy and Derek M. Yellon

Abstract Ischemic heart disease (IHD) is the leading cause of death and disability worldwide. One major consequence of IHD is an acute myocardial infarction (AMI), the treatment of which is timely myocardial reperfusion using either thrombolytic therapy or primary percutaneous coronary intervention (PPCI). Paradoxically, restoring coronary blood flow to the ischemic myocardium can in itself induce the death of previously viable cardiomyocytes—a phenomenon termed 'lethal myocardial reperfusion injury', the presence of which mitigates the full benefits of myocardial reperfusion injury and which therefore provides an important target for cardioprotection. Ischemic postconditioning, an intervention comprising the interruption of myocardial reperfusion using intermittent short-lived episodes of myocardial ischemia (discussed in Chap. 11), prevents lethal myocardial reperfusion injury and the elucidation of the underlying intracellular signal transduction pathways have resulted in the identification of several novel therapeutic approaches for pharmacologically targeting lethal myocardial reperfusion injury (termed 'pharmacological postconditioning'). In this chapter, we review novel pharmacological and non-pharmacological therapeutic strategies for preventing lethal myocardial reperfusion injury in patients presenting with an AMI undergoing PPCI, some of which may have the potential to improve clinical outcomes in patients with IHD.

Keywords Myocardial reperfusion injury • Acute myocardial infarction • Primary percutaneous coronary intervention • Cardioprotection

---

D.J. Hausenloy, B.Sc.(Hons), MBChB, MRCP, Ph.D., FESC, FACC (✉)
D.M. Yellon, D.Sc., FESC, FACC
UCL Institute of Cardiovascular Science, The Hatter Cardiovascular Institute,
University College London Hospital,
67 Chenies Mews, London WC1E 6HX, UK
e-mail: d.hausenloy@ucl.ac.uk

J.C. Kaski et al. (eds.), *Management of Myocardial Reperfusion Injury*,
DOI 10.1007/978-1-84996-019-9_12, © Springer-Verlag London 2012

Introduction

In recent years, the concept of lethal myocardial reperfusion injury as a viable target for protecting the heart from acute ischemia-reperfusion injury (IRI) has emerged [1]. The demonstration that an intervention applied at the onset of myocardial reperfusion has the ability to limit myocardial infarct (MI) size has provided convincing evidence for the existence of lethal myocardial reperfusion injury [1]. Furthermore, the recent realization that this concept can actually be translated into the clinical setting of an acute myocardial infarction (AMI) has confirmed the existence of lethal myocardial reperfusion injury in humans [2, 3]. The elucidation of the complex mechanistic pathways underlying ischemic preconditioning (IPC) and postconditioning (IPost) has not only delineated the intracellular signal transduction pathways of cardioprotection present within a cardiomyocyte but has also identified a number of targets amenable to pharmacological and non-pharmacological manipulation at the time of myocardial reperfusion (Fig. 12.1) [4, 5]. The endogenous cardioprotective strategies such as remote ischemic conditioning and ischemic postconditioning, which also target lethal myocardial reperfusion injury, are reviewed in Chap. 11.

In this chapter, we review the pharmacological and non-pharmacological therapeutic strategies for preventing lethal myocardial reperfusion injury in patients presenting with an ST elevation MI undergoing primary percutaneous coronary intervention (PPCI). It is clear that any therapeutic strategy which maintains the patency of the infarct-related coronary artery and therefore facilitates the reperfusion of ischemic myocardium, such as new developments in anti-platelet and antithrombotic therapy, thrombus aspiration and distal protection devices, is likely to reduce the microvascular component of myocardial reperfusion injury. Recent developments in these therapeutic strategies are reviewed in Chap. 10. This chapter will focus on those therapeutic strategies which are focused on protecting the myocardium from the detrimental effects of lethal myocardial reperfusion injury. In this regard, it must be appreciated that up to very recently the results have been on the whole, overwhelmingly disappointing. This apparent failure to translate cardioprotective strategies from the basic science studies to the clinical setting is multifactorial and has been the subject of recent debate (see section 'Barriers to the translation of cardioprotective therapies') [6–9].

Pharmacological Treatment Strategies

A wide variety of different pharmacological treatment strategies have been investigated as adjuncts to myocardial reperfusion. Many of the earlier therapeutic strategies, which targeted individual mediators of lethal myocardial reperfusion injury such as antioxidant therapy, calcium channel blockers, sodium-hydrogen exchange inhibitors and magnesium therapy, have produced disappointing results, and these findings are reviewed elsewhere [1]. In this chapter, we focus on the more promising and novel therapeutic strategies for reducing lethal myocardial reperfusion injury.

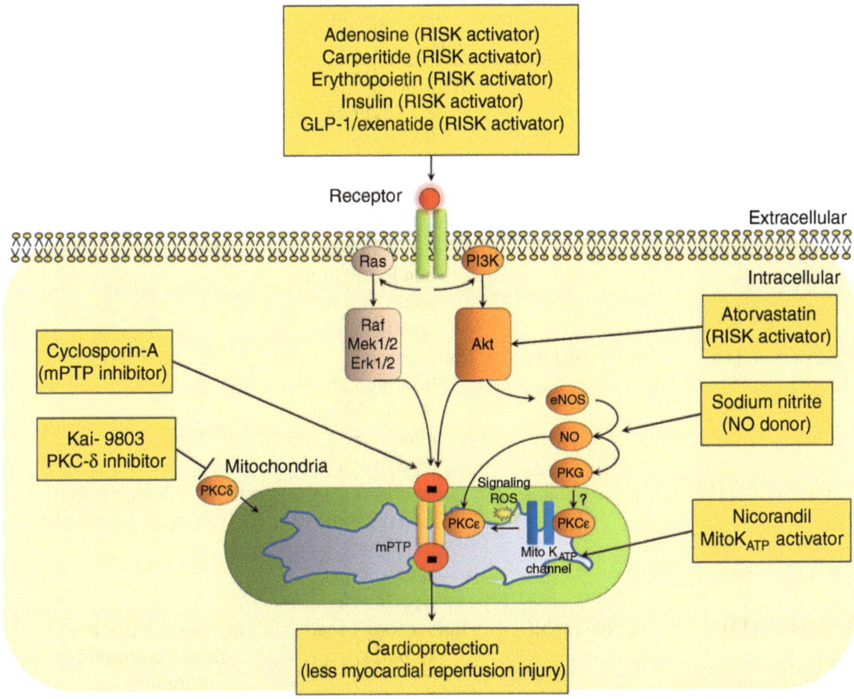

Fig. 12.1 This scheme depicts the sites of action of a number of pharmacological agents which have been or will be investigated as adjuncts to PPCI in patients. Many of the pharmacological agents (adenosine, carperitide, erythropoietin, insulin, GLP-1 and exenatide) are believed to activate receptors on the cardiomyocyte sarcolemma, which then recruits a variety of signal transduction pathways including the reperfusion injury salvage kinase (*RISK*) pathway, which comprises the pro-survival kinase cascades, Ras-Raf-MEK1/2-Erk1/2 and PI3K-Akt. For clarity, only these two major signalling pathways have been shown, but it must be noted that a number of other signal transduction pathways have also been implicated in cardioprotection. These signalling pathways then converge on the mitochondria resulting in the inhibition of the mitochondrial permeability transition pore (*mPTP*) either directly or via the mitochondrial ATP-dependent potassium (MitoK$_{ATP}$) channel and signalling reactive oxygen species (ROS). A variety of other pharmacological agents are believed to target other mediators or effectors in the signal transduction pathway such as the detrimental pro-apoptotic PKC-δ (KAI-9803), the mPTP (cyclosporin A), the MitoK$_{ATP}$ channel (nicorandil), nitric oxide (sodium nitrite) and the RISK pathway (atorvastatin)

Adenosine

Preclinical Studies

The purine nucleoside, adenosine, generated by cardiomyocytes during myocardial ischemia from the breakdown of ATP, accumulates in the myocardial interstitium resulting in a 100-fold increase in concentration [10]. Adenosine has been demonstrated to play pivotal role in cardioprotection, having been implicated as one of the first triggers of IPC [11], a mediator of IPost [12] and a cardioprotective agent in its

Table 12.1 The effect of adenosine at reperfusion in preclinical animal studies

Study	Model	Adenosine	Effects
Olaffson et al. [13]	In vivo canine	Intracoronary 3.75 mg/min for 60 min after reperfusion	↓IR, ↑radial function, ↓neutrophil infiltration, ↑myocardial blood flow
Norton et al. [14]	In vivo rabbit	Intravenous 0.1, 0.3, 0.55 mg/min for 60 min after reperfusion	↓IR,↑myocardial blood flow
Pitarys et al. [15]	In vivo canine	Intracoronary 0.15 mg/kg/min for 90 min after reperfusion	↓IR at 72 h reperfusion
Velasco et al. [16]	In vivo canine	Intracoronary 3.75 mg/min for 60 min after reperfusion	↓IR at 72 h reperfusion
Todd et al. [17]	In vivo rabbit	Intravenous 1 mg/kg bolus	↓IR, ↑myocardial blood flow, ↓neutrophil infiltration
Zhao et al. [18]	In vivo canine	Intracoronary 140 mg/kg/min for 90 min after reperfusion	↓IR at 72 h reperfusion
Zhao et al. [19]	In vivo canine	Intracoronary 140 mg/kg/min for 90 min after reperfusion	↓IR at 72 h reperfusion and less apoptosis

IR infarct to risk ratio

own right [13]. Adenosine binds to four G-protein-coupled receptor subtypes A1, A2A, A2B and A3, all of which are present in the heart except for the A2A receptor subtype. The roles the different subtypes play in cardioprotection with respect to IPC and IPost have been widely debated in the literature [10].

Whether adenosine can prevent lethal myocardial reperfusion injury when administered at the onset of myocardial reperfusion has been a contentious issue [10]. Several experimental animal studies have reported limitation in MI size with adenosine therapy administered at myocardial reperfusion [13], whereas other studies have failed to observe any beneficial effect of adenosine in the reperfused heart (Table 12.1). The reason for these disparate findings is unclear, but it may be due to the use of different animal experimental models.

In 1995, the first experimental studies to implicate adenosine as a mediator of IPC in ex vivo human atrial trabeculae and human ventricular cardiomyocytes were published by Yellon's group [20] and Ikonomidis et al. [21], respectively. Of course, the next important hurdle was to investigate adenosine as a cardioprotective agent in the clinical setting.

Clinical Studies

The seminal finding by Downey's laboratory that exogenous adenosine could mimic the infarct-limiting effects of IPC provided the stimulus for investigators to explore the role of adenosine as a mediator of IPC in the clinical setting of elective PCI. It is important to appreciate that using the setting of elective PCI in which one angioplasty balloon inflation reduces the ST-segment shift and chest pain elicited by subsequent angioplasty balloon inflations, a model which was first used in 1990 [22], is not a true model of IPC, given that there is no index lethal ischemic event. Using this clinical model of IPC, an initial study by Tomai and colleagues [23] discovered that the salutatory effects of IPC could be abolished by the A1 adenosine receptor antagonist, bamiphylline, implicating a role for this receptor in IPC protection at least in the setting of elective PCI. Leesar and colleagues [24] went onto demonstrate that a 10-min intracoronary infusion of adenosine [2 mg/min] prior to elective PCI reduced ST-segment shift with angioplasty balloon inflations and lowered chest pain. The beneficial effects of adenosine observed in the setting of elective PCI have been confirmed in subsequent studies.

STEMI Patients Undergoing PPCI

A number of clinical studies have investigated the effect of adenosine administered as an adjunct to PPCI in STEMI patients (see Table 12.2 for a summary). Overall, adenosine therapy is associated with improve myocardial perfusion following PPCI in most but not all these studies, suggesting that adenosine may be reducing coronary no-reflow (microvascular obstruction). However, the administration of adenosine at the onset of myocardial reperfusion did not reduce lethal myocardial reperfusion injury as evidenced by the absence of MI limitation [30, 36], although a post-hoc subgroup analysis did suggest that patients presenting with an anterior STEMI within 3 h of chest pain may benefit from adenosine in terms of MI size reduction [31]. The failure to observe MI size reduction with adenosine administered at the onset of myocardial reperfusion in the clinical studies may have been predicted from the inconclusive findings of the animal MI studies, an issue which is revisited in section 'Barriers to the translation of cardioprotective therapies'.

Table 12.2 The effect of adenosine as an adjunct to PPCI

Study	*N* number	Adenosine	Effects
Garratt et al. [25]	45	IV 70 μ(mu)g/kg/min plus IV lidocaine (1 mg/kg bolus then 2 mg/kg/min infusion)	Safety study
Assali et al. [26]	79	Intracoronary bolus of 24–48 μ(mu)g before and after each angioplasty inflation (total 98 ± 78 μ(mu)g/patient)	↓no reflow from 28.6% to 5.9%
Marzilli et al. [27]	54	Intracoronary bolus of 4 mg over 1 min	↓no reflow, ↓CK release, ↓Q wave MI. Improved regional wall motion
Claeys et al. [28]	79	Intracoronary 20 min infusion of dose of 60 μ(mu)g/min for the right coronary artery and 90 μ(mu)g/min for the left coronary artery	Not a randomized study. Improved ST-segment resolution
Lim et al. [29]	50	Intracoronary adenosine (24 μ(mu)g/ml) versus intracoronary adenosine + nicorandil (2 mg/ml)	Increased myocardial blush grade with combined adenosine + nicorandil compared to adenosine alone
Ross et al. AMISTAD-II [30]	2118 Anterior STEMI only	IV 3 h infusion of adenosine 50 or 70 μ(mu)g/kg/min	No difference in 6 months primary endpoint of heart failure and death. Although trend to infarct size reduction with higher-dose
Kloner et al. [31]	2118 Anterior STEMI patients presenting <3.17 h	IV 3 h infusion of adenosine 50 or 70 μ(mu)g/kg/min	Post-hoc analysis of AMISTAD-II. Those patients presenting <3.17 h of chest pain and who received thrombolysis had less mortality and a reduced primary endpoint of heart failure and death

Table 12.2 (continued)

Study	*N* number	Adenosine	Effects
Vijayalakshmi et al. [32]	150	Intracoronary bolus of adenosine (30 mg in 10 ml of heparinized saline) or bolus of verapamil (500 μ(mu)g in 10 ml of heparinized saline given over a minute)	Improved coronary flow and wall motion index with adenosine
Parikh et al. [33]	150	Intracoronary bolus of adenosine (12 μ(mu)g) or bolus of sodium nitroprusside (50 μ(mu)g)	Improved TIMI flow with combination of adenosine and sodium nitroprusside
Stoel et al. [34]	51	Intracoronary bolus of 60 mg in 10 ml NaCl 0.9% infused in 5–10 min	Improved ST-segment resolution, myocardial blush grade, TIMI frame count
Fokkema et al. [35]	448	Intracoronary 120 μ(mu)g bolus prior to thrombus aspiration and post-stent deployment	No difference in ST-segment resolution, myocardial blush grade, TIMI flow, enzyme infarct size or clinical outcome

Nicorandil

The mitochondrial K_{ATP} channel was first proposed to be a critical mediator or effector for cardioprotection elicited by ischemic preconditioning in 1997 [37, 38]. Subsequent experimental studies have implicated its role in ischemic postconditioning and pharmacological conditioning mediated by drugs such as diazoxide and nicorandil [39, 40]. Having not been cloned, the role of this channel as a mediator or effector of IPC has been heavily dependent on the effects of diazoxide (as an agonist) and 5-hydroxydecanoate (as an antagonist), pharmacological agents which are known to have non-specific actions on mitochondrial function [41]. As such, controversy surrounds the existence of this channel in mitochondria, a subject which has been debated extensively elsewhere [41, 42]. Whether diazoxide and nicorandil, purported activators of this channel, confer cardioprotection when administered at the onset of myocardial reperfusion is inconclusive [43–49].

In the clinical setting, a number of clinical studies have reported beneficial effects of nicorandil against coronary no-reflow [50] (improved myocardial perfusion, better ST-segment resolution and less LV remodelling) when administered as an adjunct to PPCI. However, a direct cardioprotective effect against lethal myocardial reperfusion injury in terms of MI size reduction and preserved cardiac function was not observed with nicorandil as an adjunct to PPCI in the large J-WIND clinical study (Table 12.3). The failure of nicorandil to reduce lethal myocardial reperfusion injury could have been again predicted by the inconclusive animal MI studies.

Atrial Natriuretic Peptide

Several experimental animal MI studies have reported a reduction in MI size with either atrial natriuretic peptide (ANP) [67] or B-type natriuretic peptide (BNP) [68] administered at the onset of myocardial reperfusion. The mechanisms underlying the cardioprotection elicited by ANP, which include the pro-survival protein kinases such as PI3K and PKG (see Fig. 12.1), have been reviewed elsewhere [69, 70]. An early clinical study by Hayashi and co-workers [71] investigated the role of ANP as a therapeutic strategy for reducing adverse LV remodelling following an AMI as opposed to having a direct cardioprotective effect against lethal myocardial reperfusion injury. These authors found that intravenous ANP administered to anterior STEMI patients following PPCI preserved LV ejection fraction and reduced LV dilatation at 1 month [71].

A subsequent large clinical study called the J-WIND study reported modest beneficial effects against lethal myocardial reperfusion injury of carperitide (an ANP agonist) administered as an adjunct to PPCI (please see Table 12.3) [65]. However, it is important to note that in 29 patients receiving this therapeutic strategy versus 1 patient receiving placebo, there was severe hypotension [65]. Whether a greater cardioprotective effect would have been observed by this therapeutic strategy in higher-risk patients is unknown and remains to be determined. In other words, by including all-comers in the J-WIND study, the cardioprotective effect of carperitide may have been diluted.

PKC-δ(delta) Inhibitors

Protein kinase C has been implicated as a critical mediator of cardioprotection elicited by both ischemic preconditioning and postconditioning [72]. The actual PKC isoform involved does vary between species and setting. However, in general, the activation of the PKC-ε(epsilon) isoform at the time of myocardial reperfusion in animal infarct studies has been reported to protect the heart against lethal myocardial reperfusion injury, whereas the activation of the PKC-δ(delta) isoform is detrimental, contributing to both apoptotic and necrotic cell death associated with lethal myocardial reperfusion injury (see Fig. 12.1) [72]. The pharmacological inhibition of PKC-δ(delta) with a small peptide inhibitor, which specifically targets the PKC-δ(delta) receptor for activated C-kinase (RACK) at the time of myocardial

Table 12.3 Recently published clinical studies investigating novel pharmacological adjuncts to myocardial reperfusion (PPCI) in STEMI patients

Study	*N* number Patient	Therapeutic strategy	Results
Atorvastatin			
Kim et al. [51] STATIN STEMI	171 STEMI <12 h treated by PPCI	Atorvastatin 80 mg versus atorvastatin 10 mg *prior* to PPCI	No effect on primary endpoint of (death, MI, revasc). No difference in MI size (CKMB max). Improved myocardial perfusion (blush grade, ST-segment resolution)
Hahn et al. [52]	173 STEMI <12 h treated by PPCI	Atorvastatin 10mg daily for 5 days initiated within 12 h of PPCI	No difference in MI size (SPECT)
Cyclosporin A			
Piot et al. and Mewton et al. [53, 54]	58 STEMI <12 h treated by PPCI	IV CsA (2.5 mg/kg) *prior* to PPCI	44% reduction in MI size (72 h AUC total CK), 20% reduction in MI size (CMR in subset of 27 patients), non-significant 13% reduction in MI size (72 h Trop I). At 6 months 28% reduction in MI size and smaller LVESV on CMR
Erythropoietin			
Lipsic et al. [55]	22 STEMI <6 h treated by PPCI	IV darbepoetin alpha 300 m(mu)g (a long-acting formulation of EPO) *prior* to PPCI	No effect on LVEF at 4 months
Ferriario et al. [56]	30 STEMI <6 h treated by PPCI	IV EPO 33,000 iU *prior* to PPCI repeated 24 and 48 h later	30% reduction in 120 h AUC CK-MB but no difference in MI size using CMR at 3 days and 6 months
Suh et al. [57]	57 Ant STEMI <12 h treated by PPCI	IV rhEPO 50 U/kg *prior* to PPCI	No beneficial effects on MI size (assessed by CK-MB and CMR at 4 days)
Ozawa et al. EPO-AMI-1 [58]	36 STEMI <24 h treated by PPCI	IV EPO epoetin-beta 12,000 iU *after* (within 24 h) PPCI	No difference in MI size or LVEF at 6 months

(continued)

Table 12.3 (continued)

Study	*N* number Patient	Therapeutic strategy	Results
Voors et al. HEBE-*III* [59]	529 STEMI <12 h treated by PPCI	IV EPO epoetin-alpha 60,000 iU *after* (within 3 h) PPCI	No difference in LVEF at 6 weeks (primary endpoint). No difference in MI size (AUC CK-MB AND Trop-T). Improved MACE (secondary endpoint)
Tanaguichi et al. [60]	35 STEMI <12 h treated by PPCI	IV EPO epoetin-alpha 6,000 iU *after* (within 3 h) PPCI repeated 24 and 48 h later	No difference in LVEF at 4 days or 6 months using SPECT
Ott et al. REVIVAL-3 [61]	138 STEMI <12 h treated by PPCI	IV EPO epoetin-beta 33,000 iU immediately *after* PPCI repeated 24 and 48 h later	No difference in LVEF at 6 months assessed by CMR (primary endpoint). No difference in MI size (5 days and 6 month CMR). Trend to increased adverse events with EPO (6-month incidence of death, recurrent myocardial infarction, stroke or target vessel revascularization)
Rao et al. REVEAL [unpublished]	138 STEMI <8 h treated by PPCI	IV EPO epoetin-beta 60,000 IU immediately *after* PPCI repeated 24 and 48 h later	No difference in MI size on CMR within 6 days and 3 months trend to increased adverse events in patients over 70 years old
Ludman et al. [62]	52 STEMI <12 h treated by PPCI	IV EPO epoetin-beta 50,000 iU *prior* to PPCI repeated 24 h later	No difference in LVEF at 6 months assessed by CMR (primary endpoint). No difference in MI size at 3 days using CMR and troponin T. doubling of incidence of MVO and increased volumes and mass acutely with EPO treatment. No difference at 4 months of CMR in any of the variables
Glucagon-like peptide-1			
Nikolaides et al. [63]	22 patients with LVEF <40% STEMI <6 h treated by PPCI	Intravenous infusion of GLP-1 (1.5 pmol/kg/min) for 72 h started 2 h *after* PPCI	Improved LVEF, better regional wall motion at 6–12 h

Lonborg et al. [64]	172 STEMI <12 h treated by PPCI	Exenatide infusion started prior to PPCI	Increased myocardial salvage (SPECT)
Atrial natriuretic peptide			
Kitakaze et al. [65] J-WIND	569 patients STEMI <12 h treated by PPCI	Intravenous carperitide infusion at 0·025 m(mu)g/kg/min for 3 days started *after* PPCI	14.7% reduction in MI size (total CK AUC). 2.5% increased in LVEF at 6–12 months
Nicorandil			
Kitakaze et al. [65] J-WIND	545 patients Ant STEMI <12 h treated by PPCI	Intravenous bolus of nicorandil (0·067 mg/kg)m followed by infusion at 1·67 m(mu)g/kg/min for 24 h for 3 days. Started *after* PPCI	No difference in MI size or LVEF
PKC-d(delta) inhibitor			
Bates et al. DELTA-MI [66]	154 Ant STEMI <6 h treated by PPCI	Intracoronary KAI-9803 at different doses (0.05, 0.5, 1.25 and 5.0 mg) administered in two divided doses prior to and after PPCI	Safe, efficacy not primary endpoint but non-significant reductions in MI size by CK-MB and SPECT

MI myocardial infarct, *STR* ST-segment resolution, *STEMI* ST elevation MI, *PPCI* primary percutaneous coronary intervention, *CMR* cardiac MRI, *AUC* area under the curve

reperfusion, has been reported to reduce MI size in both small and large animal IRI studies [72] and to improve the recovery of contractile function in human atrial trabeculae subjected to ischemia-reperfusion injury [73].

In the DELTA-MI clinical study, KAI-9803, an isozyme-specific PKC-δ(delta) inhibitor, was investigated first-in-man using a range of different doses (cohorts 1–4 with a progressive increase in dose) in anterior STEMI patients undergoing PPCI (see Table 12.3) [66]. The drug was administered via the intracoronary route with half the dose given prior to the opening of the infarct-related coronary artery and the other half given after the coronary artery had been opened. Due to difficulties in recruitment in North America (predominantly cohorts 1 and 2), the study was extended to Europe and Brazil (predominantly cohorts 3 and 4) resulting in heterogeneous patient populations and marked differences in key patient characteristics such as chest pain to PCI time and the maximum degree of ST elevation. However, despite these difficulties and bearing in mind that this study was not designed to assess efficacy of this therapeutic strategy, there were no safety issues and there was a trend to beneficial effects with this agent (see Table 12.3). However, the follow-up large phase IIb clinical study (PROTECTION AMI), which investigated the effects of peripheral intravenous KAI-9803 in the same patient group, failed to demonstrated any difference in MI size (CK-MB area under the curve) (Table 12.4).

Cyclosporin A

The immunosuppressive agent, cyclosporin A (CsA), has been pivotal in implicating the mitochondrial permeability transition pore (mPTP) as a critical mediator of cell death in the setting of ischemia-reperfusion injury [74, 75]. In 1988, Crompton and colleagues made the seminal discovery that CsA was able to inhibit the opening of the mPTP [74], a non-selective channel of the inner mitochondrial membrane, whose opening results in uncoupling of oxidative phosphorylation and ATP depletion followed by cell death (see Fig. 12.1). The observation that this phenomenon could be inhibited by CsA implicated mitochondrial cyclophilin D as an important regulatory component of the mPTP, an assertion which has subsequently been proven in genetic ablation studies [76–78].

Our laboratory and others have reported that pharmacologically inhibiting mPTP at the onset of myocardial reperfusion limited myocardial infarct size by 40–50% in small animal models [79–82] and improved recovery of contractile function in human atrial trabeculae subjected to simulated ischemia-reperfusion injury [83]. However, the larger animal infarct studies, which have investigated CsA administered at the onset of myocardial reperfusion in the pig, have been inconclusive [84–86]. Furthermore, the problem with CsA as a pharmacological inhibitor of mPTP is that it has non-specific effects through its inhibitory actions on other cyclophilins and on calcineurin. There do exist, however, a number of cyclophilin D inhibitors which do not inhibit calcineurin such as NIM811 and sanglifehrin A, but none of these have been developed for clinical use.

Table 12.4 Ongoing or planned clinical studies investigating novel pharmacological agents as adjuncts to myocardial reperfusion (PPCI) in STEMI patients

Study	*N*	Therapeutic strategy	Results
Cyclosporin A			
Ovize's group CIRCUS NCT01502774	972 patients STEMI <12 h treated by PPC	IV CsA (2.5 mg/kg) *prior* to PPCI	Death and hospitalization for heart failure
Exenatide			
Netherlands group Phase III study EXAMI (ongoing) NCT01254123	40 patients STEMI <6 h treated by PPCI	IV bolus of exenatide (5 μ(mu)g) in 30 min, followed by a continuous infusion of 20 μ(mu)g/24 h. Treatment started *prior* to PPC	Safety study. Numerous secondary endpoints including MI size, LVEF, myocardial perfusion
Denmark group Phase IV study POSTCOND II (ongoing) NCT01254123	100 patients STEMI <12 h treated by PPCI	IV infusion of exenatide (25 μ(mu)g) at 72 ml/h for 15 min, followed by 26 ml/h for 6 h. Treatment started *prior* to PPCI	Primary endpoint MI size by CMR at 3 months. Final data collection December 2009
Glucose insulin potassium			
Phase II study (ongoing) IMMEDIATE NCT00091507	880 patients All acute coronary syndrome patients treated by PPCI	Intravenous infusion of glucose insulin potassium1.5 ml/kg/h for 12 h started by paramedics in ambulance	Primary endpoint MI size
Sodium nitrite therapy			
Phase II study (ongoing) NCT00924118	STEMI <6 h treated by PPCI	Intravenous infusion of sodium nitrite (6 nmol/min/kg) for 48 h administered at time of PPCI	Primary endpoint MI size by SPECT. Study completion expected Sept. 2011
PKC-δ(delta) inhibitor			
PROTECTION AMI Phase IIb study NCT00785954	1058 Ant STEMI <6 h treated by PPCI	Intravenous KAI-9803 administered at time of PPCI	No difference in primary endpoint (area under curve CK-MB)

MI myocardial infarct, *STR* ST-segment resolution, *STEMI* ST elevation MI, *PPCI* primary percutaneous coronary intervention, *CMR* cardiac MRI, *AUC* area under the curve

Despite these issues, Piot and co-workers [53] have been able to demonstrate, in a small proof-of-concept clinical study comprising 58 patients, a significant reduction in MI size in STEMI patients administered a single intravenous bolus of CsA (2.5 mg/kg) prior to PPCI (see Table 12.3). Crucially, the beneficial effects of a single bolus of CsA administered prior to PPCI were still present 6 months later as assessed by cardiac MRI, thereby demonstrating long-term cardioprotection and the absence of adverse effects with this treatment strategy [54]. However, these findings are preliminary and need to be confirmed in large multi-centre clinical studies especially given the inconclusive large animal MI studies. In this respect, the CIRCUS (Does Cyclosporine ImpRove Clinical oUtcome in ST elevation myocardial infarction) study is a large European multi-centre randomized clinical trial designed to investigate whether CsA can improve clinical outcomes (death and hospitalization for heart failure) in PPCI patients (see Table 12.4) NCT01502774. Clearly, novel, safe and effective mPTP inhibitors need to be discovered in order to realize the potential of this therapeutic strategy for preventing lethal myocardial reperfusion injury.

Erythropoietin

The haematopoietic cytokine, erythropoietin (EPO), has been reported to reduce MI size when administered either prior to myocardial ischemia, at the onset of myocardial reperfusion or even delayed into myocardial reperfusion using both in vivo and ex vivo animal (murine, rat, rabbit and dog) MI models (reviewed in [87]). This cardioprotective effect appears to be independent of its haematopoietic effect and is mediated through the activation of EPO receptors, known to be present in cardiomyocytes, and downstream pro-survival kinase signalling pathways (see Fig. 12.1) [87]. However, it is important to note that the large animal (sheep and pig) in vivo MI studies failed to report a reduction in MI size with EPO therapy for reasons which are not clear [88–90].

Despite this, a number of clinical studies have investigated the effect of high-dose EPO as an adjunct to myocardial reperfusion in STEMI patients undergoing PPCI (these are summarized in Table 12.3). Overall, the results have been overwhelmingly disappointing with no effect on MI size and possibly detrimental effects with increased incidence of microvascular obstruction and adverse clinical outcomes. Interestingly, the use of high-dose EPO has been reported to have detrimental effects in a number of other clinical settings such as stroke and cancer. The failure to translate the effects of EPO observed in the preclinical setting into the clinical arena can be attributed to a number of different factors including the lack of consistent cardioprotection in the preclinical setting with no beneficial effect on MI size observed in the large animal MI models, the timing of EPO therapy which should have been administered prior to and not after PPCI, and potential pro-thrombotic off-target effects of EPO.

Atorvastatin

Chronic statin therapy has resulted in large reductions in cardiovascular disease risk in both patients with established coronary heart disease and in patients at risk of developing coronary heart disease [91]. The benefits of this therapy can in part be attributed to its intensive lowering of LDL cholesterol but are also due to a variety of pleiotropic effects [92]. In this regard, it has been reported in animal IRI models that the administration of a statin such as atorvastatin or simvastatin at the onset of myocardial reperfusion can reduce MI size by 40–50% [92]. This cardioprotective effect is independent of the lipid-lowering effects of the drug and is due to the activation of intracellular pro-survival kinase pathways (see Fig. 12.1) [92]. In the clinical setting, atorvastatin therapy has been reported to reduce peri-procedural myocardial injury associated with PCI in patients with stable or unstable coronary heart disease [93, 94].

High-dose atorvastatin (80 mg) therapy initiated 2–3 days following admission for an acute coronary syndrome has been reported to have beneficial effects on major cardiovascular outcomes in the MIRACL and PROVE-IT clinical studies [95, 96]. These beneficial effects were probably not due to the drug's effect on lethal myocardial reperfusion injury but may have been due to other pleiotropic effects of this therapeutic agent. However, two recently published clinical studies have failed to find any difference in MI size with atorvastatin administered at the time of PPCI (see Table 12.3) [51].

Insulin

Metabolic modulation using insulin therapy to promote glucose oxidation protects the heart during myocardial ischemia and reperfusion injury in animal MI studies. In particular, insulin therapy at the onset of myocardial reperfusion is mediated through the activation of pro-survival kinases such as PI3K-Akt (see Fig. 12.1) [97]. In small proof-of-concept clinical studies, GIK therapy has been reported to be beneficial in a number of different clinical settings of IRI including: in patients presenting with an acute myocardial infarction [98], peri-procedural myocardial injury during PCI was reduced in non-diabetic NSTEMI patients [99]; less perioperative myocardial injury in diabetic patients undergoing cardiac bypass surgery [100]; improved myocardial perfusion in STEMI patients undergoing primary PCI [101, 102]. However, in the large randomized placebo-controlled clinical trials, the results with GIK therapy as an adjunct to PPCI have been disappointing. Several large multi-centre clinical trials have failed to report any beneficial effect with GIK therapy in STEMI patients undergoing PPCI (Zwolle infarct (99), GIPS II [103], OASIS-GIK [104] and CREATE-ECLA [105]). The reason for the observed lack of cardioprotection remains unclear. The

Immediate Myocardial Metabolic Enhancement During Initial Assessment and Treatment in Emergency Care Trial (IMMEDIATE: ClinicalTrials.gov Identifier: NCT00091507) study is currently underway, which is investigating whether the administration of the GIK therapy by the paramedics in the ambulance can prevent lethal myocardial reperfusion injury.

Glucagon-Like Peptide-1

In addition to lowering postprandial blood glucose without causing hypoglycaemia, glucagon-like peptide (GLP-1, an incretin) has also been reported to confer direct cardioprotective effects in several different animal MI models through the recruitment of pro-survival kinase pathways (see Fig. 12.1) [106]. Importantly, it has been reported to reduce MI size when administered at the onset of myocardial reperfusion [107, 108]. Endogenous GLP-1 is rapidly broken down by the enzyme dipeptidyl peptidase-4 (DPP-4) limiting its role as exogenous therapy unless it is administered as a continuous infusion. This has provided an opportunity for using DPP-4 inhibitors (sitagliptin, vildagliptin, saxagliptin) or GLP-1 analogues (exenatide, liraglutide) which are resistant to DPP-4 in order to potentiate endogenous GLP-1 as novel anti-diabetic therapies. In the research setting, in which extended GLP-1 infusions have been used even in non-diabetic patients, beneficial effects on LV systolic function have been seen in patients with chronic stable heart failure [109] and in patients presenting with an acute MI and LV systolic impairment [63] (see Table 12.3). Crucially, recent preclinical animal models (mice, rat, pig) suggest that treatment with either DPP-4 inhibitors or GLP-1 analogues can also limit MI size [110, 111]. Two proof-of-concept clinical studies are currently underway investigating the GLP-1 analogue, exenatide, as an adjunct to PPCI (ClinicalTrials.gov: the EXAMI study NCT01254123 and the POSTCOND II study NCT00835848) (see Table 12.4).

Sodium Nitrite

Nitrite (NO^{2-}) can act as a reservoir for the cardioprotective molecule nitric oxide (NO), generating NO under conditions of hypoxia and ischemia (see Fig. 12.1) [112]. Several preclinical studies have demonstrated cardioprotective effects of nitrite therapy in the settings of MI (rat and canine models) [113, 114] and cardiac arrest (murine model) [115]. A number of clinical studies are now underway to investigate whether sodium nitrite therapy is beneficial when administered as an adjunct to PPCI (see Table 12.4).

Anti-inflammatory Agents

An acute myocardial infarction is associated with a marked pro-inflammatory response. Whether this inflammatory reaction actual contributes to the cardiomyocyte death induced by lethal myocardial reperfusion injury or whether it occurs as a result of the ischemia-reperfusion injury insult is unclear. A variety of anti-inflammatory therapeutic strategies have been tried in the clinical setting of an AMI including monoclonal antibodies targeted against neutrophil infiltration, complement activation, cell adhesion molecules and a fibrin-derived peptide (these are summarized in Table 12.5). However, these have on the whole been overwhelmingly disappointing. The failure to translate the findings from promising preclinical experimental studies into the clinical setting is a recurring theme and can be attributed to a number of different factors which are discussed in section 'Barriers to the translation of cardioprotective therapies'.

Mechanical Treatment Strategies

Clearly, one of the most promising mechanical therapeutic strategies from reducing lethal myocardial reperfusion injury in PPCI patients is ischemic postconditioning [123], which has been reported to limit MI size in both the short- and long term and preserved cardiac function at 1 year [2, 124]. The topic of ischemic postconditioning is reviewed elsewhere in Chap. 11. In this chapter, we will focus on two novel mechanical treatment strategies which have been investigated as adjuncts to PPCI.

Therapeutic Hypothermia

Therapeutic hypothermia is currently used to protect the myocardium from acute global ischemia-reperfusion injury sustained during cardiac bypass surgery with the use of cold blood cardioplegia. It has also been recommended for the preservation of neurological function following resuscitation for a cardiac arrest [125]. Experimental studies suggest that therapeutic hypothermia can limit MI size in animal models of IRI (reviewed in [126]). Experimental studies have shown a 10% reduction in MI size for every 1°C drop in body temperature [127]. Recently, the RAPID-MI-ICE trial investigated the beneficial effects of using the Philips Innercool Celsius Control™ System, to lower body core temperature to 35°C, and reported a 38% reduction in MI size (expressed as a percentage of the area at risk) and a 43% reduction in peak and cumulative Trop T release [128]. These initially promising results have led to the on-going CHILL-MI trial.

Table 12.5 The effect of various anti-inflammatory therapeutic strategies as adjunctive therapy to myocardial reperfusion

Study	*N* number Patient	Therapeutic strategy	Results
Baran et al. [116] LIMIT-MI	342 STEMI treated by thrombolysis	IV recombinant, humanized, monoclonal antibody to the CD18 subunit of β(beta)2 integrin adhesion receptors (rhuMAb CD18)	No beneficial effects on coronary flow, STR, MI size (SPECT 5 days later)
Faxon et al. [117] HALT-MI	420 STEMI <6 h treated by PPCI	IV monoclonal antibody to the CD18 subunit of β(beta)2 integrin adhesion receptors (Hu23F2G or Leukarrest)	No beneficial effects on TIMI frame count, MI size (SPECT 5–9 days later)
Mahaffrey et al. [118] COMPLY	943 STEMI <6 h treated by thrombolysis	IV monoclonal antibody to C5 complement (pexelizumab)	No beneficial effects on MI size (24 h AUC CK-MB) or 90-day composite incidence of death, new or worsening congestive heart failure, shock or stroke
Granger et al. [119] COMMA	960 STEMI <6 h treated by PPCI	IV monoclonal antibody to C5 complement (pexelizumab)	No beneficial effects on MI size (24 h AUC CK-MB) or 90-day composite incidence of death, new or worsening congestive heart failure, shock or stroke. However, 90-day mortality was significantly reduced
Mertens et al. [120] RAPSODY		Recombinant P-selectin glycoprotein ligand immunoglobulin (rPSGLIg), a P-selectin antagonist	No beneficial effects on MI size or ejection fraction
Armstrong et al. [121] APEX-MI	5,745 STEMI <6 h treated by PPCI	IV monoclonal antibody to C5 complement (pexelizumab)	No beneficial effects on 30-day mortality
Atar et al. [122]	234	IV FX06, a fibrin-derived peptide which reduces leukocyte migration and tissue	No beneficial effects on MI size (CMR at 5 days)
FIRE	STEMI <6 h treated by PPCI	Inflammation	

MI myocardial infarct, *STR* ST-segment resolution, *STEMI* ST elevation MI, *PPCI* primary percutaneous coronary intervention, *CMR* cardiac MRI, *AUC* area under the curve

Table 12.6 Ischemia and reperfusion in the experimental preclinical models versus the clinical setting: a critical comparison

Factor	Animal IRI model	Clinical IRI setting	Solution
Animal versus patient	Healthy juvenile animals free of co-morbid illnesses on no concomitant medication	Middle-aged patient with co-morbidities (age, diabetes, hypertension) and concomitant medication which may influence cardioprotection	Use aged animals with co-morbidities
Species variation	The susceptibility of the myocardium to IRI varies with species and is influenced by a variety of factor including collateralization	The human heart is relatively resistant to IRI and is often collateralized	Use large animals such as pigs
Ischemic time	Relatively short periods of acute myocardial ischemia ranging from 30 to 60 min. Furthermore, the animals are subjected to the same duration and severity of myocardial ischemia	Ischemic times range from 0 to 12 h. Both the duration and severity of ischemia vary between patients within the same study, factors which may influence cardioprotection	Consider selecting certain patient groups such as those presenting early after symptom onset (<3 h) or those with an anterior MI and so on
Reperfusion time	Reperfusion times are relatively short, ranging from 30 min to 3 days	Much longer periods of reperfusion, allowing time for the effects of infarct healing and LV remodelling to take place	The use of longer periods of myocardial reperfusion using echo or cardiac MRI to assess LV remodelling should be encouraged
Infarction model	In most animal studies, acute coronary occlusion is mechanically induced in healthy coronary arteries	Acute coronary occlusion is due to thrombus formation at a site of a ruptured coronary atherosclerotic plaque in a pro-inflammatory milieu	Use atherosclerotic animal hearts
Timing of intervention	The timing of the intervention in relation to the ischemic time and the onset of myocardial reperfusion is the same in all animals	The timing of the intervention should be guided by the animal infarct studies	Adjuncts of PPCI should be administered prior to myocardial reperfusion

(continued)

Table 12.6 (continued)

Factor	Animal IRI model	Clinical IRI setting	Solution
Infarct size	The infarct size for animal studies varies from 30% to 60% of the ischemic risk volume, giving a greater scope for cardioprotection	In the clinical setting, infarct sizes of 13–16% expressed as a percentage of left ventricular volume (using SPECT) appear to be the normal range, which may limit the scope for cardioprotection	Encourage the use of more accurate measurement of infarct size using delayed enhancement cardiac MRI, which can express infarct size as a percentage of ischemic risk zone in AMI patients
Endpoints of cardioprotection	Most animal studies use recovery of LV function or myocardial infarct size as their measured endpoints of cardioprotection	The clinically relevant endpoints for assessing cardioprotective benefit are clinical outcomes such as short- and long-term effects on morbidity and mortality	More robust endpoints of cardioprotection should be considered in animal studies such as long-term effects on left ventricular function and mortality

Dixon and co-workers [129] were the first to demonstrate in the proof-of-concept clinical study that mild hypothermia induced by endovascular cooling of the patient to 34.7°C was safe in STEMI patients undergoing PPCI, although no beneficial effect was seen on MI size measured by SPECT. The large COOL-MI (393 patients) [130] and ICE-T (228 patients) [131] clinical trials of PPCI patients, however, did not observe any reduction in MI size with therapeutic hypothermia, although there was the suggestion of MI limitation in those patients presenting with the large anterior STEMI. The results of the COOL-MI II clinical study (ClinicalTrials.gov Identifier: NCT00248196) are awaited to determine prospectively whether anterior STEMI patients undergoing PPCI will benefit from endovascular cooling. The clear disadvantages of this therapeutic strategy are its invasive nature and the requirement to delay PPCI.

Hyperoxemic Therapy

Hyperoxemic therapy with aqueous oxygen has been reported to reduce lethal myocardial reperfusion injury and limit MI size in experimental models of IRI [132]. Based on this principle, Dixon and co-workers [133] were the first to demonstrate in the proof-of-concept clinical study that intracoronary reperfusion with aqueous oxygen (pO_2 600–800 mmHg) administered 60–90 min after PPCI was safe in STEMI patients presenting within 24 h. The large Acute Myocardial Infarction With Hyperoxemic Therapy AMIHOT-I (269 patients) [134] clinical study comprising patients presenting with anterior or large inferior STEMI, however, did not observe any reduction in MI size with therapeutic hypothermia, although there was the suggestion of MI limitation in those patients presenting with the large anterior STEMI. The results of recently published AMIHOT-II clinical study (281 patients), which prospectively investigated hyperoxemic therapy in anterior STEMI patients presenting within 6 h, found no benefit in MI size reduction when compared to control [135]. However, these authors then performed a pooled analysis of patients recruited in both the AMIHOT-I and AMIHOT-II studies and found a significant reduction in MI size from 25% to 18% of the LV when assessed by SPECT [135]—but one has to question the validity of a pooled analysis from two different clinical studies comprising two different patient cohorts (AMIHOT-I recruited patients from Jan. 2002 to Dec. 2003, whereas AMIHOT-II recruited patients from Sept. 2005 to May 2007). As such, a further definitive clinical trial is required to confirm whether hyperoxemic therapy can limit MI size and improve clinical outcomes in PPCI patients.

Barriers to the Translation of Cardioprotective Therapies

Although a large number of therapeutic strategies have been found in the experimental setting to protect the heart against lethal myocardial reperfusion injury when administered at the point of myocardial reperfusion, the translation to the clinical setting has been hugely disappointing. The failure to translate cardioprotective therapies for patient benefit has been the subject of recent debate [1, 6, 136, 137]. To summarize, the barriers to translation of cardioprotective therapies can be divided into those factors affecting the experimental studies and those pertaining to the clinical studies (Table 12.6).

A number of specific recommendations have been issued aimed at improving the translation of future cardioprotective strategies following workshops convened by the National Heart, Lung and Blood Institute [6] and the University College London Hatter Cardiovascular Institute [9]. These include the formation of research networks (such as the multi-centre Consortium for preclinicAl assESsment of cARdioprotective therapies (CAESAR) in the USA) which systematically undertakes randomized controlled clinical trials using small and large animal in vivo IRI models to investigate novel cardioprotective strategies especially where previous animal studies have been inconclusive. Then, only if a therapeutic strategy is found to be conclusively cardioprotective should it be explored in the clinical setting. When actually proceeding to the clinical studies, it is crucial that basic science researchers work alongside clinical researchers to ensure the clinical studies have been optimally designed in terms of patient selection, the timing of the intervention and the endpoints measured [9]. Hopefully, with the implementation of these recommendations and an increased awareness of the limitations of our current approach to investigating novel cardioprotective strategies, we will be able to overcome this obstacle to translation and discover new therapeutic strategies for improving clinical outcomes in patients with CHD.

Conclusions

The recognition of lethal myocardial reperfusion injury as a viable target for cardioprotection in both the experimental and clinical settings has resulted in a resurgence in the research field of myocardial protection. Several novel therapeutic strategies discovered in the experimental setting and applicable at the onset of myocardial reperfusion have proven to be beneficial, at least in proof-of-concept clinical studies, against lethal myocardial reperfusion injury when administered as adjuncts to PPCI. The recognition that the barriers to the translation of cardioprotective therapies need to be overcome using a joined up systematic approach should further facilitate the process of identifying novel therapeutic strategies and their translation into the clinical arena. Finally, large multi-centre randomized placebo-controlled clinical trials are now required to determine whether these novel cardioprotective strategies can improve clinical outcomes for the benefit of our patients with CHD.

References

1. Yellon DM, Hausenloy DJ. Myocardial reperfusion injury. N Engl J Med. 2007;357:1121–35.
2. Staat P, Rioufol G, Piot C, Cottin Y, Cung TT, L'Huillier I, Aupetit JF, Bonnefoy E, Finet G, Andre-Fouet X, Ovize M. Postconditioning the human heart. Circulation. 2005;112:2143–8.
3. Yellon DM, Opie LH. Postconditioning for protection of the infarcting heart. Lancet. 2006;367:456–8.
4. Hausenloy DJ, Yellon DM. Reperfusion injury salvage kinase signalling: taking a RISK for cardioprotection. Heart Fail Rev. 2007;12:217–34.
5. Hausenloy DJ, Yellon DM. Preconditioning and postconditioning: united at reperfusion. Pharmacol Ther. 2007;116:173–91.
6. Bolli R, Becker L, Gross G, Mentzer Jr R, Balshaw D, Lathrop DA. Myocardial protection at a crossroads: the need for translation into clinical therapy. Circ Res. 2004;95:125–34.
7. Kloner RA, Rezkalla SH. Cardiac protection during acute myocardial infarction: where do we stand in 2004? J Am Coll Cardiol. 2004;44:276–86.
8. Ludman AJ, Yellon DM, Hausenloy DJ. Cardiac preconditioning for ischaemia: lost in translation. Dis Model Mech. 2010;3:35–8.
9. Hausenloy DJ, Baxter G, Bell R, Botker HE, Davidson SM, Downey J, Heusch G, Kitakaze M, Lecour S, Mentzer R, Mocanu MM, Ovize M, Schulz R, Shannon R, Walker M, Walkinshaw G, Yellon DM. Translating novel strategies for cardioprotection: the Hatter Workshop Recommendations. Basic Res Cardiol. 2010;105:677–86.
10. Cohen MV, Downey JM. Adenosine: trigger and mediator of cardioprotection. Basic Res Cardiol. 2008;103:203–15.
11. Liu GS, Thornton J, Van Winkle DM, Stanley AW, Olsson RA, Downey JM. Protection against infarction afforded by preconditioning is mediated by A1 adenosine receptors in rabbit heart. Circulation. 1991;84:350–6.
12. Kin H, Zatta AJ, Lofye MT, Amerson BS, Halkos ME, Kerendi F, Zhao ZQ, Guyton RA, Headrick JP, Vinten-Johansen J. Postconditioning reduces infarct size via adenosine receptor activation by endogenous adenosine. Cardiovasc Res. 2005;67:124–33.
13. Olafsson B, Forman MB, Puett DW, Pou A, Cates CU, Friesinger GC, Virmani R. Reduction of reperfusion injury in the canine preparation by intracoronary adenosine: importance of the endothelium and the no-reflow phenomenon. Circulation. 1987;76:1135–45.
14. Norton ED, Jackson EK, Virmani R, Forman MB. Effect of intravenous adenosine on myocardial reperfusion injury in a model with low myocardial collateral blood flow. Am Heart J. 1991;122:1283–91.
15. Pitarys CJ, Virmani R, Vildibill Jr HD, Jackson EK, Forman MB. Reduction of myocardial reperfusion injury by intravenous adenosine administered during the early reperfusion period. Circulation. 1991;83:237–47.
16. Velasco CE, Turner M, Cobb MA, Virmani R, Forman MB. Myocardial reperfusion injury in the canine model after 40 minutes of ischemia: effect of intracoronary adenosine. Am Heart J. 1991;122:1561–70.
17. Todd J, Zhao ZQ, Williams MW, Sato H, Van Wylen DG, Vinten-Johansen J. Intravascular adenosine at reperfusion reduces infarct size and neutrophil adherence. Ann Thorac Surg. 1996;62:1364–72.
18. Zhao ZQ, Nakamura M, Wang NP, Wilcox JN, Shearer S, Guyton RA, Vinten-Johansen J. Administration of adenosine during reperfusion reduces injury of vascular endothelium and death of myocytes. Coron Artery Dis. 1999;10:617–28.
19. Zhao ZQ, Budde JM, Morris C, Wang NP, Velez DA, Muraki S, Guyton RA, Vinten-Johansen J. Adenosine attenuates reperfusion-induced apoptotic cell death by modulating expression of Bcl-2 and Bax proteins. J Mol Cell Cardiol. 2001;33:57–68.
20. Walker DM, Walker JM, Pugsley WB, Pattison CW, Yellon DM. Preconditioning in isolated superfused human muscle. J Mol Cell Cardiol. 1995;27:1349–57.

21. Ikonomidis JS, Shirai T, Weisel RD, Derylo B, Rao V, Whiteside CI, Mickle DAG, Li RK. 'Ischemic' or adenosine preconditioning of human ventricular cardiomyocytes is protein kinase C dependent. Circulation. 1995;92 Suppl 1:1–12. Abstract.
22. Deutsch E, Berger M, Kussmaul WG, Hirshfeld Jr JW, Herrmann HC, Laskey WK. Adaptation to ischemia during percutaneous transluminal coronary angioplasty. Clinical, hemodynamic, and metabolic features. Circulation. 1990;82:2044–51.
23. Tomai F, Crea F, Gaspardone A, Versaci F, De Paulis R, Polisca P, Chiariello L, Gioffre PA. Effects of A1 adenosine receptor blockade by bamiphylline on ischaemic preconditioning during coronary angioplasty. Eur Heart J. 1996;17:846–53.
24. Leesar MA, Stoddard M, Ahmed M, Broadbent J, Bolli R. Preconditioning of human myocardium with adenosine during coronary angioplasty. Circulation. 1997;95:2500–7.
25. Garratt KN, Holmes Jr DR, Molina-Viamonte V, Reeder GS, Hodge DO, Bailey KR, Lobl JK, Laudon DA, Gibbons RJ. Intravenous adenosine and lidocaine in patients with acute mycocardial infarction. Am Heart J. 1998;136:196–204.
26. Assali AR, Sdringola S, Ghani M, Denkats AE, Yepes A, Hanna GP, Schroth G, Fujise K, Anderson HV, Smalling RW, Rosales OR. Intracoronary adenosine administered during percutaneous intervention in acute myocardial infarction and reduction in the incidence of "no reflow" phenomenon. Catheter Cardiovasc Interv. 2000;51:27–31.
27. Marzilli M, Orsini E, Marraccini P, Testa R. Beneficial effects of intracoronary adenosine as an adjunct to primary angioplasty in acute myocardial infarction. Circulation. 2000; 101:2154–9.
28. Claeys MJ, Bosmans J, De Ceuninck M, Beunis A, Vergauwen W, Vorlat A, Vrints CJ. Effect of intracoronary adenosine infusion during coronary intervention on myocardial reperfusion injury in patients with acute myocardial infarction. Am J Cardiol. 2004;94:9–13.
29. Lim SY, Bae EH, Jeong MH, Kang DG, Lee YS, Kim KH, Lee SH, Yoon KH, Hong SN, Park HW, Hong YJ, Kim JH, Kim W, Ahn YK, Cho JG, Park JC, Kang JC. Effect of combined intracoronary adenosine and nicorandil on no-reflow phenomenon during percutaneous coronary intervention. Circ J. 2004;68:928–32.
30. Ross AM, Gibbons RJ, Stone GW, Kloner RA, Alexander RW. A randomized, double-blinded, placebo-controlled multicenter trial of adenosine as an adjunct to reperfusion in the treatment of acute myocardial infarction (AMISTAD-II). J Am Coll Cardiol. 2005;45:1775–80.
31. Kloner RA, Forman MB, Gibbons RJ, Ross AM, Alexander RW, Stone GW. Impact of time to therapy and reperfusion modality on the efficacy of adenosine in acute myocardial infarction: the AMISTAD-2 trial. Eur Heart J. 2006;27:2400–5.
32. Vijayalakshmi K, Whittaker VJ, Kunadian B, Graham J, Wright RA, Hall JA, Sutton A, de Belder MA. Prospective, randomised, controlled trial to study the effect of intracoronary injection of verapamil and adenosine on coronary blood flow during percutaneous coronary intervention in patients with acute coronary syndromes. Heart. 2006;92:1278–84.
33. Parikh KH, Chag MC, Shah KJ, Shah UG, Baxi HA, Chandarana AH, Naik AM, Shah JN, Shah HD, Goyal RK. Intracoronary boluses of adenosine and sodium nitroprusside in combination reverses slow/no-reflow during angioplasty: a clinical scenario of ischemic preconditioning. Can J Physiol Pharmacol. 2007;85:476–82.
34. Stoel MG, Marques KM, de Cock CC, Bronzwaer JG, von Birgelen C, Zijlstra F. High dose adenosine for suboptimal myocardial reperfusion after primary PCI: a randomized placebo-controlled pilot study. Catheter Cardiovasc Interv. 2008;71:283–9.
35. Fokkema ML, Vlaar PJ, Vogelzang M, Gu YL, Kampinga MA, de Smet BJ, Jessurun GA, Anthonio RL, van den Heuvel AF, Tan ES, Zijlstra F. Effect of high-dose intracoronary adenosine administration during primary percutaneous coronary intervention in acute myocardial infarction: a randomized controlled trial. Circ Cardiovasc Interv. 2009;2:323–9.
36. Mahaffey KW, Puma JA, Barbagelata NA, DiCarli MF, Leesar MA, Browne KF, Eisenberg PR, Bolli R, Casas AC, Molina-Viamonte V, Orlandi C, Blevins R, Gibbons RJ, Califf RM, Granger CB. Adenosine as an adjunct to thrombolytic therapy for acute myocardial infarction: results of a multicenter, randomized, placebo-controlled trial: the Acute Myocardial Infarction STudy of ADenosine (AMISTAD) trial. J Am Coll Cardiol. 1999;34:1711–20.

37. Garlid KD, Paucek P, Yarov-Yarovoy V, Murray HN, Darbenzio RB, D'Alonzo AJ, Lodge NJ, Smith MA, Grover GJ. Cardioprotective effect of diazoxide and its interaction with mitochondrial ATP-sensitive K^+ channels. Possible mechanism of cardioprotection. Circ Res. 1997;81:1072–82.
38. Liu Y, Sato T, O'Rourke B, Marban E. Mitochondrial ATP-dependent potassium channels: novel effectors of cardioprotection? Circulation. 1998;97:2463–9.
39. Downey JM, Davis AM, Cohen MV. Signaling pathways in ischemic preconditioning. Heart Fail Rev. 2007;12:181–8.
40. Hausenloy DJ. Signalling pathways in ischaemic postconditioning. Thromb Haemost. 2009;101:626–34.
41. Hanley PJ, Daut J. K(ATP) channels and preconditioning: a re-examination of the role of mitochondrial K(ATP) channels and an overview of alternative mechanisms. J Mol Cell Cardiol. 2005;39:17–50.
42. Hanley PJ, Mickel M, Loffler M, Brandt U, Daut J. K(ATP) channel-independent targets of diazoxide and 5-hydroxydecanoate in the heart. J Physiol. 2002;542:735–41.
43. Auchampach JA, Gross GJ. Reduction in myocardial infarct size by the new potassium channel opener bimakalim. J Cardiovasc Pharmacol. 1994;23:554–61.
44. Mizumura T, Nithipatikom K, Gross GJ. Bimakalim, an ATP-sensitive potassium channel opener, mimics the effects of ischemic preconditioning to reduce infarct size, adenosine release, and neutrophil function in dogs. Circulation. 1995;92:1236–45.
45. Toyoda Y, Friehs I, Parker RA, Levitsky S, McCully JD. Differential role of sarcolemmal and mitochondrial K(ATP) channels in adenosine-enhanced ischemic preconditioning. Am J Physiol Heart Circ Physiol. 2000;279:H2694–703.
46. Vanden Hoek T, Becker LB, Shao ZH, Li CQ, Schumacker PT. Preconditioning in cardiomyocytes protects by attenuating oxidant stress at reperfusion. Circ Res. 2000;86:541–8.
47. Tsuchida A, Miura T, Miki T, Kuno A, Tanno M, Nozawa Y, Genda S, Matsumoto T, Shimamoto K. Critical timing of mitochondrial K(ATP) channel opening for enhancement of myocardial tolerance against infarction. Basic Res Cardiol. 2001;96:446–53.
48. Ohno Y, Minatoguchi S, Uno Y, Kariya T, Arai M, Yamashita K, Fujiwara T, Fujiwara H. Nicorandil reduces myocardial infarct size by opening the K(ATP) channel in rabbits. Int J Cardiol. 1997;62:181–90.
49. Imagawa J, Baxter GF, Yellon DM. Myocardial protection afforded by nicorandil and ischaemic preconditioning in a rabbit infarct model in vivo. J Cardiovasc Pharmacol. 1998;31:74–9.
50. Ito H, Taniyama Y, Iwakura K, Nishikawa N, Masuyama T, Kuzuya T, Hori M, Higashino Y, Fujii K, Minamino T. Intravenous nicorandil can preserve microvascular integrity and myocardial viability in patients with reperfused anterior wall myocardial infarction. J Am Coll Cardiol. 1999;33:654–60.
51. Kim JS, Kim J, Choi D, Lee CJ, Lee SH, Ko YG, Hong MK, Kim BK, Oh SJ, Jeon DW, Yang JY, Cho JR, Lee NH, Cho YH, Cho DK, Jang Y. Efficacy of high-dose atorvastatin loading before primary percutaneous coronary intervention in ST-segment elevation myocardial infarction: the STATIN STEMI trial. JACC Cardiovasc Interv. 2010;3:332–9.
52. Hahn JY, Kim HJ, Choi YJ, Jo SH, Kim HJ, Lee S, Ahn KJ, Song YB, Choi JH, Choi SH, et al. Effects of atorvastatin pretreatment on infarct size in patients with ST-segment elevation myocardial infarction undergoing primary percutaneous coronary intervention. Am Heart J. 2011;162:1026–33.
53. Piot C, Croisille P, Staat P, Thibault H, Rioufol G, Mewton N, Elbelghiti R, Cung TT, Bonnefoy E, Angoulvant D, Macia C, Raczka F, Sportouch C, Gahide G, Finet G, Andre-Fouet X, Revel D, Kirkorian G, Monassier JP, Derumeaux G, Ovize M. Effect of cyclosporine on reperfusion injury in acute myocardial infarction. N Engl J Med. 2008;359:473–81.
54. Mewton N, Croisille P, Gahide G, Rioufol G, Bonnefoy E, Sanchez I, Cung TT, Sportouch C, Angoulvant D, Finet G, Andre-Fouet X, Derumeaux G, Piot C, Vernhet H, Revel D, Ovize M. Effect of cyclosporine on left ventricular remodeling after reperfused myocardial infarction. J Am Coll Cardiol. 2010;55:1200–5.

55. Lipsic E. van der MP, Voors AA, Westenbrink BD, van den Heuvel AF, de Boer HC, van Zonneveld AJ, Schoemaker RG, van Gilst WH, Zijlstra F, van Veldhuisen DJ. A single bolus of a long-acting erythropoietin analogue darbepoetin alfa in patients with acute myocardial infarction: a randomized feasibility and safety study Cardiovasc Drugs Ther. 2006;20(2):135–41.
56. Ferrario M, Arbustini E, Massa M, Rosti V, Marziliano N, Raineri C, Campanelli R, Bertoletti A, De Ferrari GM, Klersy C, Angoli L, Bramucci E, Marinoni B, Ferlini M, Moretti E, Raisaro A, Repetto A, Schwartz PJ, Tavazzi L. High-dose erythropoietin in patients with acute myocardial infarction: a pilot, randomised, placebo-controlled study. Int J Cardiol. 2011;147:124–31.
57. Suh JW, Chung WY, Kim YS, Kim KI, Jeon EJ, Cho YS, Youn TJ, Chae IH, Kim CH, Choi DJ. The effect of intravenous administration of erythropoietin on the infarct size in primary percutaneous coronary intervention. Int J Cardiol. 2010;149:216–20.
58. Ozawa T, Toba K, Suzuki H, Kato K, Iso Y, Akutsu Y, Kobayashi Y, Takeyama Y, Kobayashi N, Yoshimura N, Akazawa K, Aizawa Y. Single-dose intravenous administration of recombinant human erythropoietin is a promising treatment for patients with acute myocardial infarction – randomized controlled pilot trial of EPO/AMI-1 study -. Circ J. 2010;74:1415–23.
59. Voors AA, Belonje AM, Zijlstra F, Hillege HL, Anker SD, Slart RH, Tio RA, van 't Hof A, Jukema JW, Peels HO, Henriques JP, Ten Berg JM, Vos J, van Gilst WH, van Veldhuisen DJ. A single dose of erythropoietin in ST-elevation myocardial infarction. Eur Heart J. 2010;31:2593–600.
60. Taniguchi N, Nakamura T, Sawada T, Matsubara K, Furukawa K, Hadase M, Nakahara Y, Nakamura T, Matsubara H. Erythropoietin prevention trial of coronary restenosis and cardiac remodeling after ST-elevated acute myocardial infarction (EPOC-AMI): a pilot, randomized, placebo-controlled study. Circ J. 2010;74:2365–71.
61. Ott I, Schulz S, Mehilli J, Fichtner S, Hadamitzky M, Hoppe K, Ibrahim T, Martinoff S, Massberg S, Laugwitz KL, Dirschinger J, Schwaiger M, Kastrati A, Schmig A. Erythropoietin in patients with acute ST-segment elevation myocardial infarction undergoing primary percutaneous coronary intervention: a randomized, double-blind trial. Circ Cardiovasc Interv. 2010;3:408–13.
62. Ludman AJ, Yellon DM, Hasleton J, Ariti C, Babu GG, Boston-Griffiths E, Venugopal V, Walker M, Holdright D, Swanton H, Crake T, Brull D, Moon JC, Puranik R, Muthurangu V, Taylor A, Hausenloy DJ. Effect of erythropoietin as an adjunct to primary percutaneous coronary intervention: a randomised controlled clinical trial. Heart. 2011 Oct;97(19):1560–5.
63. Nikolaidis LA, Mankad S, Sokos GG, Miske G, Shah A, Elahi D, Shannon RP. Effects of glucagon-like peptide-1 in patients with acute myocardial infarction and left ventricular dysfunction after successful reperfusion. Circulation. 2004;109:962–5.
64. Lønborg J, Vejlstrup N, Kelbæk H, Bøtker HE, Kim WY, Mathiasen AB, Jørgensen E, Helqvist S, Saunamäki K, Clemmensen P, Holmvang L, Thuesen L, Krusell LR, Jensen JS, Køber L, Treiman M, Holst JJ, Engstrøm T. Exenatide reduces reperfusion injury in patients with ST-segment elevation myocardial infarction. Eur Heart J. 2011 Sep 14. [Epub ahead of print].
65. Kitakaze M, Asakura M, Kim J, Shintani Y, Asanuma H, Hamasaki T, Seguchi O, Myoishi M, Minamino T, Ohara T, Nagai Y, Nanto S, Watanabe K, Fukuzawa S, Hirayama A, Nakamura N, Kimura K, Fujii K, Ishihara M, Saito Y, Tomoike H, Kitamura S. Human atrial natriuretic peptide and nicorandil as adjuncts to reperfusion treatment for acute myocardial infarction (J-WIND): two randomised trials. Lancet. 2007;370:1483–93.
66. Bates E, Bode C, Costa M, Gibson CM, Granger C, Green C, Grimes K, Harrington R, Huber K, Kleiman N, Mochly-Rosen D, Roe M, Sadowski Z, Solomon S, Widimsky P. Intracoronary KAI-9803 as an adjunct to primary percutaneous coronary intervention for acute ST-segment elevation myocardial infarction. Circulation. 2008;117:886–96.
67. Yang XM, Philipp S, Downey JM, Cohen MV. Atrial natriuretic peptide administered just prior to reperfusion limits infarction in rabbit hearts. Basic Res Cardiol. 2006;101:311–8.
68. Burley DS, Baxter GF. B-type natriuretic peptide at early reperfusion limits infarct size in the rat isolated heart. Basic Res Cardiol. 2007;102:529–41.

69. Baxter GF, Burley DS. Reperfusion and calculated RISKs: pharmacological postconditioning of human myocardium. Br J Pharmacol. 2008;153:1–3.
70. Burley DS, Hamid SA, Baxter GF. Cardioprotective actions of peptide hormones in myocardial ischemia. Heart Fail Rev. 2007;12:279–91.
71. Hayashi M, Tsutamoto T, Wada A, Maeda K, Mabuchi N, Tsutsui T, Horie H, Ohnishi M, Kinoshita M. Intravenous atrial natriuretic peptide prevents left ventricular remodeling in patients with first anterior acute myocardial infarction. J Am Coll Cardiol. 2001;37:1820–6.
72. Churchill EN, Mochly-Rosen D. The roles of PKCdelta and epsilon isoenzymes in the regulation of myocardial ischaemia/reperfusion injury. Biochem Soc Trans. 2007;35:1040–2.
73. Sivaraman V, Hausenloy DJ, Kolvekar S, Hayward M, Yap J, Lawrence D, Di Salvo C, Yellon DM. The divergent roles of protein kinase C epsilon and delta in simulated ischaemia-reperfusion injury in human myocardium. J Mol Cell Cardiol. 2009;46:758–64.
74. Crompton M, Ellinger H, Costi A. Inhibition by cyclosporin A of a Ca^{2+}–dependent pore in heart mitochondria activated by inorganic phosphate and oxidative stress. Biochem J. 1988;255:357–60.
75. Hausenloy DJ, Yellon DM. The mitochondrial permeability transition pore: its fundamental role in mediating cell death during ischaemia and reperfusion. J Mol Cell Cardiol. 2003;35:339–41.
76. Baines CP, Kaiser RA, Purcell NH, Blair NS, Osinska H, Hambleton MA, Brunskill EW, Sayen MR, Gottlieb RA, Dorn GW, Robbins J, Molkentin JD. Loss of cyclophilin D reveals a critical role for mitochondrial permeability transition in cell death. Nature. 2005;434:658–62.
77. Basso E, Fante L, Fowlkes J, Petronilli V, Forte MA, Bernardi P. Properties of the permeability transition pore in mitochondria devoid of Cyclophilin D. J Biol Chem. 2005;280:18558–61.
78. Nakagawa T, Shimizu S, Watanabe T, Yamaguchi O, Otsu K, Yamagata H, Inohara H, Kubo T, Tsujimoto Y. Cyclophilin D-dependent mitochondrial permeability transition regulates some necrotic but not apoptotic cell death. Nature. 2005;434:652–8.
79. Griffiths EJ, Halestrap AP. Protection by Cyclosporin A of ischemia/reperfusion-induced damage in isolated rat hearts. J Mol Cell Cardiol. 1993;25:1461–9.
80. Hausenloy DJ, Maddock HL, Baxter GF, Yellon DM. Inhibiting mitochondrial permeability transition pore opening: a new paradigm for myocardial preconditioning? Cardiovasc Res. 2002;55:534–43.
81. Hausenloy DJ, Duchen MR, Yellon DM. Inhibiting mitochondrial permeability transition pore opening at reperfusion protects against ischaemia-reperfusion injury. Cardiovasc Res. 2003;60:617–25.
82. Argaud L, Gateau-Roesch O, Muntean D, Chalabreysse L, Loufouat J, Robert D, Ovize M. Specific inhibition of the mitochondrial permeability transition prevents lethal reperfusion injury. J Mol Cell Cardiol. 2005;38:367–74.
83. Shanmuganathan S, Hausenloy DJ, Duchen MR, Yellon DM. Mitochondrial permeability transition pore as a target for cardioprotection in the human heart. Am J Physiol Heart Circ Physiol. 2005;289:H237–42.
84. Skyschally A, Schulz R, Heusch G. Cyclosporine A at reperfusion reduces infarct size in pigs. Cardiovasc Drugs Ther. 2010;24:85–7.
85. Lie RH, Stoettrup N, Sloth E, Hasenkam JM, Kroyer R, Nielsen TT. Post-conditioning with Cyclosporine A fails to reduce the infarct size in an in vivo porcine model. Acta Anaesthesiol Scand. 2010;54:804–13.
86. Karlsson LO, Zhou AX, Larsson E, Astrom-Olsson K, Mansson C, Akyurek LM, Grip L. Cyclosporine does not reduce myocardial infarct size in a porcine ischemia-reperfusion model. J Cardiovasc Pharmacol Ther. 2010;15:182–9.
87. Riksen NP, Hausenloy DJ, Yellon DM. Erythropoietin: ready for prime-time cardioprotection. Trends Pharmacol Sci. 2008;29:258–67.
88. Toma C, Letts DP, Tanabe M, Gorcsan III J, Counihan PJ. Positive effect of darbepoetin on peri-infarction remodeling in a porcine model of myocardial ischemia-reperfusion. J Mol Cell Cardiol. 2007;43:130–6.

89. Olea FD, Vera JG, De Lorenzi A, Cuniberti L, Yannarelli G, Cabeza MP, Cearras M, Laguens R, Crottogini A. High-dose erythropoietin has no long-term protective effects in sheep with reperfused myocardial infarction. J Cardiovasc Pharmacol. 2006;47:736–41.
90. Kristensen J, Maeng M, Rehling M, Berg JS, Mortensen UM, Nielsen SS, Nielsen TT. Lack of acute cardioprotective effect from preischaemic erythropoietin administration in a porcine coronary occlusion model. Clin Physiol Funct Imaging. 2005;25:305–10.
91. Baigent C, Keech A, Kearney PM, Blackwell L, Buck G, Pollicino C, Kirby A, Sourjina T, Peto R, Collins R, Simes R. Efficacy and safety of cholesterol-lowering treatment: prospective meta-analysis of data from 90,056 participants in 14 randomised trials of statins. Lancet. 2005;366:1267–78.
92. Ludman A, Venugopal V, Yellon DM, Hausenloy DJ. Statins and cardioprotection – more than just lipid lowering? Pharmacol Ther. 2009;122:30–43.
93. Di Sciascio G, Patti G, Pasceri V, Gaspardone A, Colonna G, Montinaro A. Efficacy of atorvastatin reload in patients on chronic statin therapy undergoing percutaneous coronary intervention: results of the ARMYDA-RECAPTURE (atorvastatin for reduction of myocardial damage during angioplasty) randomized trial. J Am Coll Cardiol. 2009;54:558–65.
94. Patti G, Pasceri V, Colonna G, Miglionico M, Fischetti D, Sardella G, Montinaro A, Di Sciascio G. Atorvastatin pretreatment improves outcomes in patients with acute coronary syndromes undergoing early percutaneous coronary intervention: results of the ARMYDA-ACS randomized trial. J Am Coll Cardiol. 2007;49:1272–8.
95. Cannon CP, Braunwald E, McCabe CH, Rader DJ, Rouleau JL, Belder R, Joyal SV, Hill KA, Pfeffer MA, Skene AM. Intensive versus moderate lipid lowering with statins after acute coronary syndromes. N Engl J Med. 2004;350:1495–504.
96. Ahsan CH, Shah A, Ezekowitz M. Acute statin treatment in reducing risk after acute coronary syndrome: the MIRACL (myocardial ischemia reduction with aggressive cholesterol lowering) trial. Curr Opin Cardiol. 2001;16:390–3.
97. Jonassen AK, Sack MN, Mjos OD, Yellon DM. Myocardial protection by insulin at reperfusion requires early administration and is mediated via Akt and p70s6 kinase cell-survival signaling. Circ Res. 2001;89:1191–8.
98. Diaz R, Paolasso EA, Piegas LS, Tajer CD, Moreno MG, Corvalan R, Isea JE, Romero G. Metabolic modulation of acute myocardial infarction. The ECLA (Estudios Cardiologicos Latinoamerica) Collaborative Group. Circulation. 1998;98:2227–34.
99. Yazici M, Demircan S, Durna K, Yasar E, Acar Z, Sahin M. Effect of glucose-insulin-potassium infusion on myocardial damage due to percutaneous coronary revascularization. Am J Cardiol. 2005;96:1517–20.
100. Lazar HL, Chipkin SR, Fitzgerald CA, Bao Y, Cabral H, Apstein CS. Tight glycemic control in diabetic coronary artery bypass graft patients improves perioperative outcomes and decreases recurrent ischemic events. Circulation. 2004;109:1497–502.
101. Bucciarelli-Ducci C, Bianchi M, De Luca L, Battagliese A, Di Russo C, Proietti P, Vizza CD, Fedele F. Effects of glucose-insulin-potassium infusion on myocardial perfusion and left ventricular remodeling in patients treated with primary angioplasty for ST-elevation acute myocardial infarction. Am J Cardiol. 2006;98:1349–53.
102. Van der Horst IC, De Luca G, Ottervanger JP, De Boer MJ, Hoorntje JC, Suryapranata H, Dambrink JH, Gosselink AT, Zijlstra F, van 't Hof AW. ST-segment elevation resolution and outcome in patients treated with primary angioplasty and glucose-insulin-potassium infusion. Am Heart J. 2005;149:1135.
103. Rasoul S, Ottervanger JP, Timmer JR, Svilaas T, Henriques JP, Dambrink JH, van der Horst IC, Zijlstra F. One year outcomes after glucose-insulin-potassium in ST elevation myocardial infarction. The glucose-insulin-potassium study II. Int J Cardiol. 2007;122:52–5.
104. Diaz R, Goyal A, Mehta SR, Afzal R, Xavier D, Pais P, Chrolavicius S, Zhu J, Kazmi K, Liu L, Budaj A, Zubaid M, Avezum A, Ruda M, Yusuf S. Glucose-insulin-potassium therapy in patients with ST-segment elevation myocardial infarction. JAMA. 2007;298:2399–405.

105. Mehta SR, Yusuf S, Diaz R, Zhu J, Pais P, Xavier D, Paolasso E, Ahmed R, Xie C, Kazmi K, Tai J, Orlandini A, Pogue J, Liu L. Effect of glucose-insulin-potassium infusion on mortality in patients with acute ST-segment elevation myocardial infarction: the CREATE-ECLA randomized controlled trial. JAMA. 2005;293:437–46.
106. Hausenloy DJ, Yellon DM. GLP-1 therapy: beyond glucose control. Circ Heart Fail. 2008;1:147–9.
107. Bose AK, Mocanu MM, Carr RD, Yellon DM. Glucagon like peptide-1 is protective against myocardial ischemia/reperfusion injury when given either as a preconditioning mimetic or at reperfusion in an isolated rat heart model. Cardiovasc Drugs Ther. 2005;19:9–11.
108. Bose AK, Mocanu MM, Carr RD, Brand CL, Yellon DM. Glucagon-like peptide 1 can directly protect the heart against ischemia/reperfusion injury. Diabetes. 2005;54:146–51.
109. Sokos GG, Nikolaidis LA, Mankad S, Elahi D, Shannon RP. Glucagon-like peptide-1 infusion improves left ventricular ejection fraction and functional status in patients with chronic heart failure. J Card Fail. 2006;12:694–9.
110. Sauve M, Ban K, Momen MA, Zhou YQ, Henkelman RM, Husain M, Drucker DJ. Genetic deletion or pharmacological inhibition of dipeptidyl peptidase-4 improves cardiovascular outcomes after myocardial infarction in mice. Diabetes. 2010;59:1063–73.
111. Timmers L, Henriques JP, de Kleijn DP, Devries JH, Kemperman H, Steendijk P, Verlaan CW, Kerver M, Piek JJ, Doevendans PA, Pasterkamp G, Hoefer IE. Exenatide reduces infarct size and improves cardiac function in a porcine model of ischemia and reperfusion injury. J Am Coll Cardiol. 2009;53:501–10.
112. Dezfulian C, Raat N, Shiva S, Gladwin MT. Role of the anion nitrite in ischemia-reperfusion cytoprotection and therapeutics. Cardiovasc Res. 2007;75:327–38.
113. Gonzalez FM, Shiva S, Vincent PS, Ringwood LA, Hsu LY, Hon YY, Aletras AH, Cannon III RO, Gladwin MT, Arai AE. Nitrite anion provides potent cytoprotective and antiapoptotic effects as adjunctive therapy to reperfusion for acute myocardial infarction. Circulation. 2008;117:2986–94.
114. Duranski MR, Greer JJ, Dejam A, Jaganmohan S, Hogg N, Langston W, Patel RP, Yet SF, Wang X, Kevil CG, Gladwin MT, Lefer DJ. Cytoprotective effects of nitrite during in vivo ischemia-reperfusion of the heart and liver. J Clin Invest. 2005;115:1232–40.
115. Dezfulian C, Shiva S, Alekseyenko A, Pendyal A, Beiser DG, Munasinghe JP, Anderson SA, Chesley CF, Vanden Hoek TL, Gladwin MT. Nitrite therapy after cardiac arrest reduces reactive oxygen species generation, improves cardiac and neurological function, and enhances survival via reversible inhibition of mitochondrial complex I. Circulation. 2009;120:897–905.
116. Baran KW, Nguyen M, McKendall GR, Lambrew CT, Dykstra G, Palmeri ST, Gibbons RJ, Borzak S, Sobel BE, Gourlay SG, Rundle AC, Gibson CM, Barron HV. Double-blind, randomized trial of an anti-CD18 antibody in conjunction with recombinant tissue plasminogen activator for acute myocardial infarction: limitation of myocardial infarction following thrombolysis in acute myocardial infarction (LIMIT AMI) study. Circulation. 2001;104:2778–83.
117. Faxon DP, Gibbons RJ, Chronos NA, Gurbel PA, Sheehan F. The effect of blockade of the CD11/CD18 integrin receptor on infarct size in patients with acute myocardial infarction treated with direct angioplasty: the results of the HALT-MI study. J Am Coll Cardiol. 2002;40:1199–204.
118. Mahaffey KW, Granger CB, Nicolau JC, Ruzyllo W, Weaver WD, Theroux P, Hochman JS, Filloon TG, Mojcik CF, Todaro TG, Armstrong PW. Effect of pexelizumab, an anti-C5 complement antibody, as adjunctive therapy to fibrinolysis in acute myocardial infarction: the COMPlement inhibition in myocardial infarction treated with thromboLYtics (COMPLY) trial. Circulation. 2003;108:1176–83.
119. Granger CB, Mahaffey KW, Weaver WD, Theroux P, Hochman JS, Filloon TG, Rollins S, Todaro TG, Nicolau JC, Ruzyllo W, Armstrong PW. Pexelizumab, an anti-C5 complement antibody, as adjunctive therapy to primary percutaneous coronary intervention in acute myocardial infarction: the COMplement inhibition in Myocardial infarction treated with Angioplasty (COMMA) trial. Circulation. 2003;108:1184–90.

120. Mertens P, Maes A, Nuyts J, Belmans A, Desmet W, Esplugas E, Charlier F, Figueras J, Sambuceti G, Schwaiger M, Mortelmans L, van De WF. Recombinant P-selectin glycoprotein ligand-immunoglobulin, a P-selectin antagonist, as an adjunct to thrombolysis in acute myocardial infarction. The P-selectin antagonist limiting myonecrosis (PSALM) trial. Am Heart J. 2006;152:125–8.
121. Armstrong PW, Granger CB, Adams PX, Hamm C, Holmes Jr D, O'Neill WW, Todaro TG, Vahanian A, van De WF. Pexelizumab for acute ST-elevation myocardial infarction in patients undergoing primary percutaneous coronary intervention: a randomized controlled trial. JAMA. 2007;297:43–51.
122. Atar D, Petzelbauer P, Schwitter J, Huber K, Rensing B, Kasprzak JD, Butter C, Grip L, Hansen PR, Suselbeck T, Clemmensen PM, Marin-Galiano M, Geudelin B, Buser PT. Effect of intravenous FX06 as an adjunct to primary percutaneous coronary intervention for acute ST-segment elevation myocardial infarction results of the F.I.R.E. (efficacy of FX06 in the prevention of myocardial reperfusion injury) trial. J Am Coll Cardiol. 2009;53:720–9.
123. Zhao ZQ, Corvera JS, Halkos ME, Kerendi F, Wang NP, Guyton RA, Vinten-Johansen J. Inhibition of myocardial injury by ischemic postconditioning during reperfusion: comparison with ischemic preconditioning. Am J Physiol Heart Circ Physiol. 2003;285:H579–88.
124. Thibault H, Piot C, Staat P, Bontemps L, Sportouch C, Rioufol G, Cung TT, Bonnefoy E, Angoulvant D, Aupetit JF, Finet G, Andre-Fouet X, Macia JC, Raczka F, Rossi R, Itti R, Kirkorian G, Derumeaux G, Ovize M. Long-term benefit of postconditioning. Circulation. 2008;117:1037–44.
125. Nolan JP, Deakin CD, Soar J, Bottiger BW, Smith G. European resuscitation council guidelines for resuscitation 2005. Section 4. Adult advanced life support. Resuscitation. 2005;67 Suppl 1:S39–86.
126. Tissier R, Chenoune M, Ghaleh B, Cohen MV, Downey JM, Berdeaux A. The small chill: mild hypothermia for cardioprotection? Cardiovasc Res. 2010;88:406–14.
127. Chien GL, Wolff RA, Davis RF, Van Winkle DM. "Normothermic range" temperature affects myocardial infarct size. Cardiovasc Res. 1994;28:1014–7.
128. Gotberg M, Olivecrona GK, Koul S, Carlsson M, Engblom H, Ugander M, van der Pals J, Algotsson L, Arheden H, Erlinge D. A pilot study of rapid cooling by cold saline and endovascular cooling before reperfusion in patients with ST-elevation myocardial infarction. Circ Cardiovasc Interv. 2010;3(5):400–7.
129. Dixon SR, Whitbourn RJ, Dae MW, Grube E, Sherman W, Schaer GL, Jenkins JS, Baim DS, Gibbons RJ, Kuntz RE, Popma JJ, Nguyen TT, O'Neill WW. Induction of mild systemic hypothermia with endovascular cooling during primary percutaneous coronary intervention for acute myocardial infarction. J Am Coll Cardiol. 2002;40:1928–34.
130. Stone GW, Dixon SR, Grines CL, Cox DA, Webb JG, Brodie BR, Griffin JJ, Martin JL, Fahy M, Mehran R, Miller TD, Gibbons RJ, O'Neill WW. Predictors of infarct size after primary coronary angioplasty in acute myocardial infarction from pooled analysis from four contemporary trials. Am J Cardiol. 2007;100:1370–5.
131. O'Neill WW, Dixon SR, Grines CL. The year in interventional cardiology. J Am Coll Cardiol. 2005;45:1117–34.
132. Sterling DL, Thornton JD, Swafford A, Gottlieb SF, Bishop SP, Stanley AW, Downey JM. Hyperbaric oxygen limits infarct size in ischemic rabbit myocardium in vivo. Circulation. 1993;88:1931–6.
133. Dixon SR, Bartorelli AL, Marcovitz PA, Spears R, David S, Grinberg I, Qureshi MA, Pepi M, Trabattoni D, Fabbiocchi F, Montorsi P, O'Neill WW. Initial experience with hyperoxemic reperfusion after primary angioplasty for acute myocardial infarction: results of a pilot study utilizing intracoronary aqueous oxygen therapy. J Am Coll Cardiol. 2002;39:387–92.
134. O'Neill WW, Martin JL, Dixon SR, Bartorelli AL, Trabattoni D, Oemrawsingh PV, Atsma DE, Chang M, Marquardt W, Oh JK, Krucoff MW, Gibbons RJ, Spears JR. Acute myocardial infarction with hyperoxemic therapy (AMIHOT): a prospective, randomized trial of intracoronary hyperoxemic reperfusion after percutaneous coronary intervention. J Am Coll Cardiol. 2007;50:397–405.

135. Stone GW, Martin JL, de Boer MJ, Margheri M, Bramucci E, Blankenship JC, Metzger DC, Gibbons RJ, Lindsay BS, Weiner BH, Lansky AJ, Krucoff MW, Fahy M, Boscardin WJ. Effect of supersaturated oxygen delivery on infarct size after percutaneous coronary intervention in acute myocardial infarction. Circ Cardiovasc Interv. 2009;2:366–75.
136. Downey JM, Cohen MV. Reducing infarct size in the setting of acute myocardial infarction. Prog Cardiovasc Dis. 2006;48:363–71.
137. Downey JM, Cohen MV. Why do we still not have cardioprotective drugs? Circ J. 2009;73:1171–7.
138. van der Horst IC, Zijlstra F, van 't Hof AW, Doggen CJ, Ve Boer MJ, Suryapranata H, Hoorntje JC, Dambrink JH, Gans RO, Bilo HJ. Glucose-insulin-potassium infusion inpatients treated with primary angioplasty for acute myocardial infarction: the glucose-insulin-potassium study: a randomized trial. J Am Coll Cardiol. 2003;42:784–91.

Chapter 13
Future Perspectives

Derek J. Hausenloy, Juan Carlos Kaski, Bernard John Gersh, and Derek M. Yellon

Abstract In the past, the clinical significance of myocardial reperfusion injury in man has been questioned. However, the recent discovery of therapeutic interventions, which can reduce myocardial infarct size in STEMI patients undergoing PPCI when administered at the time of myocardial reperfusion, has confirmed the existence of myocardial reperfusion injury in man and provided a new frontier for the treatment of myocardial infarction. Concurrent with these developments, recent advances in cardiac MRI have provided the ability to directly visualize the effects of myocardial reperfusion injury and assess the efficacy of novel cardioprotective strategies in PPCI patients. A number of novel cardioprotective strategies have shown promise in proof-of-concept clinical studies. Large multi-centre randomized controlled clinical trials are now required to investigate whether targeting myocardial reperfusion injury can improve clinical outcomes in patients with ischemic heart disease.

D.J. Hausenloy, B.Sc. (Hons), MBChB, MRCP, Ph.D., FESC, FACC (✉)
D. M. Yellon, D.Sc., FESC, FACC
UCL Institute of Cardiovascular Science, The Hatter Cardiovascular Institute,
University College London Hospital,
67 Chenies Mews, London WC1E 6HX, UK
e-mail: d.hausenloy@ucl.ac.uk; d.yellon@ucl.ac.uk

J.C. Kaski, DSc, DM (Hons), M.D., FRCP
Department of Clinical Sciences,
Cardiovascular Sciences Research Centre, St. George's,
University of London,
Cranmer Terrace, London SW17 0RE, UK
e-mail: jkaski@sgul.ac.uk

B.J. Gersh, MBChB, D.Phil., FRCP, Ph.D. (Hon Causa)
Division of Cardiovascular Diseases, Mayo Clinic,
First Street SW, Rochester 55902, MN, USA

Medicine Department, Mayo Clinic College of Medicine,
Rochester, MN, USA
e-mail: gersh.bernard@mayo.edu

J.C. Kaski et al. (eds.), *Management of Myocardial Reperfusion Injury*,
DOI 10.1007/978-1-84996-019-9_13,

Keywords Myocardial reperfusion injury • Cardioprotection • Primary percutaneous coronary intervention • ST segment elevation myocardial infarction

Over the years, the existence of myocardial reperfusion injury as a distinct pathological entity has been surrounded by controversy. Its existence in preclinical animal MI models has been more or less accepted with a large number of therapeutic interventions able to halve MI size when administered at the onset of myocardial reperfusion [1]. However, the clinical relevance of myocardial reperfusion injury in STEMI patients undergoing myocardial reperfusion has been unclear until very recently. The ability of ischemic postconditioning (IPost) to reduce MI size in STEMI patients undergoing PPCI by 40–50% has confirmed that myocardial reperfusion injury exists in humans and that it is clinically significant as it can contribute up to 50% of the final MI size [2–4]. The past failures to translate cardioprotective strategies from the laboratory 'bench' to the patient 'bedside' has cast a shadow on the field of cardioprotection. However, recommendations for improving the translation of cardioprotection into the clinical setting have been recently proposed and include: the use of more clinically relevant animal MI models [5], the use of preclinical multi-site randomized controlled blinded testing of potential cardioprotective strategies [6], and the better design of clinical studies [7]. The recent discovery of other therapeutic interventions (atrial natriuretic peptide [8], cyclosporine A [9], exenatide [10], and remote ischemic preconditioning [11]), which have also been reported to reducing myocardial reperfusion injury in proof-of-concept clinical studies, marks a new frontier in cardioprotection. Multi-centre randomized clinical trials with robust clinical endpoints are now needed to confirm that targeting myocardial reperfusion injury in STEMI patients undergoing PPCI can actually improve clinical outcomes.

The ability of cardiac MRI to non-invasively and safely measure myocardial salvage in STEMI patients up to 1 week after PPCI provides a reliable and accurate technique for assessing the efficacy of future therapeutic interventions for reducing myocardial reperfusion injury [12]. In addition, cardiac MRI in STEMI patients undergoing PPCI can detect the presence and extent of microvascular obstruction (MVO) and intramyocardial haemorrhage (indicators of severe myocardial reperfusion injury and key determinants of adverse prognosis), allowing the assessment of therapeutic interventions for reducing MVO. The use of CMR-determined surrogate endpoints such as myocardial salvage, MVO and LV systolic function will greatly facilitate the assessment of novel cardioprotective strategies in future clinical trials.

It is clear that despite optimal therapy, the morbidity and mortality of patients with ischemic heart disease remains significant. Although the process of myocardial reperfusion has been optimized to maximize myocardial salvage with the timely restoration of coronary blood flow in the infarct-related artery, there currently exists no effective therapy for protecting the heart muscle from the detrimental effects of myocardial reperfusion injury. Therefore, the development of novel therapeutic strategies capable of reducing myocardial reperfusion injury, when administered as adjuncts to PPCI, could result in myocardial infarct size being reduced by a further 40–50%; the consequence of which would be improved

LV systolic function, reduced incidence of heart failure and better clinical outcomes for our patients with IHD.

References

1. Yellon DM, Hausenloy DJ. Myocardial reperfusion injury. N Engl J Med. 2007;357(11): 1121–35.
2. Staat P, Rioufol G, Piot C, Cottin Y, Cung TT, L'Huillier I, Aupetit JF, Bonnefoy E, Finet G, Andre-Fouet X, Ovize M. Postconditioning the human heart. Circulation. 2005;112(14): 2143–8.
3. Thibault H, Piot C, Staat P, Bontemps L, Sportouch C, Rioufol G, Cung TT, Bonnefoy E, Angoulvant D, Aupetit JF, Finet G, Andre-Fouet X, Macia JC, Raczka F, Rossi R, Itti R, Kirkorian G, Derumeaux G, Ovize M. Long-term benefit of postconditioning. Circulation. 2008;117(8):1037–44.
4. Lonborg J, Kelbaek H, Vejlstrup N, Jorgensen E, Helqvist S, Saunamaki K, Clemmensen P, Holmvang L, Treiman M, Jensen JS, Engstrom T. Cardioprotective effects of ischemic postconditioning in patients treated with primary percutaneous coronary intervention, evaluated by magnetic resonance. Circ Cardiovasc Interv. 2010;3(1):34–41.
5. Ludman AJ, Yellon DM, Hausenloy DJ. Cardiac preconditioning for ischaemia: lost in translation. Dis Model Mech. 2010;3(1–2):35–8.
6. Schwartz LL, Kloner RA, Arai AE, Baines CP, Bolli R, Braunwald E, Downey J, Gibbons RJ, Gottlieb RA, Heusch G, Jennings RB, Lefer DJ, Mentzer RM, Murphy E, Ovize M, Ping P, Przyklenk K, Sack MN, Vander Heide RS, Vinten-Johansen J, Yellon DM. New horizons in cardioprotection: recommendations from the 2010 National Heart, Lung, and Blood Institute Workshop. Circulation. 2011;124(10):1172–9.
7. Hausenloy DJ, Baxter G, Bell R, Botker HE, Davidson SM, Downey J, Heusch G, Kitakaze M, Lecour S, Mentzer R, Mocanu MM, Ovize M, Schulz R, Shannon R, Walker M, Walkinshaw G, Yellon DM. Translating novel strategies for cardioprotection: the Hatter Workshop Recommendations. Basic Res Cardiol. 2010;105(6):677–86.
8. Kitakaze M, Asakura M, Kim J, Shintani Y, Asanuma H, Hamasaki T, Seguchi O, Myoishi M, Minamino T, Ohara T, Nagai Y, Nanto S, Watanabe K, Fukuzawa S, Hirayama A, Nakamura N, Kimura K, Fujii K, Ishihara M, Saito Y, Tomoike H, Kitamura S. Human atrial natriuretic peptide and nicorandil as adjuncts to reperfusion treatment for acute myocardial infarction (J-WIND): two randomised trials. Lancet. 2007;370(9597):1483–93.
9. Piot C, Croisille P, Staat P, Thibault H, Rioufol G, Mewton N, Elbelghiti R, Cung TT, Bonnefoy E, Angoulvant D, Macia C, Raczka F, Sportouch C, Gahide G, Finet G, Andre-Fouet X, Revel D, Kirkorian G, Monassier JP, Derumeaux G, Ovize M. Effect of cyclosporine on reperfusion injury in acute myocardial infarction. N Engl J Med. 2008;359(5):473–81.
10. Lønborg J, Vejlstrup N, Kelbæk H, Bøtker HE, Kim WY, Mathiasen AB, Jørgensen E, Helqvist S, Saunamäki K, Clemmensen P, Holmvang L, Thuesen L, Krusell LR, Jensen JS, Køber L, Treiman M, Holst JJ, Engstrøm T. Exenatide reduces reperfusion injury in patients with ST-segment elevation myocardial infarction. Eur Heart J. 2011 Sep 14. [Epub ahead of print]
11. Botker HE, Kharbanda R, Schmidt MR, Bottcher M, Kaltoft AK, Terkelsen CJ, Munk K, Andersen NH, Hansen TM, Trautner S, Lassen JF, Christiansen EH, Krusell LR, Kristensen SD, Thuesen L, Nielsen SS, Rehling M, Sorensen HT, Redington AN, Nielsen TT. Remote ischaemic conditioning before hospital admission, as a complement to angioplasty, and effect on myocardial salvage in patients with acute myocardial infarction: a randomised trial. Lancet. 2010;375(9716):727–34.
12. Eitel I, Desch S, Fuernau G, Hildebrand L, Gutberlet M, Schuler G, Thiele H. Prognostic significance and determinants of myocardial salvage assessed by cardiovascular magnetic resonance in acute reperfused myocardial infarction. J Am Coll Cardiol. 2010;55(22): 2470–9.

Index

J.C. Kaski et al. (eds.), *Management of Myocardial Reperfusion Injury*,
DOI 10.1007/978-1-84996-019-9, © Springer-Verlag London 2012

S

T

MIX
Papier aus verantwortungsvollen Quellen
Paper from responsible sources
FSC® C105338
FSC
www.fsc.org

If you have any concerns about our products,
you can contact us on
ProductSafety@springernature.com

In case Publisher is established outside the EU,
the EU authorized representative is:
Springer Nature Customer Service Center GmbH
Europaplatz 3, 69115 Heidelberg, Germany

Printed by Libri Plureos GmbH
in Hamburg, Germany